Principles of Chinese Medical Andrology

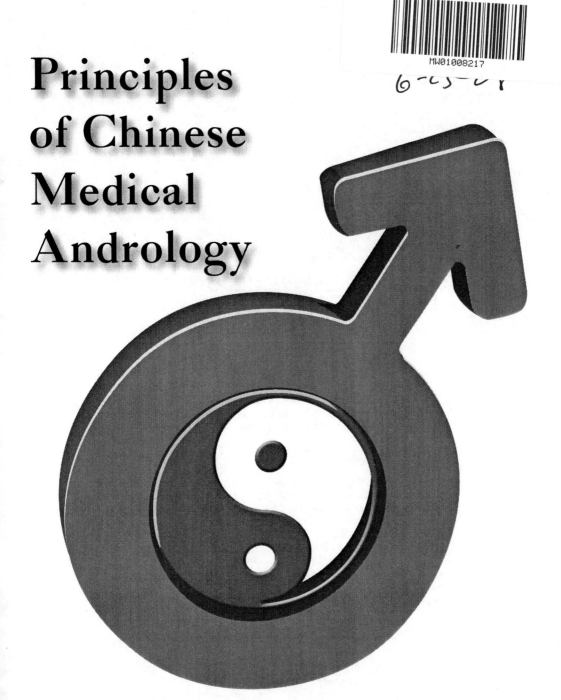

An Integrated Approach to Male Reproductive and Urological Health

by
Bob Damone

Published by:
BLUE POPPY PRESS
A Division of Blue Poppy Enterprises, Inc.
5441 Western Ave., #2
BOULDER, CO 80301
www.bluepoppy.com

First Edition, February, 2008

ISBN 1-891845-45-4
ISBN 978-1-891845-45-1
LCCN #2007942109

DISCLAIMER: The information in this book is given in good faith. However, the author and the publishers cannot be held responsible for any error or omission. The publishers will not accept liabilities for any injuries or damages caused to the reader that may result from the reader's acting upon or using the content contained in this book. The publishers make this information available to English language readers for research and scholarly purposes only.

The publishers do not advocate nor endorse self-medication by laypersons. Chinese medicine is a professional medicine. Laypersons interested in availing themselves of the treatments described in this book should seek out a qualified professional practitioner of Chinese medicine.

COMP Designation: Compilation of functional translations using a standard translational terminology plus an original work.

Cover and page layout design by Eric J. Brearton

10 9 8 7 6 5 4 3 2 1

Printed at National Hirschfeld, Denver, CO on recycled paper and soy inks.

Table of Contents

"With a depth of scholarly research that often surpasses even the Chinese source texts that inspired it, Bob Damone has created a masterpiece that weaves centuries of accumulated knowledge into one well- organized, clinically-focused reference work. The authenticity, accuracy, and utility of this text will make it the defining work in the field of Chinese medical andrology for decades to come."

—Eric Brand, M.S., L.Ac.

Preface

This book is an advanced textbook and clinical manual devoted to the treatment of andrological diseases with Chinese medicine, written for English-speaking students and practitioners of Chinese medicine. I have used both Chinese and English language andrology source literature, and interpreted these sources using my own academic perspectives and clinical experience. This book reflects the format of Chinese language andrology textbooks and clinical manuals in that the diseases it covers are discussed in both Chinese and Western medical terms. For the most part, I have gleaned the Chinese medical material in this book from professional Chinese language books and journals written by doctors who specialize in andrology (*nan ke*). However, for the Western medical information, I have almost solely relied on English language sources as they are more accessible to me and in some cases are more accurate and up-to-date.

In accordance with the format of recent Blue Poppy clinical manuals and with the layout of similarly-organized Chinese andrology texts, this book is divided into two major sections. Book 1—which introduces the foundations of Chinese andrology—begins with a short history of andrology in Chinese medicine and progresses on to discuss all of the following from an andrological perspective: 1) anatomy of the male genitourinary system; 2) the channels and network vessels; 3) the viscera and bowels; 4) disease causes and pathomechanisms; 5) Chinese andrological diseases and; 6) general treatment principles. Book 2 covers specific andrological diseases including: 1) their definition; 2) Western medical perspective; 3) causes and pathomechanisms; 4) disease and pattern discrimination; 5) treatment principles; 6) treatment with Chinese medicinals and acumoxa therapy; 7) representative Chinese research abstracts and; 8) case studies.[1] For each disease in Book 2, I have also included the major evidence-based complementary Western herbs and supplements for each condition because Western patients are often already taking them by the time they seek the help of a physician of Chinese medicine or they are interested in taking them. Further, because the reader of

---

[1] One notable exception is that Book 2 Chapter 3 on prostate cancer lacks Chinese research abstracts and case studies due to a lack of source materials. I presume that the scarcity of Chinese sources for prostate cancer research and case studies reflects the low incidence of the disease among Chinese men.

this book is most likely to be a Western English-speaking person, I have organized the material in Book 2 by Western medical disease categories, and have then reframed each Western medical disease into its constituent Chinese disease categories.

By including a chapter on Chinese andrological disease categories in Book 1, I deviate from the standard format of Chinese andrology texts so that readers may be exposed to a greater number of andrological diseases than I am able to cover in Book 2 of this text. To write a book that would be so comprehensive as to cover every known andrological disease category in depth would take a team of writers working full-time for several years rather than a solo author such as myself writing part-time between other work and family commitments. Hence, for practical reasons I cover ten major andrological diseases in detail in Book 2, and hope that I provide enough foundational knowledge in Book 1 to empower practitioners to treat diseases that are absent from Book 2.

I have included the Chinese research abstracts for each condition in Book 2 (except prostate cancer) even though the standards of some of this research can certainly be improved. Hence, I do not suggest that these research conclusions should stand unchallenged, but rather that they should establish a baseline from which future studies can flow. At the same time, these studies are very useful because they provide us with a glimpse of the current clinical protocols of Chinese experts in the field. Even though we should raise the standards of future studies in Chinese medicine, past studies—imperfect as they are—stand as qualitative records of Chinese clinical experience to date. Further, they can establish a foundation for current clinical practice and can be the starting point for future investigations. It is noteworthy that the more recent Chinese medical studies emerging from China reflect a rising research standard. Thus, the reader will notice that the more recent the study abstract, the more explicit are the standards for determining efficacy such as "cure" and "good results." Too often, however, the significance of these terms remains vague because the investigators do not report the specific criteria they used to determine efficacy.

In all fairness, I must however acknowledge that I have translated the majority of the abstracts included in this text from secondary Chinese sources that compiled andrology research and not from the primary research papers themselves. Hence, some of the lack of specific data and efficacy-determining criteria could possibly reflect the fault of the secondary reporters rather than the primary investigators. Clearly it would have been better for me to possess all of the primary papers myself. However, the sheer difficulty of acquiring the number of specialized Chinese articles I would have needed for this book from primary sources alone would have presented a formidable practical challenge.

Had I limited myself only to the primary sources I was able to gather, this book's focus would be much too narrow. I would not have been able to meet my intended goal of providing the reader with a wide professional view of the field of Chinese andrology. In most cases, I have cited the primary author's paper (rather than the source in which it was compiled) in the endnotes for that disease to give full credit to the original paper, and I have cited the secondary source in the bibliography. In some cases however, the secondary source did not cite the full title of the article and hence the citation may lack an important detail. This reflects a deficiency in the standards for source citation in Chinese medicine literature which in several cases I unfortunately perpetuate in this book because I am unable to provide a better citation than I found in the secondary Chinese sources at my disposal. In such cases, the source citation entry in the endnotes and in the bibliography reflects this reality.

Throughout this book, I have adhered to the standardized translation of Chinese medical terms as provided by Nigel Wiseman and Feng Ye's *A Practical Dictionary of Chinese Medicine* (Paradigm Publications, 1998). As comprehensive as it is, the dictionary cannot hope to provide a definition for every possible term encountered in a broad search of advanced Chinese medical clinical texts. Hence, when I have encountered terms that I could not find in the dictionary, I did my best to translate them as faithfully to the original as possible and in accordance with the translation standards established by the *Practical Dictionary*.

Although I do not support the use of threatened or endangered species in Chinese medicine, some of the clinical protocols, research formulas, and case study formulas in this book contain medicinals such as *Chuan Shan Jia* (Mantis Squama) and *Ling Yang Jiao* (Saigae Tataricae Cornu), which are derived from threatened or endangered animals. However, there are farmed sources for these medicinals available as alternatives to the wild sources. So, when we choose to use them we should verify that they are derived from a farmed source. There are some ambiguities however in that herb suppliers are not always able to provide such verification; in such cases, avoiding their use altogether by using alternatives is the more environmentally and ethically responsible choice.

Some of the formulas in the book contain toxic ingredients such as *Wu Gong* (Scolopendra) and *Quan Xie* (Scorpio). Only experienced practitioners should prescribe these medicinals, they should strictly regulate their dosage, and patients should not take them for extended periods of time without periodically abstaining.

Chinese andrology is a specialty within Chinese medicine and is usually practiced by modern Chinese doctors who with few exceptions practice integrated Chinese-Western medicine (*zhong xi yi jie he*). Thus, Chinese andrologists are dually-trained physicians of Chinese and Western urology who seek to blend the best of Chinese medicine with the best of Western medicine. In their clinical and academic work, they freely switch from the Chinese medical paradigm to the Western medical paradigm, but they strive to maintain the conceptual integrity of each. I hope to capture that same spirit in this book. Whereas we can trace the history of andrology principles in Chinese medicine at least as far back as the Ma Wang Dui texts and the *Huang Di Nei Jing* (*The Yellow*

Emperor's Inner Canon), andrology did not truly emerge in China as a recognizable clinical specialty in its own right with its own professional and systematic literature until about thirty years ago. Since its establishment, however, it has continued to develop to the degree that today there are many andrology specialists and researchers and a fair number of Chinese language andrology sources.

Whereas there is a reasonably-sized body of professional andrology literature available to the reader of medical Chinese, there is at the time of this writing no comprehensive English language Chinese andrology text extant. However, it is more and more common to see men presenting with andrological problems in clinic, to hear andrological topics presented at Western Chinese medical conferences, and papers published in English language journals of Chinese medicine. I believe this reveals a stirring of the andrology zeitgeist. I sincerely hope that this book can quicken the current in the stream that is already flowing towards a greater understanding of men's health and illness in the Western Chinese medical community.

Bob Damone, M.S., L.Ac.
Chair, Department of Oriental Medicine
Pacific College of Oriental Medicine, San Diego

The History of Chinese Andrology

Before exploring its history, I should first clarify the term Chinese andrology (*nan ke*). It refers to the specialized knowledge in Chinese medicine that describes the physiology of men, as well as the prevention, pathology and treatment of men's diseases. Chinese andrology did not officially become a medical specialty within the Chinese medical system until about thirty years ago. This is not to suggest, however, that Chinese physicians had been silent on the subject of health and diseases of men up to that point, but merely to show that there were no andrology specialists until very recently. In fact, the premodern literature is rich in andrological content. The history of Chinese andrology is the history of the fundamental source theories and clinical experiences which are recorded in the premodern literature, of which anyone interested in the practice of Chinese andrology must have a solid understanding. This data is spread widely through the premodern literature because of the historical absence of systematic manuals on andrology until the last few decades,[1] so the task of discussing the history of Chinese andrology is a formidable one. Fortunately, however, many modern Chinese andrology texts begin with a chapter on its history. Hence, my task is greatly simplified by these works, which I gratefully acknowledge as the source texts for this discussion.

As we will see, Chinese andrology has traveled a long and interesting journey from the nourishing life texts and sexual handbooks buried at Ma Wang Dui in ancient times to modern Chinese medical hospitals and clinics. Although its conceptual seeds sprouted over two thousand years ago, many of its ancient root theories still inform the daily clinical practice of modern Chinese andrologists. For the purposes of our discussion, we should be clear that modern Chinese andrologists typically are physicians who practice a species of Chinese medicine called "integrated Chinese-Western medicine (*zhong*

---

[1] I need to differentiate modern Chinese andrology from the nourishing life (*yang sheng*) tradition and especially Daoist sexual practices aimed at promoting health and attaining longevity. While these are very interesting and worthy topics which do articulate with Chinese andrology, they are not by far the main subject of this text. For an excellent coverage of the history of sexuality in China, including the Daoist tradition, see Van Gulik (1961). For translations of Daoist sexual source texts, see Wile (1992).

xi yi jie he)" and who therefore, see the objective clinical value of both modern Western medicine and Chinese medicine. As such, they are a manifestation of the medical movement that began in the 1950s whose adherents sought with varied agendas to integrate Chinese and Western medicine. While it is important to note that their aspirations are suspect in the minds of many Western and Chinese practitioners who are perhaps legitimately concerned about the loss of authenticity or purity of "classical" Chinese medicine, I do not take up this argument here. I fully acknowledge that there are certainly many philosophical, political, anthropological, and sociological factors to consider in a broader discussion of this effort at integration.[2] However, my attention in this chapter is very specifically focused on tracing the history of andrological theory in the premodern literature and not on these other factors.

The Spring-Autumn Period (722 BCE–481 BCE) and the Warring States Period (5th c. BCE–221 BCE) to the Qin (221 BCE–206 BCE) and Han (206 BCE–220 CE) Dynasties

Nourishing life (*yang sheng*) texts and other medical texts unearthed at Ma Wang Dui

In 1973, archaeologists in Chang Sha unearthed a Han dynasty noble's tomb. He was apparently an avid collector of literature because the tomb contained many books recorded on bamboo scrolls. Among the large selection of texts covering a broad range of topics, which contained material from several centuries prior, there were many medical and nourishing life (*yang sheng*) texts written on bamboo scrolls. One of the most important findings was *Wu Shi Er Bing Fang (Formulas for Fifty-Two Diseases)*, which is the earliest book on pharmacy extant in the Chinese medical literature.[3] According to Wang (2003), within this text, we find some of the earliest mentions of andrological diseases such as dribbling (*long*) and prominent mounting (*tui shan*). However, several other texts contain important discussions of male sexuality. In fact, some of these texts comprise the earliest known sexual handbooks in the world. They contain guidelines on nourishing life and promise longevity through the practice of Daoist breathing exercises, through understanding the concept of sevenfold reduction and eightfold boost (*qi sun ba yi*),[4] and through regulating one's sexual life. Within these texts, we recognize core ideas that remain central to Chinese andrology to this day. For example, in *Yang Sheng Fang (Formulas for*

---

[2] For a thorough exploration of these issues, see Scheid (2002).

[3] For a detailed discussion of this text, see Unschuld (1986).

[4] The sevenfold reduction and eightfold boost is an ancient concept in Chinese medicine that has been explained differently by different scholars at different points in Chinese medical history. For our purposes, we can adhere to the meaning in *Yang Sheng Fang*, which implies attaining harmony between yin and yang through sexual intercourse. In this light, the term "sevenfold reduction" is generally understood as a way of referring to women—whose life cycles progress in units of seven years in the *Nei Jing*, and the "eightfold boost" refers to men—whose life cycles progress in units of eight years.

Nourishing Life), the importance of moderating sexual life as a means for attaining domestic harmony is shown in the following statement, "The [sexual] union of men and women must be principled [*i.e.*, regulated]." Within the other titles, which include *He Yin-Yang Fang* (*Formulas for Uniting Yin and Yang*), *Dong Xuan Zi* ([*The Sexual Handbook of*] *Master Dong Xuan*) and *Su Nu Jing* (*Plain Woman's Canon*), there is a strong message about the power of a healthy sexual life as a means of preserving and cultivating essence.

Of great significance for understanding andrology is the emphasis these texts placed on limiting the frequency of ejaculation in order to retain essence. Wang (2003) also points out that *He Yin-Yang Fang* (*Formulas for Uniting Yin and Yang*) emphasized that men and women should make love very tenderly, and recommends ten different sexual positions that have the effect of enriching a man's essence. Here we also see a fundamental assumption of the nourishing life tradition and essential qi philosophy—that essence is the material foundation for life. According to this idea, essence is the fundamental substrate for all other aspects of human health (physical and mental), and by limiting its expenditure and cultivating it instead, one guarantees an abundant supply for nourishing and enriching the body and mind for many years into the future. Hence, the goals are to strengthen those who are vacuous, further invigorate the healthy, and cause the aged to attain longevity.

In modern andrology, we still have the core idea that men should have a healthy balance in their sexual lives, neither overindulging in sexual activity nor being overly chaste; this both preserves men's stored essence and prevents it from being retained for an abnormal length of time. Essence that is held in the essence chamber[5] for an abnormal period of time sometimes becomes vanquished essence (*bai jing*), and may become a source of disease in the same way as do other substantial evils such as blood stasis and phlegm.

Contributions of the *Huang Di Nei Jing* (*Yellow Emperor's Inner Canon*)

As in every other area of Chinese medicine, the *Inner Canon* has, since its compilation during the 1st century CE, continuously exerted a formative influence on the principles and practice of andrology. The text is rich in discussions of male anatomy and physiology, pathways and indications of acumoxa channels and points as they relate to mens' health and disease, pathomechanisms, disease categories, and treatment principles. A thorough exploration of its andrological content could consume one's entire intellectual career. We can acknowledge this fact while we take a focused look at some of its major clinically-relevant andrological features.

The importance of moderating sexual life

The *Nei Jing* contains many passages that emphasize the importance of moderat-

---

[5] The essence chamber is the structure in Chinese anatomy that is responsible for storing semen. In modern Chinese andrology, it is roughly equivalent to the prostate.

ing sexual life in order to maintain health and to avoid disease. It is clear that these ideas reflect the same sentiment as the Ma Wang Dui nourishing life texts discussed previously. It is from the nourishing life tradition and the *Nei Jing* that Chinese andrology derived its emphasis on avoiding damaging the "essential qi of the true origin (*yuan zhen jing qi*)" [*i.e.*, kidney qi] by not overindulging in sex and by avoiding sexual activity while under the influence of alcohol.

The cycles of men's lives

Chapter 1 of the *Su Wen* (*Plain Questions*) is the locus classicus for understanding the normal physiological cycles of men. It reads: "When a male is eight years old, his kidney qi is replete and development of his teeth continues. At two times eight, heavenly tenth[6] flows, essential qi overflows and drains, yin and yang are harmonious, and he can produce children. At three times eight, kidney qi is completely balanced, the sinews and bones are powerful and strong, and the true teeth develop to their utmost. At four times eight, the sinews and bones flourish [and are] exuberant, and the flesh is full and vigorous. At five times eight, kidney qi is debilitated, the hair falls out, and the teeth are desiccated. At six times eight, yang qi is debilitated above, the face is parched, and the hair at the temples turns gray. At seven times eight, liver qi is debilitated, the sinews are unmovable, heavenly tenth is exhausted, essence is scant, the kidney viscus is debilitated, and the bodily form is completely exhausted. At eight times eight, the teeth and hair fall out."

From this passage, we see that at the time of the *Nei Jing*, the kidneys had a central role in storing essence and in triggering and maintaining sexual maturation and fertility by promoting the formation of heavenly tenth. Without kidney essence, there is no heavenly tenth; without heavenly tenth, there is no sexual maturity or fertility. We also see that as men age—and according to this passage at the age of fifty-six (seven times eight)—kidney essence is scant and heavenly tenth is exhausted. In early doctors' minds, this understanding was extremely influential in establishing the importance of treating the kidneys for problems with male sexual and reproductive function. And this influence continues. For example, Wang (2003) cites a recent study by Li Biao *et al.* who examined 163 papers reporting on over 8,506 cases of male infertility and found that the most commonly used formulas were *Liu Wei Di Huang Wan* (Six-Ingredient Rehmanniae Pill) and *Wu Zi Yan Zong Wan* (Five-Seed Progeny Pill). Clearly, the influence of the *Nei Jing* on the clinical treatment of male infertility endures.

While this passage undeniably emphasizes the importance of kidney essence (kidney essential qi) in the growth and decline of men, we should be careful not to overlook its mention of the role of liver detriment and damage in the aging process. The passage states that at fifty-six (seven times eight), "the liver qi is debilitated and the sinews become unmovable." In other words, the aging process of men affects the kidneys and liver, and therefore when treating or

---

[6] According to Wiseman and Feng (1998), heavenly tenth (*tian gui*) is that which the development of the human body, sexual function, and the ability to reproduce depends.

preventing andrological problems related to aging, many modern andrology specialists emphasize the importance of enriching and nourishing liver blood and kidney essence. The theoretical basis for such an approach also derives from the *Inner Canon*, and is summarized in the dictum, "The liver and kidneys are of the same source (*gan shen tong yuan*)." Nowhere is this more clear than in the treatment of the modern Chinese andrological disease category of andropause.

Discussions of male external genitalia from the *Inner Canon*

In the text of the *Nei Jing*, the penis is referred to as the "stem (*jing*)," and the scrotum is called "[that which] hangs (*chui*)." In Chapter 15 of *Ling Shu* (*Magic Pivot*), we find the following reference to these two male anatomical features: "The stalk and [that which] hangs comprise the mechanism within the body [*i.e.*, the means by which one reproduces]; [they are] the manifestations of yin-essence, and the pathway of essence and fluid." From this passage, it is clear that at the time of the *Nei Jing*, Chinese physicians were aware that kidney essence had a direct relationship with the penis and scrotum, and that these organs had an important connection with male reproductive and urinary function.

Male secondary sexual characteristics in the *Nei Jing* (*Inner Canon*)

• The development of facial hair and initiation of ejaculatory function as indicators of male puberty

"At two times eight, heavenly tenth flows, and essential qi overflows and drains…" This line from Chapter 1 of *Plain Questions* provides an essential fact for understanding male puberty: not only women's reproductive lives are under the influence of heavenly tenth, but so are men's. As the principle of this reproductive maturity, heavenly tenth is what triggers and maintains a man's reproductive viability. The term essential qi in this passage stands for semen. Its overflowing and draining refers to ejaculation. And overflowing of essential qi is a direct indicator that heavenly tenth is in adequate supply and flowing freely. As long as heavenly tenth is in adequate supply, his reproductive potential is actualized; when it is depleted, he is no longer fertile. It is significant to note that in Chinese andrology, we owe this fundamental understanding of male puberty to this passage in *Plain Questions*.

• *Nei Jing* on the development of facial hair

In the *Inner Canon*, beard growth in young men was considered to be one of the first signs of the approach of puberty. A heavenly eunuch (*tian huan*) is a boy who did not develop secondary sexual characteristics—including facial hair—and had smaller-than-normal genitals. The reason for the beard not growing on the face of a heavenly eunuch and for his lack of genital development is explained in Chapter 65 of *Magic Pivot* as: "Insufficiency of early heaven, lack of exuberance of the thoroughfare and conception vessels (*ren mai*), and lack of formation of the ancestral sinew; he has qi, but no blood, [and] the lips and mouth lack luxuriance, so the beard cannot be engendered." So, we can see that the *Inner Canon* emphasizes that for boys to reach sexual maturity and specifically to develop facial hair, they must possess an adequate amount of early heaven essence and the thoroughfare vessel must be filled with blood.[7] In premodern Chinese medical literature, "luxuriance (*rong*)" is a term that is always associated with the nourishment and enrichment provided by blood. Tissues that are luxuriant are supple, full, exuberant, and have luster. As the fundamental source of all material nourishment in the body, and as the material foundation of blood, kidney essence is the fountainhead of male sexual maturity. In the case of heavenly eunuchs, there is an early heaven natural endowment insufficiency.

On the other hand, Chapter 65 of the *Magic Pivot* (*Ling Shu*) discusses how this process works in those who were castrated, "A eunuch [has had] his ancestral sinew removed; [thus his] thoroughfare vessel [*chong mai*] is damaged and his blood drains and cannot be transmuted, his skin binds in the interior, and his lips cannot be luxuriant; thus, his beard is not engendered." The same pathomechanism is responsible (insufficiency of essence-blood); the only difference is the disease cause. In the case of heavenly eunuchs, the cause is early heaven natural endowment insufficiency; in the case of secondary eunuchs, castration is the cause.

Selected diseases of men discussed in the *Nei Jing*

Although the *Nei Jing* is not replete with specific treatment protocols for andrological diseases, it is rich in its identification of andrological diseases, including their causes, symptoms, and pathomechanisms.[8] Some of the disease categories refer to diseases of the penis, scrotum and testicles. For example, Chapter 16 of *Su Wen* (*Plain Questions*) mentions a disease called retracted eggs [*i.e.*, testicles] (*luan shang suo*), Chapter 13 of *Ling Shu* (*Magic Pivot*) discusses retracted genitals (*yin suo*) and wringing pain in the genitals (*yin qi niu tong*), Chapter 10 of *Ling Shu* discusses testicular swelling (*gao zhong*), Chapter 49 of *Ling Shu* covers egg pain [*i.e.*, testicular pain] (*luan tong*) and stem pain [*i.e.*, pain in the penis] (*jing tong*). Other passages are concerned more with how loss of viscera-bowel regulation causes certain andrological diseases. Among these we find Chapter 1 of *Su Wen*, which mentions scanty semen (*jing shao*), and Chapter 44 of *Su Wen*, which mentions white ooze (*bai zhuo*), Chapter 8 of *Ling Shu*, which deals with spontaneous discharge of semen (*jing shi zi xia*), and Chapter 10 of *Ling Shu*, which mentions persistent erection (*zong ting bu shou*)(Guo, 1999).

The *Nei Jing* on kidney essence and essence-spirit

In the *Nei Jing*, there is no assumption that the mind and body are separated. In Chapter 8 of the *Ling Shu*, it states: "The kidney stores essence; essence is

---

[7] It is interesting to note the pathway of the thoroughfare vessel up to the face and around the lips in this regard. (See Book 1, Chapter 3: *Channels and Network Vessels in Andrology* for further explanation.)

[8] Some the disease categories differ from the modern terms, and I posit because the *Nei Jing* was compiled by different authors, some of the different disease categories overlap with each other.

the abode of spirit." The very term "essence-spirit (*jing shen*)," as it is used in *Nei Jing* is a compound word indicating the close link between essence (*jing*)—fundamental yin-substance for the mind—and spirit (*shen*)—the ethereal-yang aspect of mind. So, abundant essence is a necessity for normal male emotional life. This idea—here demonstrated to be rooted in the *Nei Jing*—is used extensively for treating the symptoms of andropause such as fearful throbbing, vexation and agitation, insomnia, and even sexual dysfunctions including yang wilt and premature ejaculation (Wang, 2003).

The *Nei Jing* on the disease causes and pathomechanisms of andrological diseases

Many of the disease causes and pathomechanisms now recognized for men's diseases were originally discussed in the *Nei Jing*. As suggested previously, one of the key andrological disease causes and pathomechanisms discussed in the text was kidney essence vacuity—either natural endowment early heaven insufficiency or later heaven detriment and damage to kidney essence caused by bedroom taxation. Other kidney-related disease causes and pathomechanisms also received generous coverage, including kidney yin vacuity, kidney yang vacuity, and insecurity of kidney qi. While it is true that these kidney discussions dominate the text, a broader look reveals that many other disease causes and pathomechanisms were also discussed including external contraction of evils and affect-mind damage. Since I have already discussed the kidney pathomechanisms to some extent, I will present some examples of the others.

• Cold, heat, and dampness

In the *Nei Jing*, cold evil is implicated as one of the main causes of mounting qi (*shan qi*), because of its contracting nature and its contracting effect on qi and blood flow in the liver channel and in the anterior yin region in general. According to Guo (1999), in addition to mounting qi, cold is discussed in the *Nei Jing* as a cause of several andrological diseases including testicular swelling, egg [*i.e.*, testicular] pain, and retracted genitals. Chapter 13 of the *Ling Shu* clearly states, "When the foot reverting yin channel is damaged by cold, there will be retracted genitals." In modern andrology, the treatment principle of warming the liver channel and dissipating cold to treat many andrological diseases is still a key clinical strategy. We owe this to the *Nei Jing*.

Heat was also implicated as the cause of many men's diseases including persistent erection (*i.e.*, priapism), prominent mounting, dribbling urinary block, and scrotal swelling.[9] For example, Chapter 13 of *Ling Shu* (*Magic Pivot*) states, "When the foot reverting yin sinew is damaged by heat, there will be persistent erection." Although nowadays practitioners generally emphasize yin vacuity fire as the cause of persistent erection, we credit the *Nei Jing* for identifying heat as the main cause of this condition. In another passage in *Ling Shu* it

---

[9] See Book 1, Chapter 6 on Chinese andrological disease categories for further information about these diseases.

states, "In channel sinew disease, heat causes sinew protraction [*i.e.*, persistent erection] and yin wilt [*i.e.*, erectile dysfunction]." Here we see heat as a cause of both priapism and erectile dysfunction. Later doctors used such passages as the theoretical basis for understanding how heat can damage original qi and fluids and can thereby cause the penis to lose its power and nourishment and to wilt. In yet another passage in Chapter 37 of *Su Wen*, dribbling urinary block is identified with heat in the bladder.

In the *Nei Jing*, dampness is repeatedly correlated with problems in the lower body. This sentiment is revealed in passages like this one in Chapter 10 of *Ling Shu*: "[In] those damaged by dampness, the lower [body] is affected first." So, dampness—alone or in combination with heat or cold—is identified as a very important cause of many andrological diseases including white ooze (*bai zhuo*), kidney sac wind (*shen nang feng*), water mounting (*shui shan*), and dribbling urinary block (*long bi*).

• Affect-mind damage
With respect to affect-mind damage as a causative factor for andrological diseases, the *Nei Jing* focuses on the liver, heart, and kidneys. The most frequently cited passage relating the liver to fear is in Chapter 8 of the *Ling Shu*, which states, "The liver stores blood and blood houses the ethereal soul. When the liver qi is vacuous, there is fear; when it is replete, there is anger." Modern andrology specialists such as Wang Qi have successfully used this passage as inspiration for basing their treatment of male sexual dysfunction on the liver.[10] Such doctors recognize that many cases of sexual dysfunction—especially those among younger men—are strongly linked with anxiety and fear, and thus with liver organ and channel pathology in terms of Chinese medicine.

There are many passages relating the kidneys and heart to fear and andrological conditions. A commonly cited one is found in Chapter 39 of *Su Wen*: "[When there is] fear, essence is eliminated. When it is eliminated, the upper burner is blocked. Blockage causes qi to return. Return causes distention in the lower burner. As a result, qi does not move." The passage brings our attention to the fact that fear damages the kidneys and leads to elimination of essence (seminal emission) and blockage of qi in the upper burner (probably referring to the heart) and in the anterior yin region. Later doctors, especially Zhang Jing-Yue in the Ming dynasty developed these ideas much further, but the seed is present in the *Nei Jing* as revealed here.

Contributions of the *Nan Jing* (*The Classic of Difficult Issues*)

Writing some years after the *Huang Di Nei Jing*—some time in the 1st century—the Eastern Han authors of the *Nan Jing* set out to clarify areas in which the *Nei Jing* was not very clear. One such area that the *Nan Jing* dealt with and was crucial to the development of andrology is the concept of the life gate (*ming men*). Life gate theory had a profound influence on the understanding of male sexual

---

[10] See Wang (2003)

and reproductive health and illness in Chinese medicine. According to the 36th difficulty of the *Nan Jing*, "The two kidneys are not both kidneys. The left one is ascribed to the kidney, and the right one is ascribed to the life gate. The life gate is the abode of all the essence-spirit, the place to which original qi is tied. In men, it stores essence; in women, it is tied to the uterus." The 39th difficulty states: "The kidneys are two viscera—the left is ascribed to the kidney, and the right is ascribed to the life gate. The qi of [the life gate] opens to the kidney." According to Guo (1999), these statements completely veered away from the concept of the life gate as it was expressed in the *Nei Jing*, and now suggested a dif- ferent view: that the life gate had a very close relationship with all the viscera and bowels, had the ability to store essence and to house the spirit, and hence played a key role in the sexual and reproductive function of both men and women. Although the *Nan Jing* itself does not develop this idea very deeply *vis-à-vis* male physiology and pathology, later doctors took note of the concept and developed it further. Of particular significance, Zhang Jing-Yue in the Ming dynasty felt that debility of life gate fire was a key cause for andrological diseases such as cold essence (*jing leng*), scanty semen, cold genitals (*yin han*), and premature ejaculation (*zao xie*). So, on the basis of the *Nan Jing's* concept of the life gate, he and other doctors favored warm supplementation of the life gate fire as a standard treatment for many male sexual and reproductive diseases.

Contributions of the *Shang Han Za Bing Lun* (*On Cold Damage and Miscellaneous Diseases*)

In Zhang Zhong-Jing's famous Eastern Han dynasty work, he discusses many andrological diseases under different headings including dribbling urinary block, inhibited urination, seminal emission, yin foxy mounting (*yin hu shan*), and cold semen and infertility (*jing leng wu zi*). In terms of disease causes, in several places throughout the text, he cites sexual taxation as a cause of men's disease. From Zhang Zhong-Jing's various discussions of andrological diseases, I have chosen three passages that have had an enduring influence on Chinese andrology.

Three of the most classic and most often cited references to male disorders appear in Chapter 6 of *Jin Gui Yao Lue* (*Essential Prescriptions of the Golden Coffer*), which is devoted to blood impediment and vacuity taxation. They state: 1) "A man with a floating and rough pulse who has no children has clear and cold essential qi."; 2) "A man who suffers from seminal loss, has stringlike urgency in the lesser abdomen, coldness at the head of the penis, dizzy eyes, hair loss, an extremely vacuous pulse [that may be] scallion-stalk or slow, [has] clear-grain diarrhea and loss of blood and semen. When the pulse is minute, moving, scallion-stalk, or minute tight, this is a man with seminal loss or a woman who dreams of intercourse. *Gui Zhi Jia Long Gu Mu Li Tang* [Cinnamon Twig Decoction Plus Dragon Bone and Oyster Shell] governs." and; 3) "The pulse is stringlike large, [and is] stringlike but reduced, and large but scallion-stalk. Scallion-stalk indicates vacuity and [that] vacuity and cold are mutually contending. This [pulse] is called drum skin. In women, this indicates miscarriage and leaking, and in men it indicates blood desertion and seminal loss."

In the first quote, we find the theoretical basis for understanding that men with yang vacuity may have clear and dilute seminal fluid and may be infertile as a result. Further, we generally interpret the pulse description—floating and rough—as an indicator of essence-blood insufficiency.

The second quote points to a more complicated scenario in which there is enduring yin vacuity with stirring of ministerial fire that leads to detriment and damage to yang and vacuous yang floating upward; this is summarized under the headings "detriment to yin affecting yang (*yin sun ji yang*)" and "vacuous yang floating astray (*xu yang fu yue*)." Eventually, there is dual vacuity of yin and yang. Hence, the signs and symptoms listed in the quote reflect a mixture of yin and yang vacuity (Chen, 2000). This is still a very useful model for understanding the pathomechanisms for men with premature ejaculation and dream emissions. The pulse descriptions included in this passage are also very useful clinically for the treatment of men. The floating rough pulse and the scallion-stalk moving pulse here indicate serious damage to yin-blood and floating of yang out to the exterior. A minute tight pulse shows vacuity cold. The seminal loss and dreaming of intercourse—the latter described as a symptom of women—may be present in men as well, and indicates noninteraction of the heart and kidneys in which sovereign fire is not moving downward to warm the kidneys and kidney yin and yang are unable to move upward to aid the heart.

For me, one of the most important and clinically-relevant gems contained within the third quote is the implied advice to carefully differentiate large pulses. Most importantly, a man may have a large pulse that is not an indication of a repletion pattern, but is instead a sign of severe vacuity. The key of course is that the pulse lacks force when pressed deeply, even if the vessel feels tight or firm on its surface. If we are not vigilant, we can easily misconstrue the largeness of the pulse as a sign of repletion and misdiagnose and mistreat the patient accordingly.

Contributions of Hua To (Hua Yuan-Hua) (2nd–3rd century CE)[11]

In his furthering of viscera-bowel theory and by systematically discriminating cold, heat, repletion and vacuity patterns, Hua To made some significant contributions to Chinese andrological theory and practice in the late 2nd or early 3rd century, during the Eastern Han dynasty. According to Guo (1999), in his treatment of andrological diseases, Hua primarily focused on the kidneys and his ideas did have a strong influence on the historical development of andrology as practiced by later practitioners. For the treatment of what he called "spontaneous seminal discharge (*jing zi chu*)," insecurity of the essence gate, and yin wilt, he emphasized the importance of warming and supplementing kidney yang with pills made from *Jiu Cai Zi* (Chinese leek, Allii Tuberosi Semen). He also felt that disease of retracted genitals was caused by cold damaging the kidneys, and that other male diseases were caused by "heat within the kidneys."

---

[11] The dates of birth and death of Hua To are uncertain, but he lived during the 3rd century and may have died in 208 CE.

The Jin Dynasty (265 CE–420 CE)

Wang Shu-He (3rd century CE)

In his famous and highly influential 3rd century (Western Jin dynasty) text on the pulse and channels—the *Mai Jing* (*Pulse Canon*)—Wang Shu-He emphasized the value of both cubit pulses for diagnosing male diseases. For example, he related a slow sinking fine pulse in the cubit to genital dampness and a slippery and floating-large in the cubit to lesser abdominal pain and fullness, inability to urinate, and pain within the penis while urinating. Further, he correlated a slow pulse within the right cubit position with rigid yang (*yang qiang*) and seminal emission. His work instilled the importance of using the inch, bar, cubit model for approaching the pulse that was emphasized in the *Nan Jing* (*Classic of Difficult Issues*), and inspired later generations of physicians to use the pulse to help diagnose andrological diseases.

Huang Fu-Mi (215–282 CE)

Huang Fu-Mi made a significant contribution to the development of acumoxa therapy and andrology with his text, *Zhen Jiu Jia Yi Jing* (*The Systematized Canon of Acupuncture and Moxibustion*). Among his discussions of treatments for various andrological diseases, he included (*Qi Jie*) ST-30 to treat yin mounting and pain in the penis and (*Li Gou*) LV-5 for swelling of the scrotum. He differentiated penile, scrotal, and testicular diseases into cold, heat, vacuity, and repletion patterns, and pointed out various disease causes and pathomechanisms of male conditions such as scrotal water swelling. This he attributed to unregulated eating and drinking and a tendency to anger, which causes fluids to flow downward into the scrotum as well as lack of free flow within the waterways. He also discussed the use of acumoxa therapy in the treatment of other male diseases including prominent mounting (*tui shan*), yin protraction, yang retraction (*yang suo*), fulminant pain in the genitals, (*yin bao tong*), yin wilt, genital sores (*yin chuang*), and genital itching and sweating (*yin yang han chu*).

Ge Hong (281–341 CE)

Ge Hong's most celebrated contribution to andrology is his Eastern Jin dynasty book, *Zhou Hou Bei Ji Fang* (*Emergency Standby Remedies*). Within the text, he discusses a number of male diseases including, male sudden swelling and pain (*nan zi yin zu tong*), sudden inward retraction of the testicles (*yin wan zu suo ru*), genital itching and sweating, pustular sores of the genitals (*yin sheng chuang nong chu*), and testicular prominence (*luan tui*). He offered a number of formulas to treat various andrological diseases. For yang wilt, he used the following medicinals: *Lu Jiao Jiao* (Cervi Cornus Gelatinum), *Ba Ji Tian* (Morindae Officinalis Radix), *Du Zhong* (Eucommiae Cortex), *Niu Xi* (Achyranthis Bidentatae Radix), *Gou Ji* (Cibotii Rhizoma), *Gan Jiang* (Zingiberis Rhizoma), and *Fu Zi* (Aconiti Radix lateralis Praeparata). For genital sweating, he used a topical application of powdered *Mu Li* (Ostreae Concha).

The Sui Dynasty (581 CE–619 CE)

Zhu Bing Yuan Hou Lun (On the Origin and Indicators of Disease) _____

By far, the most important contribution to andrology during the Sui dynasty was Chao Yuan-Fang's *Zhu Bing Yuan Hou Lun*, which was published in 610 CE. Rich in discussions of disease causes and pathomechanisms for men's diseases, the text has more than twenty entries for male conditions, some of which Chao introduced for the first time (Guo, 1999). Although the number of diseases discussed was fairly substantial, for the most part, the pathomechanisms are confined to kidney vacuity and are divided into four types: 1) vacuity taxation and detriment with "semen as clear as water; 2) kidney yang insufficiency with loss of warmth and "semen as cold as frozen iron"; 3) frequent seminal discharge leading to scanty semen and infertility and; 4) vacuity taxation and detriment and damage leading to inability to ejaculate and inability to have children due to the semen being unable to reach the uterus. Further, Chao divided seminal abnormalities into several types including: urine containing semen, hematospermia, seminal emission, dream emissions, premature ejaculation, seminal leakage, and inability to ejaculate. He also classified and described many urinary diseases as well including difficult urination (*xiao bian nan*), white turbid urine (*xiao bian bai zhuo*), post-voiding dribble (*xiao bian yu li*), and strangury. Finally, he correlated several andrological diseases with vacuity taxation disease including cold genitals, yin wilt, genital pain, genital swelling, and yin mounting. As in the categorization of many other diseases, Chao's work was extremely influential in the formation of later systems of classifying andrological diseases and understanding their pathomechanisms.

The Tang Dynasty (618 CE–907 CE)

Sun Si-Miao (581–683 CE) _____

Bei Ji Qian Jin Yao Fang (A Thousand Gold Pieces Emergency Formulary), one of Sun's major contributions to medicine, discusses over thirty andrological diseases including mounting qi, stone swelling (*ke zhong*), testicular swelling (*gao zhong*), genital pain, seminal discharge, and pain in the penis (*jing zhong tong*). In general, Sun emphasized the importance of the liver and kidneys in men's disease. However, he also advanced a unique perspective in that he identified not only vacuity patterns for kidney disease, but in addition discussed repletion kidney patterns. For example, the text states, "All [men] with a tendency to have pain in the penis while urinating have repletion heat in the kidneys." For such conditions, he recommended several different medicinals which are still in use today in the andrology department to clear repletion fire from the kidneys, including *Yu Bai Pi* (Ulmi Pumilae Cortex), *Hua Shi* (Talcum), *Tong Cao* (Tetrapanacis Medulla), *Shi Wei* (Pyrrosiae Folium), and *Dan Zhu Ye* (Lophatheri Herba) in order of importance. Sun identified excessive sexual activity damaging kidney yin as a cause of pain in the penis.

Sun is also famous for his early use of a catheter to treat male urinary retention as revealed in the following passage from *Bei Ji Qian Jin Yao Fang*: "The bladder sac belongs to the kidney and bladder; it stores liquid and humor and urine. If there is visceral heat disease, [flow in] the bladder will be rough [and there will be] urinary stoppage. This is ascribed to bladder inhibition and aggregation and liquid and humor stoppage. Use a scallion leaf with the head removed and deeply insert it into the head of the penis [to a depth of] about three *cun*. Blow into it slightly until the bladder becomes distended and there will be a great flow of liquid and humor; the condition will be cured."

Yet another unique and interesting feature of Sun Si-Miao's work on male disorders is the fact that he used a combination of therapies including medicinal formulas, acumoxa therapy, and food therapy to treat his patients. As an example, in his treatment of semen in the urine, he recommended a formula containing qi and yin supplementing medicinals made into pills with honey, thirty cones of moxa on the point beside the seventh vertebra on the back, and glutinous rice gruel made with the juice of *Jiu Cai Zi*. According to Ma and An (2001), some of his more common acumoxa point selections for men's disorders include: *Da He* (KI-12) and *Ran Gu* (KI-2) for essence spillage (*jing yi*) and upward retraction of the genitals (*yin shang suo*); *Qu Quan* (LV-8) for yin wilt; *Xing Jian* (LV-2) for toxin within the penis (*jing zhong du*) and; *Da Dun* (LV-1) for sudden mounting and fulminant pain (*zu shan bao tong*).

The Song Dynasty (960 CE–1279 CE)

During the Song dynasty, with the publication of the great formularies *Tai Ping Hui Min He Ji Ju Fang* (*Tai-Ping Imperial Grace Pharmacy*), *Tai Ping Sheng Hui Fang* (*The Great Peace Sagacious Benevolence Formulary*), and the *Sheng Ji Zong Lu* (*Sages' Salvation Records*), there was a vigorous expansion in the number of medicinal formulas available for the treatment of andrological diseases. Some of the formulas introduced in these texts became standard formulas in and of themselves, and also served as templates for other andrology formulas developed by subsequent physicians. Examples of andrological diseases addressed in these texts include yin wilt, seminal loss (*shi jing*), seminal loss in urine (*xiao bian shi jing*), dream emissions, scanty semen (*jing shao*), white turbidity (*bai zhuo*), and yin mounting.

The Jin (1115 CE–1234 CE) and Yuan (1271 CE–1368 CE) Dynasties

The Jin and Yuan dynasties are often credited with being periods in which there was a great flowering of Chinese medical theories. During these dynasties, we recognize the formation of four new schools of thought or "scholarly streams (*xue pai*)" in Chinese medicine, which are related with four physicians; they came to be known collectively as the "four great masters of the Jin-Yuan (*jin yuan si da jia*)." Their names are Liu Wan-Su, Zhang Zi-He, Li Dong-Yuan, and Zhu Dan-Xi. While each had broad and varied careers, they are individually identified with having emphasized a particular theoretical analysis of disease: Liu Wan-Su with fire as a key disease cause; Zhang Zi-He with repletion as the main disease cause and the corresponding use of the three draining methods (ejection, sweating, and precipitating); Li Dong-Yuan with the pivotal role of the spleen and stomach in health and disease and; Zhu Dan-Xi with the idea that yang is usually in superabundance and yin is usually insufficient. In fact, these are great oversimplifications, but nevertheless they are standard ways of framing the main contributions of each of these physicians. Skirting a broader analysis of the work of each of the four great masters, I will briefly outline what they contributed to the theory and practice of andrology, but by far, Zhu Dan-Xi's ideas had the most significant effect on the development of andrology.

Liu Wan-Su (1120–1200 CE)

Consistent with one of his main doctrines—the idea that "the six qi all transform from fire"—Liu emphasized the treatment of fire in his writings on andrological diseases. For example, he reasoned that many cases of strangury involved depressed heat within the bladder and he therefore stressed the importance of using cold and cool treatments for treating it. This is certainly a valuable clinical insight that still has merit in the treatment of acute and chronic prostatitis. According to Wang (2003), one of Liu Wan-Su's most famous formulas—*Fang Feng Tong Sheng San* (Saposhnikovia Sage-Inspired Powder)—was later adopted by Ming and Qing physicians for the treatment of bayberry toxin (*mei du*) [*i.e.*, syphilis].

Zhang Zi-He (1156–1228 CE)

In retrospect from the 21st century, considering his emphasis on repletion pathomechanisms of disease, Zhang Zi-He may have been extremely influential in encouraging the same for andrological conditions. He is famous for his statement, "For nourishing life, [one] should study foods that supplement, and for treating diseases [one] should study medicines that attack," which reveals his awareness that many diseases are caused by repletion. As an example, in his analysis of a pediatric case of dribbling urinary block he stated, "This is retention in the lower burner. [If one] does not use ejection or precipitation, then how can the lower burner open? [Without such methods, I] fear that rheum and water cannot be disinhibited." For this case, he successfully used *Tiao Wei Cheng Qi Tang* (Stomach-Regulating Qi-Infusing Decoction) plus *Qian Niu Zi* (Pharbitidis Semen). His treatment principle was to open the lower burner by: 1) precipitating evils from the lower burner with *Tiao Wei Cheng Qi Tang* and; 2) ejecting evils from the upper burner with *Bai Jie Zi* (Sinapis Semen). Ideas and therapeutic approaches such as this have had an enduring influence on the understanding of andrological diseases in Chinese medicine.

Li Dong-Yuan (1180–1251 CE)

The father of the so-called "earth-supplementing school," Li Dong-Yuan put forth a strong opinion that internal damage to the spleen and stomach causes "the hundred diseases." His writings contained evidence that he saw spleen-stomach vacuity as the root cause of some andrological diseases including yang wilt, seminal emission, and infertility. To understand his reasoning, I believe we should first appreciate Li's understanding of the unity of all qi in the human body as revealed in the following passage from *Pi Wei Lun* (*On the Spleen and Stomach*): "Original qi, grain qi, construction qi, clear qi, and defense qi are all [forms] of qi that are engendered from the yang that is borne upward. These six all [form when] fluid and food enters the stomach and grain qi moves upward. They are different names for stomach qi, [but] actually, they are one." Once we understand the physiology of qi in this way, we have the theoretical key that brings Li Dong-Yuan's approach to male disorders into clearer light. Further, in another passage he stated, "[If] spleen and stomach qi are already damaged, then original qi cannot be full; as a result of this, many diseases are caused." As I see it, this presupposes that the later heaven source for the engenderment of qi, blood, essence, and fluid (the spleen and stomach) enriches the early heaven source (the kidneys). So, we may conclude then that according to Li, spleen and stomach vacuity can result in kidney vacuity and hence male anterior yin diseases. This theory is still applied today in the treatment of conditions such as yang wilt and male infertility.

It is also important to note that Li Dong-Yuan's ideas explain how spleen and stomach vacuity—caused or compounded by dietary indiscretions—can result in damp-heat which pours downward and brews and binds in the lower burner. According to Wang (2003), this is a crucial pathomechanism involved in the vast majority of cases of prostatitis, orchitis, and many other andrological diseases.

Zhu Dan-Xi (1281–1358 CE)

Zhu Dan-Xi's ideas had a profound influence on the understanding of male physiology and pathology in Chinese medicine. His basic notion—an elegant expression of yin-yang theory—is that yin governs quietude and yang governs stirring and movement. One of the most famous phrases from his writings which reveals how he saw yin and yang interacting in pathology is: "yang is usually in superabundance and yin is usually insufficient." In *Ge Zhi Yu Lun* (*Further Treatises on the Properties of Things*), he stated, "That which governs blockage and storage is the kidneys; that which manages coursing and discharge is the liver. Both of these possess ministerial fire and are tied to the heart in the upper [body]. The heart is ascribed to sovereign fire and is easily stirred by emotional matters. When the heart stirs, ministerial fire also stirs. When it [*i.e.*, ministerial fire] stirs, semen spontaneously moves. [Hence] when the tranquility of ministerial fire is stirred up, even in the absence of intercourse, [semen] is coursed and discharged, and flows in the dark [*i.e.*, during the night]." He went on to say that for this reason it is important to nourish the heart and control one's desires to avoid damaging one's essence.

Based on this understanding, it is apparent why Zhu Dan-Xi advocated enriching kidney yin and downbearing yin vacuity fire for many men's diseases. One of his most famous formulas, *Da Bu Yin Wan* (Major Yin Supplementation Pill), nourishes kidney yin and downbears yin vacuity fire. Dan-Xi used it to treat dream emissions and seminal efflux among other andrological diseases. This formula and others that Zhu Dan-Xi created (and perhaps even more importantly the theory they are based on), became firmly embedded in the minds of subsequent Chinese doctors and remain extremely influential to this day.

The Ming (1368 CE–1644 CE) and Qing (1644 CE–1912 CE) Dynasties

During the Ming and Qing dynasties, mirroring the rich development within Chinese medicine in general, and in accordance with the expression of divergent opinions and the development of many different specialties, there was a corresponding expansion in andrology. There were significant improvements in the understanding of male physiology, and in andrological disease nomenclature, causation and pathomechanisms. We cannot undertake a detailed study of all the various developments within andrology that occurred during the Ming and Qing dynasties, but we can cover a few significant points.

Zhang Jing-Yue (1563–1640 CE) and his expansion of kidney theory

Certainly Zhang Jing-Yue was one of the most famous physicians of the Ming dynasty. His understanding of the roles of the kidneys in male physiology had a deep influence on andrology. Based on his detailed study of the *Nei Jing*, and on his clinical experience, he wrote extensively about the kidneys in male physiology and pathology, and especially focused on the unity and interactions of yin and yang. In *Lei Jing Fu Yi* (*Wings to the Classified Canon*), he stated, "Yin cannot exist without yang; without qi, form cannot be engendered. Yang cannot exist without yin; without yang, form cannot be carried. So, substance is engendered because yang engenders it, and substance is formed because yin forms it. This is so-called original yin and original yang and is also called true essence and true qi." In another section of the same text, he explained further: "Early heaven causes qi to transform [into] form; [this] is yang engendering yin. Later heaven is form transforming [into] qi; [this] is yin engendering yang. Form is essence and essence is water. Spirit is qi and qi is fire. The two qi—yin and yang—most importantly should not be imbalanced. If they are not imbalanced, qi is harmonious and can engender substance. If they are imbalanced, qi is disharmonious and kills substance."

Zhang followed through with those ideas in his formula construction, as exhibited in two of his most famous formulas: *Zuo Gui Wan* (Left-Restoring [Kidney Yin] Pill) and *You Gui Wan (Right-Restoring [Life Gate] Pill)*. The former—for nourishing and enriching kidney yin and essence—also has some yang-supplementing action, and the latter—for warming and supplementing kidney yang—also has some yin and essence-enriching action. He explained, "Those who are good at treating essence are able to make qi be engendered from within essence; those who are good at treating qi are able to make essence be engendered from within qi. This follows the mysterious use of [the fact that yin and yang] are separate but indivisible," and "Those who are good at supplementing yang, must seek yang within the midst of yin; thus yang is helped by yin, so that its engendering and transformation is not impoverished. Those who are good at treating yin, should seek yin within the midst of yang; thus yin is engendered by yang and its source is not exhausted."

Finally, as we follow Zhang's work to its logical conclusion about the interactions between kidney essence and kidney yang at puberty and as long as a man remains fertile, we see that at two times eight years of age and continuously from that point forward until old age, there must be adequate kidney yin-essence and kidney yang qi in order for heavenly tenth to be engendered and to flow. In other words, the initiation and continuous transformation of kidney yin-essence into heavenly tenth requires kidney yang, and kidney yang in turn transforms out of kidney yin-essence. This represents a deeper explanation of the original ideas found in Chapter 1 of *Su Wen* that we explored earlier, and continues to be applied by modern physicians in their treatment of many different male diseases.

Clarification of Andrological Disease Nomenclature

With the accumulated experiences of physicians recorded over the several preceding dynasties, doctors of the Ming and Qing dynasties had access to a greater wealth of written material and clinical experience than any previous generation of Chinese physicians. This spawned what is sometimes called the "golden age of Chinese medicine." In terms of andrology, Ming and Qing efforts—some of which were government-driven—produced ever more finely detailed definitions and differentiations of diseases such as seminal emission, dribbling urinary block, strangury-turbidity, and mounting qi. Medical historians believe that it is during this period that syphilis entered China; hence we see discussions of bayberry toxin in the medical literature of this period, most notably by Li Shi Zhen (1518–1593 CE) in his massive work, *Ben Cao Gang Mu* (*Herbal Foundation Compendium*).

Further Development of External Medicine (*wai ke*)

During the Qing dynasty, the field of external medicine underwent a great expansion. Texts from this period contain detailed descriptions of male external diseases. Among these are Xu Ke-Chang and Hua Fa-He's *Wai Ke Zheng Zhi Quan Shu* (*Compendium of External Medicine, Patterns and Treatment*), published in 1831, and the *Wai Ke Xin Fa Yao Jue* (*A Heart Approach to External Medicine*) section of the *Yi Zong Jin Jian* (*The Golden Mirror of Medicine*), which was compiled and edited by Wu Qian in 1742. Within these two texts, there are detailed discussions of the causes, pathomechanisms, and treatments of many andrological external diseases including suspended welling-abscess (*xuan yong*), crotch-boring sore (*chuang dang fa*), lower *gan* sore (*xia gan chuang*), genital wind sore (*yin feng chuang*), penis head sore (*yin tou chuang*), penis head pain (*yin tou tong*), genital welling-abscess (*yin nong*), and kidney sac wind (*shen nang feng*).

The Nationalist Period (1911 CE–1949 CE) and the People's Republic of China (1949 CE–present)

After the fall of the Qing dynasty, the newly empowered Nationalist party aspired to modernize China to bring it into step with the modern Western world. They adopted sweeping changes in many areas of Chinese life including medicine. Generally speaking, party officials did not look very favorably upon traditional medicine. They viewed it as a remnant of prescientific China, and it was therefore targeted for major reform. Hence, headstrong factions within the party actually strove to outlaw it, and they came very near to succeeding in the early years of their reign. However, in the final hour the traditional doctors organized themselves politically, and in concession to the modernization agenda agreed to add Western medical courses to the traditional medicine curriculum. Reactions to this concession varied among traditional doctors from outright resentment of what were perceived as the unnecessary interloping concepts of Western medicine to acceptance of the new ideas in a spirit of exchange. A prime example of the latter was Zhang Xi-Chun (1860–1933 CE), author of *Yi Xue Zhong Zhong Can Xi Lu* (*Records of Chinese Medicine with Reference to Western Medicine*), a series of seven handbooks which were published between 1918 and 1934. According to Wang (2003), these texts contain many discussions of andrological conditions and Zhang Xi-Chun's ideas reflected the ferment of Chinese and Western medicine that characterized the times in which he lived and worked. He attempted to integrate some Western medical ideas and practices with his traditional ones. In this light, we can view Zhang as an early pioneer of modern Chinese andrology, which is a manifestation of what eventually came to be known—in the People's Republic of China—as "integrated Chinese-Western medicine (*zhong xi yi jie he*)."

After the establishment of the People's Republic of China in 1949, in response to many different factors, the government gave more active support to Chinese medicine by establishing many colleges and hospitals, and by promoting research and development within the field on a huge scale. Following in the footsteps of the concessions made to the Nationalist government, the Chinese medicine curriculum at these new institutions included a substantial amount of Western medicine, and research was conducted according to Western scientific principles. On the other hand, many Western doctors were also required to take some course work in Chinese medicine, and thus were exposed to the traditional knowledge as well as the modern. From within this fertile milieu, there emerged a body of practitioners and researchers that sought to integrate ideas and practices from both Chinese and Western medicine and to use Western science to test and validate Chinese medicine. This gave rise to unique and interesting hybrid doctors such as oncologists who treated the side effects of chemotherapy and radiation with Chinese medicine, hepatologists who used Chinese medicine to treat their hepatitis patients—and most central to the task of this book—urologists who integrated modern urology with traditional knowledge about men's health and disease. Gradually, as these practitioners gathered their research and experience and published their findings, a new speciality within integrated Chinese-Western medicine emerged. In Chinese, the title of the department in the hospitals and clinics where these specialists worked came to be known as *nan ke*—here translated as andrology.

As is typical in the pluralistic environment of Chinese medicine, the knowledge ratio (Western medicine to Chinese medicine) varies for any given andrology specialist; hence, his clinical skills and emphasis vary in direct relationship to that ratio. Thus, the modern Chinese andrology textbooks, and published clinical research and case study collections all reflect this reality. For example, in the same text I often find detailed discussions of Western medical physiology and pathology alongside thorough explorations of the premodern understanding of the same phenomena. In clinical practice, although modern diagnostic techniques may be used to detect and assess a patient's enlarged prostate, he may solely receive Chinese medical treatment. This text is designed to reflect the current state of the field as it has historically evolved in China, though my own emphasis is weighted much more heavily on the Chinese medical side than on the Western. Although I fully embrace modern Western medical knowledge, I do this for two reasons—I am not a Western-trained urologist and there are excellent Western urology textbooks available in the English language. Further, I am a physician of Chinese medicine and there are currently no systematic English language texts on Chinese andrology extant.

This text is designed to reflect the current state of the field as it has historically evolved in China, though my own emphasis is weighted much more heavily on the Chinese medical side than on the Western. Although I fully embrace modern Western medical knowledge, I do this for two reasons—I am not a Western-trained urologist and there are excellent Western urology textbooks available in the English language. Further, I am a physician of Chinese medicine and there are currently no systematic English language texts on Chinese andrology extant.

Functional Male Anatomy: Correlating Chinese and Western Medicine

It is well-known that the growth of premodern Chinese anatomy was stunted by Confucian beliefs in ancestor worship and the sanctity of the human body which made dissection taboo. We often overlook the fact that in the 1st century CE, the authors of the *Nan Jing* (*Classic of Difficult Issues*)[1] provided elementary anatomical descriptions of the organs of the human body. However, Chinese anatomy never really progressed any further than that, despite periodic efforts by physicians and the government to promote its advance. Prominent among these efforts were those of Wang Qing-Ren, who in his Qing dynasty text—*Yi Lin Gai Cuo* (*Corrections of Errors in Medical Classics*)[2]— criticized physicians who attempted to practice medicine or write medical treatises without grasping anatomy when he stated: "To write a book without knowing thoroughly the internal organs—is it not comparable to a man speaking in a dream? To treat a disease without knowing thoroughly the internal organs—how does it differ from a blind man groping in the dark?" (Wong and Wu, 1985, p. 199). Unfortunately, although Wang made many attempts to personally visualize or examine the internal organs of the human body by attending public executions and by traveling to areas in which epidemics had occurred and corpses were available, he made no major contributions to Chinese anatomy. Of course, he did advance our understanding of blood stasis and designed several effective formulas which are still in use today.

This is not to say that Chinese physicians completely ignored anatomy, but merely to suggest that it remained fairly unsophisticated until Western medicine began to make significant inroads into Chinese medicine during the 19th century. In terms of male anatomy, centuries before the arrival of Western medicine, Chinese physicians developed their own specific terms to describe the male external genitalia—which of course were readily observable without dissection. Among these we find terms for the scrotum (*yin nang*), the testes (*shen zi*), and the penis (*yin jing*). And there were also terms for internal structures that were invisible without dissection, which were vaguer

---

[1] The *Nan Jing* was published in the 1st century CE, during the Eastern Han dynasty.
[2] *Yi Lin Gai Cuo* was written by Wang Qing-Ren in 1830, during the Qing dynasty.

and more functional than structural; these included the essence chamber (*jing shi*), the essence gate (*jing guan*), and the seminal pathway (*jing dao*). In some of these latter examples, Chinese physicians surmised that such structures must exist and described them as functional entities, even without having personally visualized their specific morphology.

Although there is no shame in acknowledging the inferiority of Chinese anatomy in comparison to Western anatomy, at the same time we should be confident that Chinese medicine's underdeveloped understanding of the individual morphological structure of the organs and tissues is somewhat offset by its early and sophisticated grasp of the unity and interactions among organs and tissues. In this light, the holism of Chinese medicine and the reductionism of Western medicine complement each other. Once we accept this premise our task as practitioners of modern Chinese andrology is to make intelligent and clinically useful correlations between functional male anatomy as understood by both Chinese and Western medicine.

Since andrology specialists in China are generally dually trained in Western and Chinese medicine, all Chinese textbooks of andrology contain a section devoted to male anatomy and physiology according to Western medicine. There are many English language texts that contain excellent presentations of these facts, and in much greater detail than I will provide here. Nevertheless, any textbook of Chinese andrology should have at least a brief review of the functional anatomy of the male urogenital system according to Western medicine, and should show how these anatomical structures are labeled in Chinese medicine. Further, as a form of integrated Chinese-Western medicine, modern Chinese andrology attempts to treat Western-defined diseases such as prostatitis and epididymitis, even though there are no premodern texts that specifically mention the prostate or epididymis. It can only do so by reframing the Western disease into Chinese medical disease categories[3] and by reframing the Western-defined anatomical structures into the closest-known Chinese one. So, for these reasons I present a brief review of the functional anatomy of the male genital system and correlate the Western names with the Chinese ones.

The Scrotum

Chinese medicine

There are many names for the scrotum in Chinese medicine including the "sac" (*nang*), the "kidney sac" (*shen nang*), and the "yin sac" (*yin nang*).

Western medicine

Anatomy

According to Western anatomy, the scrotum is a pouch of loose skin and fascia that is evaginated from the abdominal wall. There is a ridge or raphe which

[3] See Book 1, chapter 6 on Chinese medical disease categories for more on this subject and the introduction to each disease in Book 2.

divides the scrotum into two lateral sections. The spermatic cord—which suspends the testes within the scrotum—is longer on the left side than on the right. This makes the lateral left portion of the scrotum and the left testis hang lower than the right. The dartos, involuntary muscle fibers that lie within the superficial fascia of the scrotum, contract or relax in response to temperature changes. When the scrotum becomes cold, the dartos contract and the scrotum pulls up, wrinkles, and becomes firm; when the scrotum becomes warm, the dartos relax and the scrotum elongates and becomes flaccid in response. The left and right compartments of the scrotum are established by the dartos and superficial fascia. In each of these two compartments lies a testis, its epididymis, and all other related structures.

Physiology

The main functions of the scrotum are to: 1) house and protect the testes and all their associated structures and; 2) maintain optimal temperature for sperm production and vitality by keeping testicular temperature 2°C cooler than the abdominal cavity.

The Testes and Epididymis

Chinese medicine

In Chinese medicine, the testes and the epididymis are grouped together under various names including *shen zi* and *luan zi*, meaning "kidney seed" or "kidney child" and "eggs" literally. The epididymis was not discussed as a separate anatomical structure until the modern era, after Western medicine had exerted its influence over andrology. Hence, I am aware of no traditional anatomical term for it.

Western medicine

Anatomy

The testes are situated within the left and right compartments of the scrotum. In a normal male, the testes should be symmetrical in size and ovate, though it is normal for the left testis to hang lower than the right because the spermatic cord is longer on the left than on the right. According to Crouch (1978), the average length of each testis is 4–5 cm and the average weight ranges from 10.5–14 grams. The testes are housed within the abdominal cavity during the early part of fetal life, but then descend downward through the inguinal canal into the scrotum before birth. Thereafter, they are housed within the scrotum. It is during their descent that they become covered with various microscopic layers which are derived from the abdominal wall, and which include the outermost layer—the tunica vaginalis—under which there is a fibrous membrane called the tunica albuginea. Fibrous septa extend inward from the tunica albuginea and divide each testis into numerous compartments. Each of these compartments contains from 1–3 seminiferous tubules, which each average from 70–80 cm in length. Amazingly, given the vast number of seminiferous tubules contained within each testis, the total length of these tubules contained within one testis exceeds a half of a mile. They comprise about two-thirds of the total volume of each testis (Bhasin and Jameson, 2007). Each of these tubules eventually straightens and collectively forms a network of tubes called the rete testis, which then join with the head of the epididymis through the efferent ductules.

At the posterior aspect of each testis, on a surface that is not covered by the tunica vaginalis, lies the epididymis. It is an elongated and flattened structure which is highly tortuous. If straightened, its length would be roughly equal to that of the small intestine (6–7 meters). The upper end of the epididymis is known as the head (caput epididymidis), the lower end is known as the tail (cauda epididymidis), and the section between these two is called the body (corpus epididymidis). The head of the epididymis joins with the efferent ductules from the testis and thus directly receives semen and sperm. The tail of the epididymis becomes less and less tortuous and eventually straightens out to become the vas deferens (ductus deferens). The basement membrane of the epididymis is lined with a thin layer of smooth muscle which contracts during ejaculation and conveys semen and sperm into the vas deferens.

On the posterior surface of the testis, arteries enter and veins leave, comprising the testicular circulatory loop. There are many more veins than arteries supplying the testis. These veins are very tortuous and rather large; they gather together to form the pampiniform plexus. A varicocele—a major cause of male infertility—is essentially a varicosity within this venous plexus which raises the temperature within the testis and sometimes causes male infertility by causing poor-quality semen and sperm.

Physiology

Testicular function is controlled by the gonadotropin hormones secreted by the anterior pituitary such as luteinizing hormone (LH) and follicle stimulating hormone (FSH). LH stimulates testosterone synthesis by acting on specialized testicular cells within the seminiferous tubules called Leydig cells. FSH serves to stimulate spermatogenesis by acting directly on yet another specialized testicular cell within the seminiferous tubules called the Sertoli cell. Anterior pituitary gonadotropin release is in turn influenced by gonadotropin-releasing hormone (GnRH), which is secreted from the hypothalamus. The actions and interactions of these hormones with each other, with other hormones including testosterone and estrogen, and enzymatic pathways is a complex and interesting dance which is well-documented in existing English language textbooks on physiology. A more detailed exploration is beyond the scope of this text and arguably outside the clinical realm of a Western practitioner of Chinese andrology.

The main functions of the testes are to produce sperm and to secrete the male sex hormone testosterone. According to Bhasin and Jameson (2007), 95% of circulating testosterone in the adult male body is secreted in the testes. Testosterone functions to promote: 1) spermatogenesis; 2) the development of male secondary sex characteristics; 3) the growth and development of subsidiary male sex organs; 3) normal libido and sexual vigor and; 5) anabolism (constructive metabolism).

The main functions of the epididymis are to: 1) store sperm (primarily in the tail of the epididymis [cauda epididymidis]); 2) provide a place for sperm to mature; 3) phagocytize and reabsorb those sperm that have not been ejaculated or have disintegrated and; 4) convey semen and sperm forward and outward to the vas deferens when contracting during ejaculation.

The Vas Deferens and the Seminal Vesicle

Chinese medicine

In Chinese medicine, the vas deferens and the seminal vesicle are somewhat loosely referred to as the "seminal pathway" (*jing dao*).

Western medicine

Anatomy

The vas deferens (ductus deferens)—which is essentially a tube that delivers sperm from the testis—is really a continuation of the epididymis and is separated from it only in name. It begins at the tail of the epididymis as it gradually becomes less tortuous and straightens out, and then travels upward into the groin on the lateral side of the abdomen and enters the pelvic cavity. It crosses between the ureter and the bladder at the posterior aspect of the urinary bladder, eventually meets the seminal vesicle and terminates at the ejaculatory duct, which empties into the prostatic urethra (the portion of the urethra surrounded by the prostate). Roughly midway toward its termination, the vas deferens widens and forms the ampulla of the vas deferens. In a vasectomy, the vas deferens is either severed from the scrotum or tied in order to achieve permanent birth control by preventing the delivery of sperm via ejaculation. The traveling vas deferens, along with the arteries, veins, lymphatic vessels, and nerves that accompany it, comprise the spermatic cord.

The seminal vesicle is pressed against the latero-posterior aspect of the bladder and the upper part of the prostate. The seminal vesicle and the vas deferens meet at the superior aspect of the prostate and form the ejaculatory duct which passes into the prostate and empties into the prostatic urethra.

Physiology

The main functions of the vas deferens are to: 1) deliver sperm from the testis to the urethra and; 2) store and lubricate sperm, especially within the ampulla.

The main function of the seminal vesicle is to secrete an alkaline fluid which combines with the fluid secreted within the vas deferens and comprises the bulk of semen. This fluid reduces the acidity of vaginal mucus to ensure the viability and motility of sperm.

The Prostate

Chinese medicine

The most commonly used premodern Chinese anatomical term for the prostate is the "essence chamber" (*jing shi*). However, some texts refer to it as part of the "life gate" (*ming men*), most notably the *Nan Jing* (*Classic of Difficult Issues*).

Western medicine

Anatomy

The prostate is a walnut-shaped gland which is situated inferior to the bladder and anterior to the rectum, and surrounds the superior end of the urethra and the ejaculatory duct. The fact that it is superior to the rectum allows it to be palpated via digital rectal examination (DRE) to assess its size and morphology when prostatic hyperplasia, inflammation, infection, or cancer is suspected. The fact that it surrounds the urethra accounts for the high incidence of urinary outlet obstruction symptoms in prostatic disease. Further, the fact that it surrounds the ejaculatory duct accounts for the high incidence of sexual dysfunction such as premature ejaculation and painful ejaculation in prostatic diseases, especially in chronic prostatitis. The prostate is surrounded on its outside by fibrous connective tissue and smooth muscle fibers which protrude into the gland itself and divide it into five lobes: the anterior lobe; two lateral lobes; the central lobe and; the posterior lobe.

Physiology

The prostate is the largest male sex gland and its main physiological function is to secrete alkaline prostatic fluid which, along with the secretions from within the epididymis and seminal vesicle, is one component of semen. This relatively alkaline secretion serves as a buffer to the acidic vaginal secretions and thereby improves the viability and activity of sperm. During ejaculation, smooth muscle fibers within the prostate contract helping to propel sperm forward as the prostate adds its secretion to the semen.

The Bulbourethral Glands (Cowper's Glands)

Chinese medicine

There is no known specific premodern anatomical term for the bulbourethral glands in Chinese medicine. Their secretions, however, can logically be considered a manifestation of essence since they comprise an aspect of semen.

Western medicine

Anatomy

The bulbourethral glands are two pea-sized mucus-producing glands that lie superior to the bulb of the urethra bilaterally, within the fascia of the urogenital diaphragm. They empty into the cavernous urethra (the portion of the urethra traveling through the corpus cavernosum of the penis) via the bulbourethral duct.

Physiology

When the penis becomes erect and during ejaculation, the ensuing pressure these glands are subjected to causes them to secrete their fluid which serves to lubricate the mucosal surface of the urethra.

The Spermatic Cord

Chinese medicine

In Chinese medicine, the spermatic cord is called "the seminal tie" (*jing zi xi*).

Western medicine

Anatomy

The spermatic cord is the rope-like tissue which suspends the testes and other tissues within the scrotum. It arises from within the groin and moves diagonally outward passing through the groin and enters the scrotum connecting with the testes at their posterior aspect. The spermatic cord arises from the testicular tissue, and comprises the internal artery of the vas deferens, external spermatic cord artery, spermatic cord artery, pampiniform veins, spermatic cord nerves, lymphatic vessels, and fascia. Testicular torsion—a surgical emergency because it obstructs normal blood and lymphatic circulation to the testis—occurs when the testis becomes twisted on its spermatic cord. It presents with an acutely painful, tender, and swollen testis that is retracted upward into a red and edematous scrotum.

Physiology

Since the spermatic cord contains the arteries, veins, nerves, and lymphatics that supply the testes, it is intimately related with their blood supply, nervous system control, lymphatic drainage, and tissue metabolism.

The Penis

Chinese medicine

In Chinese medicine, the penis is known as the "stem " (*jing*), the "ancestral sinew" (*zong jing*), and the "jade stem" (*yu jing*). In Chinese medicine, the penis is divided into three sections; distally to proximally, they are the turtle head, the body, and the root or foot of the penis.

Western medicine

Anatomy

The penis is divided into three cavernous or erectile bodies: the left and right corpus cavernosum and the corpus spongiosum urethrae. These three bodies are supported by connective tissue and are "wrapped" together by Buck's fascia. They are richly supplied with a sponge-like network of spaces and tortuous arteries which dilate and hence become engorged with blood during erection. When the deeper veins within the corpus cavernosum and corpus spongiosum constrict, the blood is trapped in these spaces and in these arteries. The increased pressure that results from this trapped blood pressing against the fibrous sheaths surrounding these corpora stiffens the penis. Normally, after ejaculation or sexual excitation otherwise wanes, arterial contraction and venous relaxation causes blood to drain out of the penis and it becomes flaccid. In priapism, for various reasons, blood remains in the penis causing persistent painful erection unaccompanied by sexual excitation. Untreated and persistent priapism leads to permanent loss of erectile function due to damage to erectile tissue and arteries and veins within the penile corpora, and even to gangrene of the penis in the most serious cases.

The thin layer of loose skin on the outside of the penis expands and contracts in accordance with temperature and the presence or absence of erectile response. In the uncircumcised male, this loose skin forms a hoodlike fold (the foreskin or prepuce) which covers the glans penis at the distal end of the penis; it retracts spontaneously during erection and can be manually pulled back proximally over the glans penis when the penis is flaccid. Circumcision involves the surgical removal of the foreskin.

Physiology

Erection of the penis is elicited by sexual excitation from visual, olfactory, mental, and tactile stimuli. The three physiological events that must occur for normal erectile function include: 1) sufficient engorgement of arterial blood within the corpus cavernosum and the corpus spongiosum; 2) constriction of the deeper veins within these same corpora in order for blood to remain trapped within them and; 3) constriction against the pressure caused by the trapped blood within the skin and fascia surrounding the spongy tissue. These are important to keep in mind when evaluating men with sexual dysfunction, as any disease process that interferes with normal blood flow to and from the penis may cause erectile dysfunction (Beers and Porter *et al.*, 2006).

Of course, the penis is also a urinary organ in that the cavernous urethra (the portion of the urethra that passes through the corpus cavernosum) passes through the penis.

The Channels and Network Vessels in Andrology

Herbal medicine and acumoxa therapy are arguably the two most prominent treatment modalities of Chinese medicine. Each of these is firmly based on its constituent cognitive structure which guides practitioners through the clinical encounter.[1] Herbal medicine is primarily infused with viscera-bowel theory and acumoxa therapy with channel and network vessel theory. At first glance, these cognitive structures might appear to be separate and distinct. In this view, herbal medicine is purely informed by viscera-bowel theory and acumoxa therapy solely by channel and network vessel theory. However, when we closely examine the early premodern texts of Chinese medicine such as *Huang Di Nei Jing* (*The Yellow Emperor's Inner Canon*),[2] viscera-bowel theory and channel and network vessel theory are clearly integrated in a sophisticated way. While acknowledging this integration, I do think it is equally important to grasp that the rational structure of Chinese herbal medicine is dominated by viscera-bowel theory and that of acumoxa therapy was originally dominated by channel and network vessel theory. Hence, while both modalities can be combined together clinically, medicinals excel at rectifying pathomechanisms of the viscera and bowels (which then affect their constituent channels and network vessels) and acumoxa therapy excels at treating pathomechanisms of the channels and network vessels (which then affect their constituent viscera and bowels). In the unified human body depicted in *Nei Jing*, the same clinical problems can theoretically be treated from either direction, though clinical experience often reveals that one or the other (or a combination of both) yields better results in specific circumstances.

Anyone who has studied Chinese medicine in China or who has lived for any length of time in the People's Republic of China or on Taiwan is acutely aware that herbal medicine dominates modern Chinese medicine on its home turf. In fact it does so to the extent that in those places a doctor of Chinese medicine is first and foremost a doctor of herbal medicine who more often than not never even touches a needle or moxa stick in

---

[1] I do not suggest, however, that the clinician should only be guided by rationalism. Indeed, successful clinicians also exhibit highly developed affective and psychomotor skills.

[2] *Huang Di Nei Jing* was written in the 1st century CE, during the Han dynasty.

clinical practice. This is so regardless of how Western acumoxa therapists feel about it or whether or not we wish it were otherwise.

In my experience, many students of Chinese medicine return from internships in China or Taiwan with a new appreciation for the preeminent place of herbal medicine within the edifice that is Chinese medicine in China. Many are perplexed by this fact in comparison to the relative dominance of acumoxa therapy in the West. In trying to understand this reality, some are tempted by overly simplistic and erroneous assertions that this is purely a post-Maoist development and that in some prior "golden age" of Chinese medicine, acumoxa therapy was dominant. Some may even feel that we should strive to reinstall the more "energetic" or "spiritual" channel theory-based acumoxa therapy to its rightful place ahead of the more base, materialistic, and viscera-bowel theory based herbal medicine. I do not espouse this position and make no such argument here.[3] I do, however, assert that to understand the traditional use of acumoxa therapy in andrology, and indeed at all, we must first understand channel and network vessel theory.

I am very interested in the fact that although acumoxa therapy generally dominates the minds of practitioners in the West, its practice is generally defined and (I argue) confined by the cognitive structure of Chinese herbal medicine (viscera-bowel theory) rather than that of acumoxa therapy (channel and network vessel theory). Hence, like Chinese medicinals, acumoxa points are assigned certain "actions" which supposedly embody the full range of their clinical applications. Students memorize these actions in order to pass their acupuncture college and licensing examinations and more often than not do not attempt to relate these actions to channel and network vessel theory.[4] To illustrate this point, I have observed that when asked to provide the rationale behind their point selection in clinic, students usually completely bypass channel and network vessel theory and instead cite the actions of the points as the primary reason for using them. Indeed, teaching and learning acumoxa point application in this context can be a useful way of helping students and practitioners remember facts about the clinical use of points and can be used as a bridge back to channel and network vessel theory. However, if left isolated

---

[3] In all fairness, we should recognize that a thorough exploration of these issues would surely involve a detailed analysis of historical, anthropological, and sociopolitical factors. Clearly, this is not the focus of our discussion here.

[4] As Deadman and Al-Khafagi (1998) argue, while describing acumoxa points as having a particular action is predominantly a twentieth century phenomenon, we can indeed find examples of this practice in premodern texts. What a closer examination of the theoretical underpinnings of assigning actions to points reveals is that sometimes the use of a point for a particular purpose is explained well by viscera-bowel theory, sometimes it is explained by the physical pathway of its channel, sometimes by its record of empirical effectiveness for a certain condition, at times it is used purely based on its anatomical proximity to the tissue of concern, and at yet other times it is explained by other theories unique to acumoxa therapy such as assignment of points according to five phase theory, five stream point theory, stem and branch theory, etc.

from its rational backbone—channel and network vessel theory—only teaching point actions has a tendency to transmit a flat and nondynamic understanding of acumoxa therapy, one that isolates acumoxa points from their constituent channels and network vessels and thus divorces the clinical use of acumoxa therapy from its rational basis.

What do I mean by channel and network vessel theory? Channel and network vessel theory in Chinese medicine comprises the descriptions of all the pathways, networks, organ and tissue connections, relative balance of qi and blood within, and physiological and pathological manifestations of all the various channels and network vessels within the human body. If I accept channel theory, it means that I actually believe that our predecessors' understanding of the pathways of and connections among the various channels and network vessels in the body has clinical validity. It further implies that I believe that knowing these pathways should have a direct impact on my daily practice of acumoxa therapy, and that this knowledge enhances my ability to diagnose and treat my patients. While some clinicians might be quite comfortable and effective in the clinic by only selecting points according to assigned therapeutic actions and/or viscera-bowel theory, this does not represent the fullest expression of acumoxa therapy as the clinical art form originally described in *Huang Di Nei Jing* nor does it mean that it should only be taught and practiced in this way. If we do so, we run the risk of transmitting our ignorance and bias against channel and network vessel theory on to our students and of driving acumoxa students and practitioners—who find acumoxa therapy that is divorced from channel and network vessel theory fundamentally unsatisfying—away from Chinese acumoxa therapy.

In my opinion, acumoxa channel and network vessel theory needs to be understood as a perception of the body unique to Chinese medicine which is neither separate and distinct from viscera-bowel theory nor subservient to it. In unsophisticated descriptions of the Chinese medical body—especially as they are presented in basic acumoxa textbooks and academic courses on Chinese medicine—the viscera and bowels appear to be more important than the channel system. As such, channel theory is usually not given much more than lip-service as something to memorize for exams and forget in the clinic in favor of choosing points purely based on viscera-bowel physiology and pathomechanisms. The implicit message is that the channels should be subjugated to the viscera and bowels in clinical practice. In other words, one should use a particular acumoxa channel or point primarily or even solely because of its association with a specific viscera or bowel and not because of its channel pathway, its particular place in the continuum of qi and blood flow through the body, or the tissues and regions that it traverses. Acumoxa points occur along the course of channels and these channels have certain trajectories. Unless one rejects Chinese medicine's channel theory, knowing the pathways of the channels—including what structures and tissues they pass through—provides a practical link to applying acumoxa points in clinical practice. For example, once we know that the liver channel "skirts" the genitals, we understand why points along that channel are used to treat disorders of the testes and penis.

Applying this logic to other channels and disorders provides us with similar connections.

To be clear, I do not assert that there is anything inherently "wrong" with choosing acumoxa points according to their therapeutic actions or to viscera-bowel theory, but only that we should also acknowledge that channel theory provides a conceptual and clinical link to the theory underlying point actions and to the use of certain channels and points that would not otherwise appear on our clinical "radar screen."

In this chapter, I briefly discuss the role of the channels and network vessels in male anatomy, physiology, and pathology. In point of fact, almost all of the Chinese andrology texts I have gathered and examined in my research for this book are written by herbalists. Further, the very practice of modern Chinese andrology in China is usually carried out by practitioners of integrated Chinese-Western medicine (*zhong xi yi jie he*) who tend as a group to be much more positively disposed towards herbal medicine, more oriented towards Western scientific views of the body, and therefore often less interactive with traditional acumoxa channel theory. Hence, the discussions of acumoxa channel theory and therapy I encounter in these texts are fairly limited and when such a text contains acumoxa treatment protocols for specific conditions (which is only in the minority of cases), they are generally in the style of choosing points according to viscera-bowel theory. In this chapter, I have chosen to cast my net wider however, and to provide information that encourages historically-based and broader insights without injecting my own independent ideas that lack any historical or clinical precedent. Also, I aim to encourage a perspective of the human body as a complex network of linkages among the viscera and bowels and the channels and network vessels, which I believe is closer to the original one revealed in the *Huang Di Nei Jing* and other texts in the literate stream of Chinese medicine.

On a practical note, this chapter provides the theoretical basis for reasoning through the acumoxa point combinations I offer in the treatment section of this text, as I do not explain those point combinations in each individual chapter.

The Twelve Regular Channels and Their Branches and Networks

The lung channel

Pathways

As I see it, there are four main theoretical bridges between the lung channel and the clinical practice of Chinese andrology: 1) the links between the lung channel and its network vessel and the large intestine; 2) the fact that *Lie Que* (LU-7) is the confluent point of the conception vessel; 3) the lung governs qi and; 4) the lung is the upper source of water and moves fluids. The connection between the lung channel and the large intestine channel, along with its clinical ramifications for andrology, will also be discussed in the large intestine channel section in the following pages. Similarly, the pathways and indications of the conception vessel will also be discussed in its corresponding section.

Briefly, however, the lung channel's links with the large intestine channel and bowel and with the conception vessel are clinically significant. The large intestine's function of "governing liquid" links the large intestine channel with the bladder's function of qi transformation, which of course is the direct source of the power to store and excrete urine. The conception vessel is physically linked with the male anterior yin region by virtue of the course of its pathways through the anterior yin region. So, since the lung channel nets with both of these other channels, we have a stronger theoretical basis for seeing the lung channel as having a physiological role in maintaining normal urinary function, in distributing liquid more widely in the body, and in helping to maintain free flow of qi and blood to the anterior yin region. Finally, the facts that the lung governs qi, is the upper source of water, and moves fluids, are more logically connected to viscera-bowel theory than to channel and network vessel theory, and are therefore, discussed more fully in the chapter on the viscera and bowels in andrology.

Indications

Some of the channel theory-based clinical indications of the lung channel are revealed when we consider a wider view of lung channel points such as *Chi Ze* (LU-5), *Lie Que* (LU-7), and *Yu Ji* (LU-10). *Chi Ze* (LU-5) is recommended for frequent urination in *Zhen Jiu Da Cheng* (*The Great Compendium of Acupuncture and Moxibustion*).[5] Wang Zhi-Zhong recommended *Lie Que* (LU-7) in combination with *Shao Fu* (HT-8) and *Yin Ling Quan* (SP-9) for genital pain in his famous Song dynasty text *Zhen Jiu Zi Sheng Jing* (*Life-Promoting Acumoxa Canon*).[6] And in *Zhen Jiu Jia Yi Jing* (*The Systematized Canon of Acupuncture and Moxibustion*),[7] *Yu Ji* (LU-10) is used for dampness and itching of the genitals. Without the channel pathway links described above, these clinical indications make less sense unless we see them simply as descriptions of empirical experiences with those points.

The large intestine channel

Pathways

As suggested in the lung channel section above, the netting of the large intestine channel with the lung channel and viscus—the upper source of water—makes a strong theoretical connection between the large intestine channel and fluid physiology and therefore fluid pathology. The role of the large intestine in fluid metabolism—which in *Nei Jing* is summarized under the heading of "The large intestine governs liquid"—is better explained with viscera-bowel

---

[5] *Zhen Jiu Da Cheng* was written by Yang Ji-Zhou in 1601, during the Ming dynasty.

[6] *Zhen Jiu Zi Sheng Jing* was published by Wang Zhi-Zhong in 1220, during the Song dynasty. It is a combination of many references to preceding acumoxa texts and Wang's own personal clinical experiences with acumoxa therapy.

[7] *Zhen Jiu Jia Yi Jing* is attributed to Huang Fu-Mi and was written in about 259 CE, during the Three Kingdoms period.

theory rather than with channel and network vessel theory. Nevertheless, there is a link between the large intestine channel and the physiology and pathology of fluids and it reveals itself in the clinical indications of some points on the course of the large intestine channel.

From the perspective of the quantity of qi and blood within individual channels, yang brightness channels carry an abundance of qi and blood and hence their pathways are important for maintaining the nourishment and normal function of the entire body, as well as for ensuring that there is a relative balance of qi and blood (and therefore yin and yang) throughout the whole body, including within the male anterior yin region. In this light, the large intestine channel is theoretically also important for maintaining male sexual, urinary, and reproductive functions,[8] though the emphasis in the premodern and modern literature is clearly on the foot *yang ming* stomach channel in this regard.

Indications

In modern Chinese medicine, we often overlook the connection between large intestinal function and liquid (*jin*). The idea that the large intestine "governs liquid" first appears in chapter 10 of *Ling Shu* (*Magic Pivot*)[9] where it states that the large intestine is "the governor of diseases caused by [lack of] of engendering of liquid." Further, in chapter 12 of *Lei Jing* (*The Classified Canon*)[10] Zhang Jing-Yue relates this function of the large intestine with the lungs when he states: "The lung and large intestine [stand in] exterior-interior [relationship]. The lung governs qi and fluids because of its qi transformation [action]. So, whenever there is a large intestinal [disease] such as diarrhea or bound stool, it is a disease resulting from [abnormalities] of fluid and [hence] resides within the large intestine." In some modern texts, the large intestine's function of governing liquid stands for its action of absorbing liquid from stool, which it sends to the bladder for excretion (Wang, 2001, p. 234). The list of symptoms related to the large intestine channel and liquid distribution are usually confined to problems occurring along the course of the channel in the upper body, namely the teeth, face, moustache, etc., and within the large intestine bowel (as related to diarrhea and bound stool). However, there are reflections of this connection in relation to urination and sweating revealed in the clinical use of certain points on the large intestine channel such as *Pian Li* (LI-6), which is a well-known point for treating inhibited urination and water swelling, and *Xia Lian* (LI-8), which treats yellowish urine and small intestinal insufficiency.[11]

---

[8] See also the section on the foot yang brightness stomach channel.

[9] *Ling Shu* is the second section of *Nei Jing*. Generally speaking, it provides more in-depth information about the channels and network vessels than does the first section (*Su Wen*).

[10] *Lei Jing* was written by Zhang Jing-Yue in 1601, during the Ming dynasty.

[11] This is a direct quote from *Zhen Jiu Da Cheng* (*The Great Compendium of Acupuncture and Moxibustion*). I must conclude that here we are referring to the function of the small intestine in urination, as after it separates the clear and the turbid (*i.e.*, liquid and solid in this context), it sends fluid to the bladder for excretion.

The large intestine channel is ascribed to hand yang brightness, and yang brightness channels contain an exuberant amount of qi and blood. Although theoretically this might mean that the large intestine channel would be useful for qi and blood vacuity or repletion patterns, by far the clinical emphasis is placed on using the large intestine channel for repletion patterns.[12] So, the large intestine channel is usually employed when there are andrological conditions such as acute and chronic prostatitis, yang wilt, and scrotal abscess manifesting as repletion patterns such as damp-heat pouring downward, exuberant fire-toxin, etc. In this context, we see points such as *He Gu* (LI-4) and *Qu Chi* (LI-11) recommended.

The stomach channel

Pathways

One of the most interesting aspects of the stomach channel pathway in terms of its relationship to andrology is the fact that its external and internal pathways converge at the abdominal "qi thoroughfare (*qi jie*)." Chapter 52 of *Ling Shu* describes the qi thoroughfare in the abdomen as follows: "Qi that is within the abdomen terminates at the back transport points, at the thoroughfare vessel, and at the "stirring vessels (*dong mai*)" to the left and right of the umbilicus."[13] The qi thoroughfare then is arguably very important for the free flow of qi and blood within the abdomen and in the anterior yin region downstream. Recalling that the thoroughfare vessel originates in the lesser abdomen and is the "sea of blood" further strengthens the link between qi and blood flow within the stomach channel and within the lesser abdomen and anterior yin region.

Another interesting fact about the stomach channel is that it is connected with three of the four seas[14]—the sea of qi within the chest, the sea of water and grain (located in the upper abdomen), and the sea of blood (located in the lower abdomen). The sea of qi within the chest is the source of all qi within the body, the sea of water and grain is the source of the engendering and transformation of qi and blood, and the sea of blood [*i.e.*, thoroughfare vessel] is responsible for governing the flow of qi and blood throughout the whole body. Through its connections with these seas, the stomach channel indirectly affects the quantity and free flow of qi and blood throughout the whole body.

---

[12] Also see the connection between the foot yang brightness stomach channel and yang wilt.

[13] There are four qi thoroughfares (*qi jie*) described in chapter 52 of *Ling Shu*. They are located in the chest, the abdomen, the head, and the lower leg. They represent bodily regions within which there is an especially concentrated flow of qi and blood within the channels and network vessels.

[14] Chapter 33 of *Ling Shu* describes four seas (*si hai*), namely, the sea of marrow, the sea of blood [*i.e.*, the thoroughfare vessel], the sea of qi, and the sea of water and grain [*i.e.*, the stomach]. Similar to the four qi thoroughfares, these four seas represent areas of concentration of qi, blood, and fluids which in turn have an important role in engendering and maintaining the flow of qi.

The stomach sinew channel accumulates at the genitals before it spreads upward into the abdomen. Therefore it helps to maintain normal genitourinary function.

Indications

As does the foot yang brightness channel, the stomach channel contains an exuberance of qi and blood. Because of their abundant supply of qi and blood, yang brightness channels are typically recommended for treating wilting pathoconditions (*wei zheng*). Although this is widely applied in the realm of poststroke recovery, we must remember that yang wilt (*yang wei*) is also a wilting pathocondition. Therefore, the stomach channel is used to treat yang wilt[15] and many other andrological conditions such as swelling and pain of the penis, testicular pain, and mounting qi pain (Huang and Zhan, 1999).

Because of the importance of the connection between the abdominal qi thoroughfare and the stomach channel, and because *Qi Chong* (ST-30) is a powerful point located in the region of the lesser abdomen, it is an excellent point for andrological diseases. The fact that this point and the abdominal qi thoroughfare connect with the thoroughfare vessel further strengthens its effect in anterior yin disorders. *Zhen Jiu Da Cheng* specifically mentions that this point is useful for treating yin wilt [*i.e.*, yang wilt], and penile and testicular pain.

As mentioned above, points along the stomach channel are connected with three of the four seas. With the general exception of *Ren Ying* (ST-9), these points are all useful in andrology disorders due to either qi and blood vacuity or to stagnation of qi and stasis of blood. The remaining points of the four seas that lie along the stomach channel are *Qi Chong* (ST-30) and *Zu San Li* (ST-36), and *Shang Jia Xu* (ST-37) and *Xia Ju Xu* (ST-39).

Because the stomach sinew channel gathers at the genitals, we have another reason to use points along the stomach channel to treat andrological conditions such as mounting qi, dribbling urinary block, and pain and swelling in the testes and scrotum.

The spleen channel

Pathways

In chapter 10 of *Ling Shu*, perhaps the most significant fact about the course of the spleen channel *vis-à-vis* andrology is that after it ascends upward along the anterior border of the medial aspect of the thigh, it enters the abdomen. It is then that it joins with the spleen and nets with the stomach. On its way to the spleen and stomach, as it travels through the abdomen, however, it brings luxuriance to the tissue and organs in the abdomen, including to the lesser abdomen

---

[15] This connection was first suggested to me by Fan Jian-Min (personal communication, 2001).

(*shao fu*)[16] and the anterior yin region. This helps explain how the spleen viscera and channel comprise a unified means of nourishing the penis, the testes, and the scrotum with construction qi. Chapter 10 of *Ling Shu* further describes that the spleen sinew channel accumulates at the genitals; hence, its pathway also helps to link the spleen with normal male genitourinary function.

In discussing the role of the spleen channel in andrology, we also cannot overlook the fact that the spleen channel unites with the liver and kidney channels at *San Yin Jiao* (SP-6), thus reinforcing the connections between these three channels. The fact that these three yin channels also unite with the conception vessel in the lesser abdomen clarifies even further the role of the spleen channel in male sexual and reproductive function.

In our attempt to simplify acumoxa therapy and in the subjugation of channel theory to viscera-bowel theory, we often overlook the spleen great network vessel (*da luo*) in modern clinical practice. The pathway described in chapter 10 of *Ling Shu* mainly involves its spreading through the chest and rib-side, but this pathway may have an important and underused role in maintaining the smooth flow of qi and blood through the smaller network vessels in that it serves as a center for coordinating their flow (Ni, 1996).

Indications

Due to the fact that the spleen channel travels through the lesser abdomen, and unites with the liver and kidney channels and with the conception vessel, it is clinically useful for treating male urogenital disorders such as mounting qi (*shan qi*), infertility, seminal efflux, yang wilt, inhibited urination and strangury (*lin zheng*), and genital pain. Also, as mentioned above, since the spleen sinew channel accumulates at the genitals, this further reinforces our understanding of the clinical utility of the spleen channel in treating male genital disorders. The clinical indications of the spleen great network vessel described in chapter 10 of *Ling Shu* include generalized pain as well as slackness in the "hundred joints (*bai jie*)."[17] Because of its association with the movement of qi and blood in the smaller network vessels, this channel may be useful in the treatment of andrological conditions due either to qi and blood vacuity or to qi stagnation and blood stasis patterns.[18]

---

[16] According to Wiseman and Feng (1998), the lesser abdomen (*shao fu*) is almost synonymous with the smaller abdomen (*xiao fu*), which is the section of the abdomen that is below the umbilicus. Sometimes the term lesser abdomen also comprises the lateral sides of the smaller abdomen, depending on the context within which the term is used.

[17] This is simply a collective term for all the joints within the body (Li *et al.*, 1975).

[18] I must admit to a certain degree of speculation on my part here. Most typical Chinese sources, such as Huang and Zhan (1999), limit the clinical use of the spleen great network vessel to indications such as rib-side distention and pain, generalized pain, slackness and lack of strength in the limbs, cough and panting, and chest pain.

The heart channel

Pathways

For andrology, the pathways of the heart channel do not reveal any major links with the anterior yin region other than the fact that the internal pathway of the heart channel descends downward through the diaphragm and joins with the small intestine in an exterior-interior (*biao-li*) pair. This suggests that the heart channel may have a role in promoting the smooth flow of qi and blood to the small intestine and to the lesser abdominal and anterior yin regions overall. Although this link does not appear to be that strong—judging from the fact that there are not very many andrological indications described for heart channel points—it is certainly worth mentioning. It should be clear from my discussion of the physiological role of the heart viscus in the chapter on the viscera and bowels, however, that conceptualizing the heart as the great ruler of the five viscera and six bowels and as the residence of essence-spirit is more revealing about its role in normal andrological function than focusing on the physical pathways of the heart channel. That being said, the heart network vessel provides the physical linkage between the heart and small intestine channels. If we recall the role of the small intestine in maintaining normal urinary function through its action of separating the clear and turbid, then this physical linkage provides an additional theoretical explanation for using heart channel points for urinary disorders.

Indications

As stated above, the link between the heart viscus and the physiology of the male anterior yin region is more visible than that of the heart channel. But that is not to say that points along the heart channel are not used to treat andrological conditions. It merely implies that the powerful functions of the heart viscus provide a stronger explanation for the use of such points than do the physical pathways of the heart channel.

The pathology listed for the heart channel in texts such as *Nei Jing, Zhen Jiu Jia Yi Jing*, and *Nan Jing* (*The Classic of Difficult Issues*)[19] tends to focus on the results of the heart failing to govern the vessels. Often cited are signs of either lack of blood engendering or nonfree movement of blood within the vessels (blood stasis) such as lack of normal facial color and sheen and a soot-black facial complexion. In modern Chinese andrology (which is an expression of integrated Chinese-Western medicine), heart channel points such as *Shen Men* (HT-7) are used to treat erectile dysfunction. The reasoning behind the use of these points represents a combination of both Chinese and Western medical knowledge. On the Western side, there is the fact that erectile dysfunction is often due to functional or organic vascular diseases, and on the Chinese side exists the concept that the heart governs the blood and the blood vessels. Because of the interior-exterior relationship between the heart and small intes-

---

[19] *Nan Jing* was written by unknown authors, and published during the 1st century (Eastern Han dynasty).

tine channels, which is strengthened by the physical pathway of the heart net-work channel, *Tong Li* (HT-5) is used for urinary problems such as dribbling urinary block and urinary incontinence. Also, *Shen Men* (HT-7) is indicated for urinary incontinence, *Shao Fu* (HT-8) is used for genital itching and pain, inhibited urination, and urinary incontinence.

The small intestine channel

Pathways

The physical pathway of the small intestine channel—like that of the large intes-tine channel—does not specifically link with the anterior yin region. Therefore, it is viscera-bowel theory (rather than channel theory) which better explains the link between the small intestine channel and the treatment of male anterior yin problems. The channel does of course link with the small intestine bowel, which according to *Nei Jing*, "separates the clear and the turbid." In terms of urinary function, the clear and turbid refers to water and solid. In other words, the small intestine separates the water and solids it receives from the stomach, and then sends the waste water to the bladder for excretion.[20] In terms of movement and transformation of water and grain (primarily the role of the spleen), the small in-testine separates the clear (usable) and the spleen raises the clear to the lungs and heart. Through the coordinated actions of the stomach, spleen, small intestine, lungs, and heart, qi, blood, and fluids are engendered. Of course, it is qi, blood, and fluids which power and nourish the male anterior yin region. Considering these facts, it is not difficult to see that for normal male functioning, the small intestine channel provides an additional means of supporting its corresponding bowel's function in maintaining normal urinary and digestive physiology. More often than not, however, when these physiological functions of the small intes-tine go awry, they are rectified by treating the spleen. While this is especially true for herbal medicine, it is also largely the case in acumoxa therapy.[21]

We find a more channel-based understanding of the role of the small intestine channel in normal male emotional life in the interior-exterior relationship be-tween the heart and small intestine. This link between the small intestine and the heart is provided by the small intestine channel divergence and network ves-sel. This is important because these channels carry construction qi to the heart and because of the small intestine's role in engendering qi, blood, and fluids which—as an arm of splenic movement and transformation—power, nourish, and enrich the heart. When the heart qi is sufficiently powered, when heart blood is adequately nourished, and when heart fluids are ample, the heart can store the spirit and male psychological and physiological functions are normal.

We should also not overlook the link between the small intestine channel and the governing vessel. The governing vessel links with the brain, which is the

---

[20] For a detailed explanation of this, see the small intestine section in Book 1, chapter 4 on the viscera and bowels.

[21] An exception to this is that *Xiao Chang Shu* (BL-27) is used to treat digestive disturbances such as diarrhea and constipation.

palace of the original spirit.[22] Through its linkage with the governing vessel, the small intestine channel helps to nourish the brain. Since at least the time of *Nei Jing*, the brain has been assigned an important role in the emotional and psychological function of human beings.

Indications

Given the connection between the small intestine channel and urinary function, we might expect to find more clinical applications of it for urinary problems. However, while *Qian Gu* (SI-2) and *Hou Xi* (SI-3) are often used for reddish urine and rough urination (complaints men can experience with acute and chronic prostatitis), there are not many other points on the channel which are used for such problems.[23]

Considering the physiological role of the small intestine bowel in male physiology (as described above), the small intestine channel is sometimes used to treat emotionally-based male anterior yin problems such as yang wilt and premature ejaculation. While premodern and modern texts do not usually list these andrology complaints as specific indications for small intestine channel points, they do widely recommend points on the small intestine channel for psychological problems such as visceral agitation (*zang zao*),[24] mania-withdrawal (*dian-kuang*),[25] heart vexation, fear, and sadness. It is not too far a stretch of the imagination to see that in a channel-based approach to acumoxa therapy, small intestine points can be useful for treating some of the emotional manifestations of male sexual dysfunction. *Hou Xi* (SI-3), *Zhi Zheng* (SI-7), and *Xiao Hai* (SI-8) are the most important points on the small intestine channel for these purposes.

The bladder channel

Pathways

There are a few pathways of the bladder channel revealed in chapter 10 of *Ling Shu* that are especially important when we are trying to understand its role in the physiology and pathology of men. The first significant fact is that

---

[22] Although there is by no means universal agreement on this, original spirit (*yuan shen*) is the aspect of the spirit associated with the brain in some premodern Chinese sources. As such, it is associated with consciousness, memory, and vision. In chapter 34 of *Ben Cao Gang Mu* (*Herbal Foundation Compendium*), Li Shi-Zhen refers to the brain as "the palace of the original spirit."

[23] *Xiao Chang Shu* (BL-27) is also used to treat bladder conditions such as inhibited urination and dribbling urinary block.

[24] Visceral agitation (*zang zao*) was originally discussed in Zhang Zhong-Jing's Han dynasty classic—*Jin Gui Yao Lue Fang Lun* (*Essentials of Prescriptions of the Golden Coffer*)—as a woman's disease. However, some men do experience similar symptoms due to similar pathomechanisms; hence, this disease category can also be used for men with depression and anxiety disorders either as a cause or result of sexual dysfunction.

[25] Mania-withdrawal (*dian-kuang*) is a Chinese medical disease category in which the patient vacillates between an extremely depressed state and a manic state. The closest modern Western psychiatric condition is bipolar affective disorder.

one of the internal branches of the bladder channel—after passing upward through the forehead and to the vertex of the head—links with the governing vessel and the brain. Second, as we might expect, another internal branch of the bladder channel enters the interior of the body at the level of the second lumbar vertebra (L2) and links with the bladder and kidney organs. Further, as the bladder channel travels down the posterior aspect of the body, three body inches (*cun*) lateral to the governing vessel, it links with all the viscera and bowels through their respective transport (*shu*) points. Finally, as the bladder channel flows through the lumbosacral and anterior yin region, free-flowing qi within this part of the channel is crucial to normal male function.

Because of the linkages between the bladder channel and the governing vessel and brain, the bladder channel provides another means of guaranteeing that clear yang qi is supplied to the head and brain. The head is sometimes referred to as "the clear sky" in premodern Chinese medical sources. When the bladder channel is free and open, the clear sky is bright and clear; hence, the brain—considering its important role in regulating emotion and sensation—is also free and open. This is important for men in that when there is free flow within the bladder channel, one's mind, thoughts, and emotions are clear; this supports normal male sexual and urinary functions. Further, the bladder channel divergence links with the heart and supports its normal functions. Since the heart governs the spirit, including all psychological activity, the bladder channel divergence provides an additional means of supplying construction qi to the heart. This maintains a balanced mental outlook (*jing shen*) and thus normal male urinary and sexual functions.

The links between the bladder regular channel and the bladder and kidney organs are of great significance for male physiology. It is also noteworthy that these links are further strengthened by the bladder channel divergence and the bladder network vessel. Free flow within these channels helps to maintain kidney and bladder qi transformation, which is responsible for normal fluid metabolism throughout the entire body, and especially for normal urinary function. For men, this of course means that free flow within the bladder channel is essential for normal urination. Further, because of this link between the bladder channel and the kidney viscus—which stores essence and governs growth and reproduction—free-flowing bladder channel qi supports normal male sexual and reproductive functions.

The bladder channel is distinguished from other channels by its possession of transport points that are associated with all of the viscera and bowels. This means that the bladder channel plays a key role in maintaining the physiology of all the viscera and bowels, and by extension their associated orifices and tissues. From the standpoint of andrology, when one has abundant and freely-coursing bladder channel qi he is more likely to have abundance and free flow of qi within all the other viscera and bowels. This is not only important for male urinary function but is also crucial for all other male physiological functions—psychological, sexual, and reproductive.

Indications

Since the bladder channels net with the brain, the governing vessel, and the heart, we find many bladder channel points that are useful for treating the psychological aspects of men's diseases. Among them we find points on the head, along the back (the transport points), and on the lower limbs. Useful points on the head include *Qu Cha* (BL-4), which is recommended in *Zhen Jiu Da Cheng* for "heart vexation and fullness in the heart," and *Luo Que* (BL-7), which is often used for insomnia and poor memory (Huang and Zhan, 1999). We often choose the back transport points on the bladder channel in accordance with whichever viscera's spirit aspect is involved in any particular case (Ni, 1996). For example, when a man has premature ejaculation from liver depression and depressed fire which is in turn due to enduring anger and indignation disturbing the ethereal soul (*hun*), *Gan Shu* (BL-18) is useful along with liver channel points, and when a man has erectile dysfunction from fright and fear damaging the heart-spirit and kidney-will, *Xin Shu* (BL-15) and *Shen Shu* (BL-23) are chosen in addition to points from the heart and kidney channels, etc. Bladder channel points on the lower limbs that have spirit-calming effects useful in men's diseases include *Kun Lun* (BL-60), *Pu Can* (BL-61), *Shen Mai* (BL-62), and *Jing Gu* (BL-64).

As we might expect, many points along the course of the bladder channel are used for normalizing male kidney and bladder qi transformation and/or for treating andrological problems related to the kidneys in terms of essence, growth, and reproduction. I have established earlier that this is in part explained by the bladder channel's links with the kidney and bladder organs and in part explained by viscera-bowel theory pertaining to the bladder and kidneys. Most bladder channel points with such indications are either located in the lumbosacral region or on the lower extremity. Most prominent among them are *San Jiao Shu* (BL-22), *Shen Shu* (BL-23), *Da Chang Shu* (BL-25),[26] *Xiao Chang Shu* (BL-27), *Pang Guang Shu* (BL-28), *Shang Liao* (BL-31), *Ci Liao* (BL-32), *Xia Liao* (BL-33), *Cheng Fu* (BL-36), *Wei Yang* (BL-39), and *Jin Men* (BL-63).[27]

The back transport points associated with all of the viscera and bowels are used for treating all aspects of male pathology, whether directly or indirectly related to the bladder and kidney organs. Many are used for andrological complaints that are either related to that viscera or bowel's physiological function according to viscera-bowel theory and/or to the pathway of its associated channel. For example, *Fei Shu* (BL-13) is used for dribbling urinary block and

---

[26] While it seems counterintuitive that the large intestine back transport point *Da Chang Shu* (BL-25) would be used for urinary problems, Sun Si-Miao's famous 7th century (Tang dynasty) text, *Qian Jin Yao Fang* (*A Thousand Gold Pieces Prescriptions*) recommends it for both bowel and urinary problems. For what Dr. Sun's reasoning might be based on in terms of channel theory, see the large intestine channel section in this chapter.

[27] As the cleft point (*xi xue*) of the bladder channel, *Jin Men* (BL-63) is useful for fulminant mounting qi pain.

inhibited urination because of the lungs' role as the "upper source of water," in "moving fluids," and as the "regulator of the waterways [*i.e.*, the triple burner]" in viscera-bowel theory, and because of the lung channel's connections described previously. Further, *Xiao Chang Shu* (BL-27) is used for inhibited urination, urinary incontinence, and mounting qi (*shan qi*) pain both because of the physiological function of the small intestine *vis-à-vis* urination, and because of the pathways of its channel. Carrying on with this logic would help clarify the specific usage of each of the back transport points. However, having set the stage here for seeing the andrological use of the back transport points explained by both viscera-bowel theory and channel theory, we do not need to explore each of them at this juncture. Rather, readers can refer to Book 1, chapter 4 on viscera-bowel theory, and to the section within this chapter which discusses the corresponding channel theory related to each organ.

The kidney channel

Pathways

As described in chapter 10 of *Ling Shu* and chapter 2 of *Zhen Jiu Jia Yi Jing*, after beginning beneath the little toe and traveling to the sole of the foot and then up the inner thigh, the kidney channel passes through the spine and then joins with the kidneys and nets with the bladder. Chapter 2 of *Zhen Jiu Jia Yi Jing*, describes the connections between the kidney channel and the governing vessel (*du mai*), which provides an additional link between the course and indications of these two channels. It is also noteworthy that chapter 38 of *Ling Shu* describes the course of the lower branch of the thoroughfare vessel (*chong mai*) as flowing into the "great network (*da luo*)" of the kidney channel (presumably at *Da Zhong* [KI-4]), providing linkage between the pathways and thus the clinical indications of the kidney channel and the thoroughfare vessel.

Indications

When considering the many andrological indications of the kidney channel, the pathway of the kidney channel itself does not provide any dramatic new insights that we would not surmise given a solid knowledge of the physiological functions of the kidney viscus-channel complex[28] alone. Rather, it is what we know about the paramount importance of the kidney viscus-channel complex in the storage of essence, in governing growth and reproduction, and in fluid metabolism, and what we know about the connections between the kidney channel and other channels that speaks louder to me about the usefulness of the kidney channel in andrology.[29] As mentioned above, the fact that the thoroughfare vessel (*chong mai*) joins with the kidney channel at the "great network (*da luo*)" of the kidney channel, and that the kidney channel passes through the spine and links with the governing vessel at *Chang Qiang* (GV-1)

---

[28] I have taken the liberty of coining the term "viscus-channel complex" to represent the inseparability of a given viscera from its associated channel.

[29] For a detailed discussion of the physiology of the kidney viscus, see Book 1, chapter 4 on the viscera and bowels as well as Damone (2006).

is quite significant. In the case of the thoroughfare vessel, chapter 44 of *Su Wen* states that it "unites with the ancestral sinew [*i.e.*, the penis]." Logically then, if the kidney channel and the thoroughfare vessel are connected, we have yet another way of understanding why the kidney channel can be used to treat disorders of the penis. Further, chapter 2 of *Zhen Jiu Jia Yi Jing*, after describing the connection between the governing vessel and the kidneys, points out that the governing vessel in males "follows the penis to the perineum." In addition to clarifying the use of the governing vessel for all disorders of the penis, including yang wilt, premature ejaculation, pain in the penis, etc., this of course can also reinforce our understanding of the use of the kidney channel for those same disorders.

The pericardium channel

Pathways

There are three significant facts about the pathway of the pericardium channel in terms of the practice of andrology: 1) chapter 10 of *Magic Pivot* states that the pericardium channel is governed by the heart; 2) chapter 71 of *Magic Pivot* states that the pericardium regular channel nets with the heart channel and chapter 10 of *Magic Pivot* states that the pericardium network vessel connects with the "heart tie (*xin xi*)" [*i.e.*, heart system] and; 3) the pericardium channel divergence homes to the triple burner (here used as a means of dividing the body into three regions—upper, middle, and lower) and therefore connects with all three burners.

In the first two cases, these channel connections reinforce the close relationship between the heart and pericardium. In short, the pericardium channel enhances the physiological relationship between the heart and pericardium. Hence, free and adequate flow of qi and blood within the pericardium channel helps the heart viscus and channel to perform their functions. As for the heart, this means governing the blood and blood vessels and storing the spirit; as for the pericardium, this means protecting the heart. In the third case, the pericardium channel helps to provide free qi and blood flow to all three burners. Of special note here, and most significant to andrology, is that the pericardium channel connects with the lower burner, which includes the anterior yin region.

Indications

Because of the close links between the pericardium channel and the heart channel, in andrology, the pericardium channel is used in similar situations as the heart channel. Usually, the pericardium channel—and especially *Nei Guan* (PC-6)—is used to treat men who have mental-emotional symptoms either as a cause or as a result of their andrological problem. According to chapter 6 of *Mai Jing* (*The Pulse Canon*),[30] indicators of pericardium channel disease in-

---

[30] *Mai Jing* was written by Wang Shu-He in the 3rd century CE, during the Western Jin dynasty.

clude heart vexation and great thudding of the heart [*i.e.*, rapid and forceful heartbeat]. In chapter 10 of the same text, a tendency to be angry is listed as an indicator of pericardium channel disease. In this light, the pericardium channel becomes useful for treating men with sexual dysfunction, infertility, and andropause because men with these conditions often experience emotional symptoms such as these.

Because the heart governs the blood and the blood vessels, and because the pericardium channel links with the heart tie [*i.e.*, system], points along the pericardium channel are useful in treating yang wilt and male infertility when they are related to disorders of the blood. The pathomechanisms—alone or in combination—include blood vacuity failing to nourish the anterior yin region, phlegm obstructing the network vessels, and blood stasis obstructing free flow of blood to the anterior yin region. Ni (1996) cites *Jian Shi* (PC-5) as a good point for treating hypercholesterolemia and atherosclerosis. No explanation is provided, though this point is widely known to be useful for treating phlegm disorders. Further, as yang wilt is one of the manifestations of hypercholesterolemia and atherosclerosis, the use of *Jian Shi* (PC-5) may extend to treating yang wilt of circulatory origin, though this is admittedly speculative.

Because the pericardium channel divergence links with the lower burner (including the anterior yin region), and because the pericardium channel connects with the heart (which stands in exterior-interior relationship with the small intestine channel), certain points along the pericardium channel are used for treating the Chinese disease categories of dribbling urinary block, strangury, and inhibited urination. When we reframe these Chinese disease categories into modern Western andrological diseases, we find that they correlate with benign prostatic hyperplasia (BPH) and acute and chronic prostatitis.[31] Thus, points such as *Jian Shi* (PC-5) and *Da Ling* (PC-7) are sometimes used for men who have these conditions.

The triple burner channel

The triple burner is an ambiguous concept in Chinese medicine. Scholars have argued for centuries over the nature and functions of the triple burner as they wrestled with the descriptions of the triple burner handed down to them in the *Nei Jing* and *Nan Jing*. One of the key points of debate was whether or not the triple burner has "form" [*i.e.*, its own individual morphological structure]. Placing these debates aside, in this section I focus on generally agreed upon notions about the triple burner channel and how they relate to the practice of Chinese andrology.

Pathways

As discussed in Book 1, Chapter 4 on the viscera and bowels, there are three

---

[31] For more information on this, see the chapters devoted to these diseases in Book 2 of this text.

main features of the triple burner: 1) it is the "special courier of original qi";[32] 2) it is the pathway of water and grain and; 3) it holds "the office of the sluices and manifests as the waterways."

According to the first and second features of the triple burner described above, the triple burner channel is a key element of the channel system because it facilitates free flow of qi throughout the entire body and supports the movement and transformation of water and grain essence and the excretion of waste through urine and stool. As holder of the "office of sluices" and as the "waterways," the triple burner channel is associated with supporting normal fluid metabolism. This includes the functions of all the organs concerned with the formation, distribution, and excretion of fluids, and especially the lungs, spleen, stomach, kidneys, small intestine, large intestine, and bladder. These are important functions for maintaining the health and treating diseases of men.

One of the most important links between the triple burner channel and all of its functions is provided by an internal pathway of the triple burner channel and its channel divergence that descends downwards from within the chest and connects with all three burners. Most significantly for our discussion, these channels link with the lower burner and thus with the male anterior yin region. Here they support normal male anterior yin function and have an especially close relationship with bladder qi transformation and thus with urination. Further, this internal branch and divergence provides the rationale for how the triple burner channel helps to support large intestinal conduction and conveyance and therefore the smooth and efficient expulsion of stool. Because the large intestine is the largest bowel in the lower burner, free flow within it strongly encourages free flow within the anterior yin region as a whole.

Another channel connection worth noting in this discussion is the confluence between the triple burner channel and the yang linking vessel at *Wai Guan* (TB-5). The yang linking vessel has a very strong physiological function of balancing all yang qi within the body because it connects all six yang channels with the governing vessel, which is "the sea of all yang qi." So, the confluence of the triple burner channel with the yang linking vessel provides additional rationale for the triple burner channel's broad effects on qi function within all three burners as "the special courier of original qi."

Yet another link between the triple burner channel and other channels germane to the topic of andrology is that between the triple burner channel and the urinary bladder channel at *Wei Yang* (BL-39). This further strengthens the relationship between the triple burner channel and bladder qi transformation.

---

[32] In this context, the term original qi (*yuan qi*) is generally taken as a collective term for all physiological qi within the body and is similar to other collective terms for qi including right qi (*zheng qi*) and true qi (*zhen qi*).

Finally, since the triple burner channel network vessel links with the pericardium channel, it supports the functions of the pericardium *vis-à-vis* andrology as described previously in the pericardium channel section.

Indications

There are many upper body musculoskeletal indications for the triple burner channel that are not especially related to andrology. However, tucked in among these there are also some more systemic and even lower burner indications for triple burner points such as *Wai Guan* (TB-5) and *Zhi Gou* (TB-6) that are clinically significant for andrology. For example, TB-5 is indicated for abdominal pain and bound stool, which are common symptoms associated with various male anterior yin diseases including prostate diseases, yang wilt due to repletion patterns, and scrotal diseases. Similarly, TB-6 has an even stronger effect on bound stools and can be used instead of, or in addition to, TB-5 for the same diseases.

Some of the indications of the triple burner channel, and especially of TB-5 are better understood in light of the confluence between the triple burner channel and the yang linking vessel. These include binding of heat in all of the viscera and bowels (Deadman and Al-Khafagi, 1998, p. 396–397). As mentioned previously and discussed further in the section on the yang linking vessel, the yang linking vessel links the six yang channels with the governing vessel. Its clinical indications include various conditions in which there is an imbalance between yin and yang, and especially when yang is either replete or insufficient. This covers a broad selection of male disorders. Although most textbooks do not usually specifically mention this use of TB-5, some authors indicate that the yang linking vessel (and TB-5 as its confluent point) can be used for disorders of yang repletion or vacuity (Ni, 1996, p. 131).

Chapter 2 of *Ling Shu* (*Magic Pivot*) shows a very clear relationship between *Wei Yang* (BL-39), the lower associated point [*i.e.*, lower he-sea] of the triple burner channel, and urinary diseases such as urinary dribbling and block (when there is repletion) and enuresis (when there is vacuity). This exhibits the usefulness of *Wei Yang* (BL-39) for andrological conditions such as benign prostatic hyperplasia (BPH) and acute and chronic prostatitis which manifest with these urinary symptoms.

In part because of the close relationship between the triple burner channel and the pericardium channel, and in part because of the importance of the triple burner channel in maintaining normal fluid metabolism, *Tian Jing* (TB-10) is a very useful point for treating phlegm-related emotional disorders including those that accompany andrological conditions, including emotional depression and anxiety like that experienced by men with sexual dysfunction and infertility. It can be used for phlegm patterns accompanied by either repletion or vacuity patterns of other viscera and bowels including the heart, spleen, liver, stomach, and gallbladder.

The gallbladder channel

Pathways

The four most significant facts about the gallbladder channel to consider for our discussion of the channels and network vessels in andrology are: 1) the gallbladder channel stands in interior-exterior relationship with the liver channel; 2) the gallbladder divergent channel links with the heart; 3) the gallbladder channel possesses the alarm point of the kidneys—*Jing Men* (GB-25) and; 4) the gallbladder channel crosses with the girdle vessel.

To better understand the andrological role of the gallbladder channel as the exterior paired channel to the liver, refer to the section on the liver channel in the following pages. This connection is of course provided by the gallbladder network vessel. In short, the gallbladder channel helps to guarantee the smooth flow of qi and blood in the liver channel, which encircles the genitals. Hence, normal male anterior yin function depends in part on free-flowing gallbladder qi.

The connection between the gallbladder divergent channel and the heart is important because it helps the heart's functions of storing the spirit and ruling the activities of the entire body. According to *Nei Jing*, as the sovereign viscus, the heart governs the physiological activities of all the viscera and bowels. As explained in Book 1 chapter 4 on the viscera and bowels, this includes the functions of the male anterior yin region. So, by encouraging free flow of qi and blood to the heart, the gallbladder divergent channel encourages the heart to be able to both store the spirit and to properly govern the physiological functions of the anterior yin region.

Since *Jing Men* (GB-25) is the alarm point of the kidneys, and is thus a point that has an especially strong influence on the kidneys, the patency and strength of qi and blood flow within the gallbladder channel has a significant influence on the kidney channel and viscus. As the viscus which stores essence, governs growth and reproduction, and governs the qi transformation of water, the kidneys have an essential role in male anterior yin function. For further explanation of the physiological role of the kidney channel and viscus in male anterior yin function, see their respective sections in this chapter.

Since *Dai Mai* (GB-26), *Wu Shu* (GB-27), and *Wei Dao* (GB-28) are the only acumoxa points that occur along the course of the girdle vessel, the gallbladder channel becomes important for maintaining its physiological functions. These include supporting the functions of the kidney and binding and regulating qi within the longitudinally-flowing channels passing through the lower abdominal and lumbar region. Hence, the gallbladder channel is an important link between the girdle vessel and the anterior yin region.

Indications

By virtue of the gallbladder channel's linkage with the liver channel, the heart viscus, and the girdle vessel, it is sometimes used for treating male anterior yin problems such as scrotal pain, mounting qi, enuresis, itching and dampness of the scrotum, pain in the lesser abdomen, and yang wilt. Points with such clinical indications include *Jing Men* (GB-25), *Dai Mai* (GB-26), *Wu Shu* (GB-27), *Wei Dao* (GB-28), *Huan Tiao* (GB-30), *Qiu Xu* (GB-40), and *Zu Lin Qi* (GB-41).

The liver channel

Pathways

In chapters 31 and 39 of *Su Wen*, in chapters 10 and 52 of *Ling Shu*, and in chapters 2 and 7 of *Zhen Jiu Jia Yi Jing*, the liver channel is described as either encircling, skirting, netting, or gathering at the genitals, joining with the sinews, and arriving at the lesser abdomen before it eventually reaches the liver viscus. In chapter 10 of *Ling Shu* it states, "The liver [channel] unites with the sinews and the sinews gather at the genitals." This description of the pathway of the liver channel reveals a link between the sinews and the penis (the "ancestral sinew" [*zong jin*] or "sinew gathering," depending on how we translate the word "*zong*"). This helps explain why the liver channel is often used to treat diseases of the penis.

Indications

Several chapters of *Su Wen*, including chapters 39, 41, and 63, and similarly chapter 10 of *Ling Shu*, provide us with the clinical indications of the liver channel. In chapter 39 of *Su Wen*, pain in the lesser abdomen is attributed to cold evil settling into the liver channel causing blood to "weep" and hypertonicity of the channel. Chapter 10 of *Ling Shu*, correlates two types of mounting pathoconditions (*shan zheng*)—bulging mounting (*tui shan*) and foxy mounting (*hu shan*)—with the liver channel, and also offers urinary incontinence, urinary block, and urinary dribbling as indications of the liver channel.[33] Commonly used points include *Da Dun* (LV-1), *Xing Jian* (LV-2), *Tai Chong* (LV-3), *Li Gou* (LV-5), and *Qu Quan* (LV-8).

The Eight Extraordinary Vessels and Their Branches and Networks

The governing vessel

Pathways

Although there are at least four main pathways described for it, there are a few facts about the governing vessel that are especially important for the study of andrology. First, one branch of the channel arises deeply from within the lesser abdomen, nets with the genitals and unites with the perineum (where it nets with the conception vessel), and then travels up the sides of the coccyx to connect with the kidney and bladder channels, and then eventually connects with the kidneys. Secondly, one of the branches of the channel follows the

---

[33] For a detailed discussion of mounting disease, see Book 1, Chapter 6 on Chinese medical disease categories.

spinal column up to the region of *Feng Fu* (GV-16), and then enters the brain. Finally, since the governing vessel is mainly distributed along the yang aspect of the body (the back) and connects with all of the six regular yang channels at *Da Zhui* (GV-14), it is also called the sea of all yang qi.

It should be clear then that since the governing vessel nets with the genitals, travels to the perineum, and nets with the conception vessel, this channel exerts a strong influence over the flow of qi and blood in these areas, and thus over the functioning of the male anterior yin region. As noted above, the governing vessel connects with the brain. In Chinese medical literature dating as far back as the *Nei Jing*, the brain is considered the palace of the original spirit (*yuan shen*), and thus has a major role in the normal functioning of the essence-spirit and arguably the male anterior yin organs as well, since spirit (*shen*) is what governs all the physiological activities of the entire body.[34] The fact that the governing vessel is the sea of all yang qi within the body is enormously helpful in pointing out the importance of this channel in maintaining all the warming and transforming functions of the viscera and bowels and their associated tissues, as well as the functions of the male anterior yin region in general such as maintaining urinary flow, engendering and activating sperm, and powering erection and ejaculation.

Indications

Because the governing vessel nets with the genitals and the perineum and since it unites with the kidney and bladder channels, points along this channel are very useful in the treatment of all male anterior yin disorders including but not limited to yang wilt, premature ejaculation, acute and chronic prostatitis, prostate cancer, dribbling urinary block, and pain and swelling of the penis and scrotum. Since the governing vessel connects with the brain, it is useful for treating the mental emotional aspects of male anterior yin disorders as well as the physical aspect of such problems. These include anxiety accompanying sexual dysfunction such as yang wilt and premature ejaculation, and emotional manifestations of andropause. The governing vessel—as the sea of all yang qi within the body—is very useful in the treatment of all male anterior yin disorders resulting from either too little or too much yang qi such as yang wilt, premature ejaculation, male infertility, low libido, dribbling urinary block, and acute and chronic prostatitis. Prominent points for these indications include *Chang Qiang* (GV-1), *Ming Men* (GV-4), *Yao Yang Guan* (GV-3), and *Da Zhui* (GV-14).

The conception vessel

Pathways

The most significant aspects of the conception vessel to the practice of andrology are: 1) in men, the conception vessel begins from deep within *Guan Yuan* (CV-4) and then joins with *Hui Yin* (CV-1) and together with the governing

---

[34] For more specifics on spirit in this context, see the section on heart physiology in Book 1, Chapter 4 on the viscera and bowels.

vessel passes through the coccyx and enters the spinal column; 2) the conception vessel is distributed over the anterior portion of the body and connects with all yin channels, directly or indirectly; hence, it regulates all yin qi throughout the entire body; 3) the connecting vessel of the conception vessel nets with the governing vessel, which is the sea of all yang qi within the body and; 4) the conception vessel passes over all three burners and is distributed through the abdomen; hence, it indirectly connects with all the viscera and bowels and regulates their functions.

The significance of the pathways of the conception vessel to andrology is that it distributes yin qi through the anterior yin region, including the penis, testes, and scrotum, and thus has an important role in maintaining nourishment and enrichment of these organs. By doing so, the conception vessel supports healthy male sexual, reproductive, and urinary functions. Also, in the process of distributing yin qi, it ensures that yin evils do not collect, accumulate, or bind in the anterior yin region. Free flow within the conception vessel is essential in order to prevent the seven mounting qi (qi shan) diseases from occurring.[35]

According to chapter 65 of the Ling Shu (Magic Pivot), the conception vessel and the thoroughfare vessel collectively comprise "the sea of the channels and network vessels." As revealed in this chapter of the Ling Shu, they specifically function to nourish the ancestral sinew [i.e., the penis]. We generally relate this back to the fact that the conception vessel converges with all the yin channels and is thus central to providing substantial nourishment to the anterior yin region. By "substantial" nourishment, I mean enrichment in the form of blood, essence, and fluids.

By netting with the governing vessel—the sea of all yang qi—the network vessel of the conception vessel (which is sometimes called the sea of all yin qi) strengthens the coordination and balance of yin and yang throughout the anterior yin region, and by extension within the entire body. In doing so, it supports normal male physiology as described above.

The conception vessel travels through the abdomen and connects with all the viscera and bowels. Most of the alarm points occur along its course. It directly or indirectly connects with all the viscera and bowels and provides them with substantial nourishment. Further, it helps to regulate the balance of yin and yang within them.

Indications

Because of the course of the conception vessel through the perianal region and the lesser abdomen, and its central role in the enrichment of the penis, testes,

---

[35] This link between the conception vessel and the seven shan (qi shan) is first discussed in Chapter 60 of Ling Shu. For a definition and more detailed discussion of mounting qi, see Book 1, Chapter 6 on Chinese disease categories.

essence chamber, and scrotum, points along the conception vessel are widely used in the treatment of andrological conditions such as yang wilt, premature ejaculation, acute and chronic prostatitis, male infertility, and scrotal diseases. Commonly used points include *Hui Yin* (CV-1), *Qu Gu* (CV-2), *Zhong Ji* (CV-3), *Guan Yuan* (CV-4), *Shi Men* (CV-5), *Qi Hai* (CV-6), and *Yin Jiao* (CV-7).

As previously stated, the conception vessel's role in distributing yin qi through the anterior yin region extends to ensuring that yin evils do not accumulate. Points along its course are essential for treating the seven mounting qi diseases, some of which result from yin evil accumulation, especially water-mounting (*shui shan*), cold mounting (*han shan*), and blood mounting (*xue shan*). Also, this extends to the use of conception vessel points for male urinary disturbances such as those that occur with acute and chronic prostatitis and benign prostatic hyperplasia (BPH). Commonly used points include *Hui Yin* (CV-1), *Qu Gu* (CV-2), *Zhong Ji* (CV-3), *Guan Yuan* (CV-4), *Shi Men* (CV-5), *Qi Hai* (CV-6), *Yin Jiao* (CV-7), *Shen Que* (CV-8), and *Shui Fen* (CV-9).

On a broader note and as previously established, the wider course of the conception vessel through the abdomen links it with all the viscera and bowels. The presence of many of the alarm points ("collecting points" of the associated viscus or bowel) along its course make it a vital link in the normal qi and blood flow through all the viscera and bowels, and especially in ensuring they are sufficiently supplied with substantial nourishment (Wiseman and Feng, 1998, p. 7). As the physiological transforming functions of the qi of any given organ depends on it being adequately nourished, by providing yin material nourishment to a given organ, the conception vessel supports its yang functions. This is revealed below in the andrological indications of the alarm points along the conception vessel.

In terms of andrological uses of alarm points, consider the following: 1) *Zhong Ji* (CV-3), as the alarm point of the bladder is commonly used for urinary symptoms of prostate diseases as well as other male urological conditions such as urethritis; 2) *Guan Yuan* (CV-4), as the alarm point of the small intestine, is used for similar urinary conditions as CV-3; 3) *Shi Men* (CV-5), as the alarm point of the triple burner, is indicated for andrological problems related to nonregulation of the waterways, including signs such as inhibited urination, enuresis, and water swelling; 4) *Zhong Wan* (CV-12), as the alarm point of the stomach, is an extremely important point for all vacuity andrological diseases because it helps to support free flow of qi and blood to the stomach bowel. The stomach is "the sea of water and grain, and qi and blood." To help the decomposition function of the stomach is to increase the quantity of raw material available to the spleen, lungs, and heart for engendering and transforming qi, blood, and fluids that ultimately power and nourish the male anterior yin region and; 5) *Shan Zhong* (CV-17), as the alarm point of the pericardium, theoretically supports the heart functions of governing the physiological activities of all the viscera and bowels, of storing the spirit, and its role in normal male physiology as indicated in Book 1, Chapter 4. In terms of its actions on the pericardium and heart, however, we usually see more resonance with CV-17 and the fact that it is the meeting point of qi than we do with the fact that it is the alarm point of the pericardium.[36]

The thoroughfare vessel[37]

Pathways

For andrology, the three most important facts about the pathways of the thoroughfare vessel are: 1) it begins from deep within *Guan Yuan* (CV-4), travels to the perineum and meets with *Hui Yin* (CV-1), and then emerges at *Qi Chong* (ST-30), the qi thoroughfare point in the lower abdomen. From there it mainly follows the course of the kidney channel upward on the abdomen and eventually reaches the face, lips, and mouth; 2) Chapter 44 of *Su Wen* states: "The thoroughfare vessel is the sea of the channels and vessels; it governs seeping and pouring into streams and valleys. Together with the yang brightness [channel], it unites with the ancestral sinew [*i.e.*, the penis]," and; 3) After beginning from deep within CV-4, it passes backwards towards the spine and courses through the spine following the pathway of the governing vessel up the back.

From the first description, we have the means to understand why the thoroughfare vessel is so important to the physiology of the male anterior yin region. Recalling that the qi thoroughfare in the lower abdomen is an area of great concentration of qi and blood, it follows that when the thoroughfare vessel contains an abundance of blood and has free-flowing qi, it would have a significant effect on the qi and blood flow within the entire anterior yin region, including the penis, testes, and scrotum. So, the thoroughfare vessel plays a key role in maintaining the physiological functions of the male anterior yin region.

The relationship between the thoroughfare vessel and the male anterior yin region is further strengthened by the quote from chapter 44 of *Su Wen* cited above. It clearly states that there is a link between the thoroughfare vessel and the penis. Thus, free-flowing qi and blood within the thoroughfare vessel is essential for normal erectile and ejaculatory functions, as well as for male fertility. As the "sea of the channels and vessels," and the "sea of blood," the thoroughfare vessel provides substantial nourishment to the male anterior yin region.

I find another interesting link between the thoroughfare vessel and the penis in chapter 65 of *Ling Shu* which states: "Eunuchs have had their penises removed and have [suffered] damage to their thoroughfare vessel. [Their] blood drains but is not returned, their skin is bound in the interior, and their lips and mouth lack luxuriance. This is why their beard does not grow." This quote establishes both the relationship between the thoroughfare vessel and the penis and once

---

[36] This points to another perspective on the conception vessel as an important channel for treating all qi disorders. The presence of *Qi Hai* (CV-6) and *Shan Zhong* (CV-17)—the lower and upper sea of qi—on the conception vessel, is an especially important link to this view of the conception vessel.

[37] The thoroughfare vessel is more frequently known as the *chong mai*.

again establishes the pathway of the thoroughfare vessel up the abdomen and to the face, mouth, and lips.[38]

The connections between the pathway of the thoroughfare vessel and the spine and governing vessel strengthens the physiological interactions between these two channels. Through this interaction, the thoroughfare vessel supports all the actions of the governing vessel as cited in its section in the preceding pages.

Indications

Because of the channel pathways discussed above, the thoroughfare vessel is an important channel for the treatment of many andrological diseases. As this channel has no acumoxa points of its own, we access it through its crossing points on other channels and through the points corresponding to the sea of blood.

Because the thoroughfare vessel travels with the kidney channel up the abdomen, *Heng Gu* (KI-11) through *Huang Shu* (KI-16) are commonly-used points for andrological conditions such as yang wilt, infertility, and pain in the penis, scrotum, and testicles, especially when these conditions manifest with either a blood vacuity or blood stasis pattern. *Qi Chong* (ST-30), the point of the qi thoroughfare in the lower abdomen has a very strong action on the thoroughfare vessel because it is a major crossing point between the thoroughfare vessel and the stomach channel. Hence, it has the same andrological indications as those cited for the kidney channel crossing points.

Within the most influential premodern acumoxa text (*Ling Shu*), the thoroughfare vessel is repeatedly referred to as "the sea of blood." In chapter 33 for example, the following points are identified as points of the sea of blood (the thoroughfare vessel): *Da Zhu* (BL-11), *Shang Ju Xu* (ST-37), and *Xia Ju Xu* (ST-39). In fact, as the sea of blood, the thoroughfare vessel and the sea of blood points are useful for all male anterior yin problems caused by blood vacuity and blood stasis.

Of course, the confluent point of the thoroughfare vessel—*Gong Sun* (SP-4)— is also an important point for regulating its physiology. It is well-known as a gynecological point, but because of its strong association with the thoroughfare vessel, modern acumoxa practitioners sometimes use it for male anterior yin diseases such as yang wilt, mounting qi pain, and infertility, though textual documentation of such use is lacking in premodern and modern works on Chinese andrology. SP-4 seems to have a stronger link with the portion of the thoroughfare vessel that travels through the abdomen and up to the head and face rather than with the portion that travels through the lower body and the anterior yin region. Practitioners may have to test this in their own clinical practices.

---

[38] From the standpoint of modern Western medicine, when the testicles are removed in castration male androgen production is drastically curtailed and this is the primary cause for feminization and lack of masculinization (including the lack of growth of facial hair) among eunuchs.

Hui Yin (CV-1) is also an important crossing point with the thoroughfare vessel and does have many well-documented andrological indications including yang wilt, inhibited urination, enuresis, scrotal swelling and pain, genital itching, and mounting qi pain. How many of these are related directly to the thoroughfare vessel and how many to the conception vessel is difficult to determine. Nevertheless, this is a major point for treating the thoroughfare vessel and it does have andrological indications.

The girdle vessel

Pathways

Regarding how the pathway of the girdle vessel is related to andrology we may first read the following quote from Book 10, Chapter 4 of *Zhen Jiu Jia Yi Jing*: "All the yin and yang [channels] meet at the ancestral sinew [and go on to] meet at *Qi Chong* (ST-30), and the yang brightness [channel] is the chief [of all of them]. They are all ascribed to the girdle vessel and join with the governing vessel." It is clear from this quote that the girdle vessel is connected with the ancestral sinew (the penis) and with both the foot yang brightness channel and the governing vessel, which we have already seen are central to the physiology of the male anterior yin region. So, how does the girdle vessel come in to play? Because it encircles the body at the waist, the girdle vessel joins with all the channels that course through the trunk. Thus, free flow of qi and blood within the girdle vessel supports free flow within all of these other channels. And the girdle vessel's connections with the foot yang brightness stomach channel and the governing vessel are of special importance in supplying the ancestral sinew with qi and blood.

Indications

While there is a strong resonance between the girdle vessel and the treatment of gynecological disorders, and especially abnormal vaginal discharge (note that the word *dai* also means vaginal discharge, as in the word *"dai xia"*), it is also sometimes used in the treatment of andrological conditions. In *Mai Jing* (*The Pulse Canon*), Wang Shu-He recommends the girdle vessel for men who suffer from lesser abdominal hypertonicity and seminal emission.

Since the girdle vessel does not possess any points of its own, it can only be accessed by its crossing points: *Dai Mai* (GB-26); *Wu Shu* (GB-27) and; *Wei Dao* (GB-28). The main andrological indications of these points are lesser abdominal pain and mounting qi pain, which commonly accompany prostatitis and BPH. While theoretically we might see a possible use for the girdle vessel for yang wilt (erectile dysfunction), from reviewing the andrology literature, it seems that Chinese practitioners rarely use it that way.

The yin and yang linking vessels

Pathways

The pathways of the yin and yang linking vessels—as their names implies—link together all the yin and yang channels. For andrology, they are helpful in regulating and harmonizing yin and yang throughout the body, including within the anterior yin region. When there is adequate supply of enriching and nourishing yin qi, the anterior yin region is nourished, and all the channels and their corresponding viscera and bowels involved with normal male physiological activity are also nourished. When there is sufficient power and movement within the yang channels, the anterior yin region as well as all the channels and viscera and bowels associated with it are similarly powered and activated.

Indications

Since the physiological functions of the yin and yang linking vessels are rather general, it is hard to find specific andrological uses for these channels. In andrology, if points along these channels are used, they usually serve as supportive channels for secondary symptoms and not for the primary disease. For example, *Zhu Bin* (KI-9)—the cleft point of the yin linking vessel—can be used as a point to facilitate calming the spirit, as the yin linking vessel passes through the chest and has a strong influence on the heart. This is of benefit for men with anxiety or depression related to challenged sexual performance, and for andropausal men, especially when there is an insufficiency of yin-blood and essence. And *Jin Men* (BL-63)—the cleft point of the yang linking vessel—can be used when there is sudden and severe mounting qi pain that might accompany acute prostatitis.

The yin and yang springing vessels
Pathways

Since the yin and yang springing vessels connect with all the yin and yang channels respectively, similar to the yin and yang linking vessels, they have an important role in regulating yin and yang throughout the body. There is an especially close link between the yin springing vessel and the kidney channel. Hence, since the yin springing vessel unites with the kidney channel at *Zhao Hai* (KI-6)—its confluent point—free and abundant flow of qi and blood within the yin springing vessel supports the same in the kidney channel, which as established previously has substantial links with the male anterior yin region. And *Jiao Xin* (KI-8)—the cleft point of the yin springing vessel—also has a strong physiological effect on nourishing the male anterior yin region.

Indications

There is a strong resonance between *Zhao Hai* (KI-6)—the confluent point of the yin springing vessel—and the male anterior yin region. Traditional andrological indications for this point include itching of the genitals, seminal emission, and mounting qi pain. Also, of special note is the use of this point cited in *Zhen Jiu Jia Yi Jing* for "sudden erection." This symptom is clearly due to a hyperactivity of yang qi and can be balanced by increasing the quantity of yin qi coursing to the penis and through the kidney channel by using the yin springing vessel.

Jiao Xin (KI-8), as the cleft point of the yin springing vessel, has several andrological indications cited in premodern texts including genital pain, swelling and pain of the testes, sweating of the genitals, qi strangury (a disease pattern commonly seen in men with BPH and prostatitis), and lesser abdominal pain (also found in many andrological conditions).

Viscera-Bowel Physiology and Pathology in Relation to Andrology

The Roles of the Viscera and Bowels in Andrology

In this section, I do not provide a thorough coverage of visceral manifestation theory[1] in general, as would be covered in a basic textbook on the fundamentals of Chinese medicine. Instead, I am focusing on the roles of the various viscera and bowels in male physiology and pathology. I offer this section with the presumption that the reader is fully educated in the fundamentals of Chinese medicine.[2] I have chosen passages from premodern sources that contain quintessential though lesser-known aspects of each viscera and bowel's physiology and pathomechanisms and I relate them to the clinical practice of Chinese andrology.

I assume that early Chinese medical literature represents the only known written record of the evolution of Chinese medicine as it was molded and changed by doctors and scholars during different dynasties. It therefore served as the academic and clinical fountainhead for our predecessors and can continue to be the source of new insight. The premodern texts are the essential written repositories of Chinese medicine and are necessary to the intellectual vigor of many aspects of Chinese medicine, including clinical practice, research, education, and publication. These passages contain insights which are essential to the clinical practice of both andrology and general internal medicine.

By taking this approach, I deliberately continue in the tradition of text-based scholarship within Chinese medicine. This is an important process which should be both responsive to and influential on the prosecution of actual clinical practice. I also briefly explain the pathomechanisms which result from failed physiology. In Book 1, Chapter 6 on Chinese andrological diseases and in the appropriate sections of Book 2 of this text, the reader will find definitions and more detailed discussions of the andrological disease categories which are mentioned here in the context of pathomechanisms.

---

[1] Visceral manifestation theory (*zang xiang xue shuo*) is the premodern term used to refer to the Chinese medical understanding of the anatomy and physiology of human organs.

[2] For an audio presentation containing a thorough review of the physiology and pathomechanisms of the viscera and bowels, see Damone (2005).

The Five Viscera

The heart

Premodern references

Chapter 44 of *Su Wen* (*Plain Questions*) states: "The heart governs the body's blood vessels."

Chapter 10 of *Su Wen* states: "All blood belongs to the heart."

Chapter 71 of *Ling Shu* (*Magic Pivot*) states: "The heart is the great monarch of the five viscera and the six bowels; it is the residence of essence-spirit."

Explanation

These are commonly cited references to the physiology of the heart from *Nei Jing* (*Inner Canon*).[3] The first two reveal the Chinese medical conception of the heart as the ruler of all blood and blood vessels in the human body. The Chinese literature on the fundamentals of Chinese medicine often stress the importance of the heart in not only moving blood throughout the body but also in engendering blood. The last premodern reference above reveals the Chinese medical assumption that the heart "governs spirit" and that spirit is a force intrinsic to human life which directs all the physiological activities of the entire body, including those of the male reproductive and urinary systems.

The role of the heart in engendering blood is described in premodern literature as a process of "red transformation (*hua chi*)." This concept is rooted in five phase theory in that the heart belongs to the fire phase which corresponds to the color red, and "fire is the flaming upward." Thus, the physiological role of the heart in the human body is analogous to the phenomenon of fire and therefore to warmth, radiation, and activation. The heart's sovereign fire (*jun huo*) is one of the motive forces within the body which power the transformation of water and grain essence and clear qi into red-colored and life-giving blood. And it is blood which nourishes, moistens, and enriches the entire body. Further, blood provides material nourishment to all the viscera and bowels and the essence-spirit, and in doing so enables them to function normally. Thus, when blood is ample, both qi and essence-spirit are abundant, and when blood is vacuous, both viscera-bowel physiological functions as well as essence-spirit diminish.

In order to grasp the relationship between essence-spirit (*jing shen*) and viscera-bowel function, consider that spirit (*shen*) directs all physiological activities within the body. Seen in this light, spirit is akin to "life force" in a more general way, even though this translation is still saddled with other nuances and is

---

[3] *Nei Jing* was published in the 1st century CE.

therefore still unsatisfying. Wang (2001) is quite clear in his assertion that the mutual transformations among qi, blood, essence, and fluids are all under the dominion of spirit and therefore are controlled by the heart.

In my opinion, we must not limit our understanding of the concept of spirit (*shen*) in Chinese medicine to spirit in the sense of "spirituality" or "consciousness." I believe such an understanding reveals New Age perceptions—and perhaps misconceptions—of Chinese medicine as a purely spiritual medicine. Sometimes this leads to the logical if not mistaken assumption that spirit problems cannot be treated through physical means—such as supplementing and nourishing qi and blood for example—and that the highest form of treatment in Chinese medicine is a spiritual treatment. Furthering this logic, some assert that physical treatments are banal and not esoteric enough to treat the spirit.

Although spirit in Chinese medicine is without a doubt inextricably connected with consciousness and emotion, it is at the same time rooted in and derived from physical substance with which it is locked in yin-yang unity. I assert that conceiving of spirit as a purely ethereal and nonphysical phenomenon requires the underlying Western assumption that the mind and body are divided. Upon careful review of the premodern and modern literature, however, I find that the core of Chinese medicine is devoid of any such mind-body division.

What specific significance do these physiological functions of the heart have for the principles and practice of Chinese andrology? First, since blood nourishes the entire body, including the penis, scrotum, testes, prostate, and all other male sexual, reproductive, and urinary tissues, it follows that the heart—as the viscus that governs blood—plays an essential role in men's health and illness. Further, since spirit holds dominion over all physiological and psychological phenomena occurring in a man's body, including all his sexual and reproductive functions, it too is central to men's physiology. So when we truly understand the implications of the fact that the heart governs spirit, we see more clearly that normal heart function is essential to the vigor of men in the view of physicians of Chinese andrology.

Pathology

If the heart fails to function normally—either because it suffers diseases of repletion or those of vacuity—various male diseases can occur. For example, normal male erectile function requires that qi and blood enter and remain in the penis long enough to satisfy himself and/or a responsive partner. As we have seen above, the heart plays a central role in the formation of blood and in the movement of blood to the penis, and spirit is the life force that is behind blood formation and movement. If there is heart qi vacuity or heart blood vacuity, then the anterior yin region will be underpowered and undernourished and yang wilt may occur. Yang wilt may also result when hyperactive heart fire scorches and consumes blood. Further, when hyperactive heart fire stirs ministerial fire, it harasses the essence chamber;[4] thus, dream emissions and hematospermia may occur. Though more detailed discussions of the pathomechanisms of men's diseases are presented in their corresponding chapter, this short discussion should provide some basic examples of how heart dysfunction plays a central role in male anterior yin diseases.

The lung

Premodern references

Chapter 10 of *Su Wen* states: "All qi belongs to the lung."

Chapter 21 of *Su Wen* states: "The lung is the upper source of water."

Chapter 21 of *Su Wen* states: "The lung governs the movement of water."

Chapter 21 of *Su Wen* states: "The lung regulates the waterways and transports [fluids] down to the bladder."

Chapter 21 of *Su Wen* states: "The lung faces the hundred vessels."

Explanation

In exploring the role of the lung in men's health and illness, I find these classical statements of special significance. "The lung governs qi" is not an empty phrase to memorize in fundamental theory class and forget. Grasping the deeper significance of this aspect of lung function enables us to see the role of the lung in maintaining normal male sexual, reproductive, and urinary functions. These functions require adequate quantity and free flow of qi, and therefore the lung (as governor of qi) is directly involved with both. The latter two statements above establish the roles of the lung in: 1) providing emollience and nourishment to the entire body, including the male anterior yin organs and; 2) maintaining normal urinary function. According to Wang (2001):

> "When ancestral qi reaches the heart, it becomes heart qi. When it reaches the spleen, it becomes spleen qi. When it reaches the liver, it becomes liver qi. When it reaches the kidney, it becomes kidney qi. When it is in the vessels it becomes construction qi. When it is outside of the vessels, it becomes defensive qi. Although it may change in name, all of this qi originates in the lung. It is a result of the combination of qi from respiration (lung) and the fluid and grain essence from the spleen" (p. 179).

This passage reveals the importance of the lung in the formation of ancestral qi and its logical connection with the fact that the lung governs the qi of the entire body. We may carry this line of thinking to its logical conclusion: "when it [*i.e.*, ancestral qi] reaches the penis, it becomes penile qi; when it reaches the scrotum,

---

[4] The essence chamber (*jing shi*) is the place where semen is stored, see Wiseman and Feng, (1998).

it becomes scrotal qi, etc." In other words, the functions of all male anterior yin organs and tissues—along with all the other organs and tissues that comprise the human body—ultimately rely on lung qi in order to function normally.

To see the interconnectedness between ancestral qi and the qi of each of the individual viscera and bowels is to see the body as one unified system. Thus, I conclude that the classification of qi into different types (*i.e.*, construction, defense, and viscera-bowel) is simply a tool that the original framers of Chinese medicine used to draw attention to specific aspects of qi function. In this light, if we supplement lung qi with *Ren Shen* (Ginseng Radix) or *Huang Qi* (Astragali Radix), then we supplement the qi of the entire body, not only lung qi. In fact, when we supplement spleen qi, we enhance the spleen's ability to absorb and transport the essence of water and grain up to the lung, which will in turn increase the quantity of lung qi and stimulate its formation of ancestral qi. Thus, when lung qi is "harmonious," in that it possesses sufficient strength, it "governs qi"; it thus optimizes male anterior yin physiology.

While the statements that the lung "moves water" and "regulates the waterways" emphasize the role of the lung in the movement of fluids throughout the body, according to Wang (2001), the dictum "the lung is the upper source of water" more specifically refers to another aspect of lung function—providing moisture and enrichment. The lung spreads and distributes fluids—one of the material bases of life—to the rest of the body. This of course includes the male anterior yin organs.

In *Lei Jing* (*The Classified Canon*),[5] we find the following statement: "Free flow in the channels must derive from qi. Qi is governed by the lung and so [the lung] is the meeting place of the hundred vessels." We generally understand this aspect of lung physiology in terms of how the lung—through its close association with ancestral qi—aids the heart in its movement of blood. Since blood is one of the substantial sources of nourishment for the male anterior yin, lung qi helps the heart to move blood and thus plays a role in normal male urological and reproductive function *vis-à-vis* movement of blood.

Pathology

If the lung fails to govern qi, and therefore inadequately forms ancestral qi, then various male anterior yin diseases may result including yang wilt, premature ejaculation, and decreased libido. When the lung fails to move water or to regulate the waterways, then conditions such as dribbling urinary block, inhibited urination, and urinary incontinence may occur. If the penis and testes suffer a lack of nourishment as a result of the lung failing in its role as the upper source of water, then conditions such as yang wilt, infertility, and scanty semen may occur.

As seen above, when the lung "faces the hundred vessels" it helps the heart to

---

[5] *Lei Jing* was written by Zhang Jing-Yue and published in 1604, during the Ming dynasty.

propel the blood. It follows then that lung disease may lead to blood stasis. And blood stasis plays an important role in the pathomechanisms of male diseases such as infertility, yang wilt, and dribbling urinary block.

The spleen

Premodern references

Chapter 21 of *Su Wen* states: "The spleen governs the movement and transformation of water and grain essence."

Chapter 21 of *Su Wen* states: "The spleen moves and transforms water-damp."

Chapter 21 of *Su Wen* states: "Spleen qi dissipates essence upwards to the lung."

Jing Yue Quan Shu (Jing-Yue's Complete Compendium)[6] states: "The initiation of human life relies on the engendering of essence-blood. Continued human life relies on nourishment from water and grain. Without essence-blood, there is no foundation for establishing the physical body. Without water and grain, the physical body cannot be invigorated... The sea of water and grain is rooted and reliant on the governance of early heaven. And the sea of essence-blood is also reliant on investment from later heaven."

Explanation

When we consider the applicability of the above-quoted dictums pertaining to the spleen, the first two emerge as bridges to understanding the digestive role of the spleen as well as its part in the metabolism of fluids. In pointing to the upbearing role of the spleen, the third statement reveals that the spleen has an important role in maintaining the upbearing and downbearing aspect of the body's qi dynamic. Lastly, Zhang Jing-Yue's discussion of the relationship between the spleen and kidney in his statement above invites us to challenge our understanding of the interaction between earlier and later heaven and how that affects our diagnosis and treatment of male anterior yin disease.

In the *Pi Wei Lun (On the Spleen and Stomach)*,[7] Li Dong-Yuan explains the vital role of the spleen and stomach in the maintenance of health. From his work, one may draw the conclusion that splenic movement and transformation of water and grain essence—as the later heaven source of qi, blood, and fluids—provides the foundation for the normal physiological functions (of qi) and the material resources for the human body (including blood, marrow, fluids, and essence). In the absence of healthy splenic movement and transformation, the function and nourishment of the male anterior yin will suffer. In clinical practice, this gives rise to conditions such as infertility and yang wilt.

---

[6] *Jing Yue Quan Shu* was written by Zhang Jing-Yue (a.k.a Zhang Jie-Bin) in 1624, during the Ming dynasty.

[7] *Pi Wei Lun* was written by Li Dong-Yuan and published in the 13th century, during the Jin-Yuan dynasty.

Generally, we use the phrase "the spleen moves and transforms water-damp" to emphasize the function of the spleen in fluid metabolism. This refers to the active and transforming functions of spleen qi (or spleen yang) in its movement of yin-fluid throughout the body. This function of the spleen helps to ensure that the movement of water-damp is sufficiently powered and thus prevents the collection of water-damp and the subsequent development of male anterior yin diseases such as testicular phlegm node (scrotal mass), water mounting (scrotal hydrocele), and yin stem phlegm node (Peyronie's disease).

When the spleen raises the clear, it automatically helps the stomach to downbear the turbid and to maintain the normal qi dynamic within the body. Although this aspect of splenic function is responsible for carrying the essence of water and grain—as well as fluids—up to the lung, it also arguably has a role in maintaining normal containment within the anterior and posterior yin; thus, center qi fall causes male anterior yin diseases such as seminal emission, prostatic hyperplasia, frequent urges to urinate, and dribbling urinary block. Further, posterior yin conditions such as hemorrhoids and enduring unremitting perineal rashes and sores may occur when the spleen fails to raise the clear and qi then falls downward and becomes depressed in the lower body, giving rise to heat and dampness.

Too often the English language literature in Chinese medicine fails to address an issue of subtlety that is quite clear in the Chinese language source literature.[8] Such is the case with its presentation of the relationship between early heaven (the kidney) and later heaven (the spleen). I frequently find the overly simplistic understanding of this relationship entrenched in the minds of Western practitioners of Chinese medicine: that there is no way to affect one's inherited constitution because it is delivered from one's parents at the moment of con-

---

[8] I would like to emphasize here that there are many historical and sociopolitical factors why this is so. The vast majority of the first-generation American students of Chinese medicine lacked personal access to the Chinese language source material, and failed to grasp the centrality of Chinese language to the accurate transmission of Chinese medicine. Although many of these pioneers proceeded with a great degree of earnest and have served key roles in the transmission of Chinese medicine to the West, as the first generation of American teachers of Chinese medicine, they have understandably passed on their ignorance along with their knowledge. As a result, we have a few generations of practitioners and teachers—completely reliant on secondary English sources—who often unknowingly misrepresent and transmit idiosyncratic and nonconsensus views to Chinese medical students. As a result, Chinese medical discourse in the West is not anchored to any standardized body of literature and experience as it is in China and other East Asian countries. The premodern source texts are the anchors. They have undoubtedly been the repository of academic exchange among Chinese doctors since at least the Han dynasty. It should come as no surprise that exposure to a broad range of these texts would season one's ability to think and do Chinese medicine. The best ways to rectify our shortcomings and have a lasting impact on the transmission of Chinese medicine to the West are to support the study of Chinese language in Chinese medical educational institutions in the West, and to encourage the publication and study of accurate and clinically-useful translations.

ception and is therefore unalterable. From this perspective, all that one can do is to limit the rate of loss of early heaven essence. However, from Zhang Jing-Yue's statements above, it is clear that there is more to the story. Surplus later heaven essence may be added to one's natural endowment of early heaven essence. The physiological and thus clinical implications of this aspect of spleen and kidney physiology are significant. For example, clinicians often adopt a spleen-supplementing strategy for treating kidney vacuity patterns, as seen in the classic formula *Huan Shao Dan* (Rejuvenation Elixir).[9] It follows then that spleen vacuity can also lead to kidney vacuity as the early heaven root then lacks sufficient support and investment from later heaven. In men, spleen vacuity may thus play a role in the development of conditions such as infertility, yang wilt, and scanty semen.

The liver

Premodern references

Chapter 10 of *Ling Shu* states: "The liver is the uniting place of the sinews. Its sinews gather at the yin organs [*i.e.*, the penis and scrotum] and its vessel nets at the root of the tongue."

Zhen Jiu Jia Yi Jing (*The Systematized Canon of Acupuncture and Moxibustion*)[10] states: "During sleep, blood returns to the liver. When the liver receives blood, one can see. When the feet receive blood, one can walk. When the hands receive blood, one can grasp."

Ge Zhi Yi Lun (*Further Treatises on the Properties of Things*)[11] states: "The liver manages free coursing." In another chapter (*Xiang Huo Lun, On Ministerial Fire*) of the same text it states that ministerial fire is "that [fire] which is possessed by humans [and which] resides in two locations—[in both] the liver and kidney."

Chapter 1 of *Su Wen* states: "The kidney receives essence from the five viscera and six bowels and stores it. The essential qi that is stored within the kidney is reliant on liver blood to nourish and maintain its fullness. Kidney essence and liver blood—if one is luxuriant, then so is the other; if one [suffers] detriment, then so does the other. Their effulgence and debility are one and the same. They are bound by a common cause [in that they] mutually enrich and engender each other and mutually convert into one another. [Thus,] kidney essence

---

[9] The ingredients of *Huan Shao Dan* (Rejuvenation Elixir) are *Shan Yao* (Dioscoreae Rhizoma), *Niu Xi* (Achyranthis Rhizoma), *Fu Ling* (Poria), *Shan Zhu Yu* (Corni Fructus), *Xiao Hui Xiang* (Foeniculi Fructus), *Xu Duan* (Dipsacus Radix), *Tu Si Zi* (Cuscutae Semen), *Du Zhong* (Eucommiae Radix), *Ba Ji Tian* (Morindae Radix), *Rou Cong Rong* (Cistanches Rhizoma), *Wu Wei Zi* (Schizandrae Fructus), *Yuan Zhi* (Polygalae Radix), and *Shu Di Huang* (Rehmanniae Radix preparata).

[10] *Zhen Jiu Jia Yi Jing* was written by Huang Fu-Mi in 259 CE, during the Three Kingdoms period.

[11] *Ge Zhi Yu Lun* was written by Zhu Dan-Xi, and published during the Jin-Yuan dynasty.

nourishes the liver and transforms into blood and liver blood enriches the kidney and transforms into essence. So, it is said that 'the liver and kidney are of the same source' and 'essence and blood are of the same source.'"

Explanation

The first passage above establishes that the liver channel has an especially close relationship with the normal structure and functioning of the anterior yin. While Chapter 3 on the channels and network vessels contains a more detailed discussion of the pathways and functions of the liver channel *vis-à-vis* andrology, a few important facts are worth repeating here. Note the direct relationship between the fact that the liver unites with the sinews and that the penis and scrotum are a uniting place for sinews. It follows logically then that the nourishment and functioning of the penis and scrotum is directly linked to the liver channel, which, in turn, is in direct contact with the liver viscus. In physiology, free flow within the liver channel and ample liver blood are essential to normal male function.

The famous and often repeated passage from *Zhen Jiu Jia Yi Jing* quoted above very succinctly establishes the dependence of functional abilities—such as seeing, walking, and grasping—on nourishment provided by substance (in this instance, blood). The functioning of the male anterior yin must receive the nourishment provided by blood—which is "stored" in the liver—in order to function properly.[12] In *Jing Yue Quan Shu*, Zhang Jie Bin states: "Humans have a yin and yang [aspect], which are qi and blood. Yang governs qi, so when qi is complete, spirit is effulgent; yin governs blood, so, when blood is exuberant, the bodily form is strong." As part of the bodily form, the normal function of the penis, scrotum, and testes requires exuberant blood.

As Zhu Dan-Xi reminds us above in the quote from *Ge Zhi Yi Lun* both the liver and kidney posses ministerial fire. Clarifying this further, the very yang and therefore active functions of the liver—free coursing and orderly reaching—require the steaming and quickening of the ministerial fire. Wang (2001) summarizes the functions of liver yang (or ministerial fire acting through the liver) as: 1) keeping blood from becoming cold; 2) managing the upbearing and effusion of qi dynamic and; 3) maximizing the effectiveness of free coursing. Normal male function clearly depends on all of these.[13]

The statements that "the liver and kidney are of the same source," and "essence and blood are of the same source," comprise a very important repository of Chinese medical analysis of liver and kidney physiology. These statements mean that

---

[12] The liver "stores" blood for both its own nourishment and for that of the rest of the body as well. It therefore plays a role in ensuring that blood—as the material foundation for function—is properly distributed to all the organs, tissues, orifices, etc.; it is these structures that make up the "bodily form" (Wang, 2001).

[13] For an insightful coverage of the physiology and pathology of the liver in Chinese medicine, including physiological liver yang, see Qin, B.W. (1997).

liver blood and kidney essence are mutually convertible. That is, when there is sufficient liver blood, it can be stored as kidney essence, and when there is insufficient
liver blood, kidney essence can be transformed into liver blood to compensate. To
comprehend this, we must challenge any existing notion we may harbor in our
Chinese medical mind of kidney essence as a fixed and immutable phenomenon as
either immature or at best incomplete. When the dust from such an inquiry settles,
the vision of a more dynamic liver and kidney physiology emerges—one in which
the ratio between liver blood and kidney essence is relative and changeable. We
must conclude then that any clinical strategy which supplements blood—such as
supplementing the spleen for example—may result in increased storage of essence,
and conversely that any clinical strategy which enriches essence may result in a
supplementation of blood. This is clear when we analyze the fact that many medicinals and formulas which enrich kidney essence also nourish liver blood; in this
light one may consider *Lu Rong* (Cornu Cervi Pantotrichum), *Shu Di Huang*
(Rehmannia Radix preparata), and *You Gui Wan* (Right-Restoring [Life Gate]
Pill). Further, many formulas which enrich kidney essence contain the therapeutic
strategies of fortifying the spleen and supplementing spleen qi; witness the presence of *Shan Yao* (Disocorea Radix) and *Fu Ling* (Poria) in *Liu Wei Di Huang
Wan* (Six-Ingredient Rehmannia Pill), *Jin Gui Shen Qi Wan* (Golden Coffer Kidney Qi Pill), and *Huan Shao Dan* (Rejuvenation Elixir).

Pathology

When there are conditions such as liver depression, liver blood vacuity, depressed liver fire conducting downward through the liver channel, or damp-
heat pouring downward into the liver channel, the male anterior yin is often
affected. Thus, liver channel pathology is a frequent contributor to andrological conditions such as rigid yang (priapism), acute and chronic prostatitis, inability to ejaculate, and hematospermia. As such these factors should remain
accessible in the practitioner's mind when making a differential diagnosis.

If there is insufficiency of liver blood, the male anterior yin will be undernourished. This can lead to conditions such as yang wilt, scanty semen, mounting
qi, and genital retraction. The basic pathomechanism in all of these instances
would be insufficient liver blood to nourish the penis, testes, and scrotum.

If there is debility of liver ministerial fire, there is usually also debility of kidney ministerial fire; indeed, the kidney is usually the root of the problem. As a
result of these pathomechanisms one may develop male diseases such as yang
wilt, retracted genitals, premature ejaculation, and cold genitals. It is important to note here that although the medicinals used to warm liver yang are
generally those that warm kidney yang, one also chooses certain other warm
medicinals which specifically enter the liver channel and rectify qi and dissipate cold. I suggest when seeking out such medicinals that one use the clinical
indication of mounting qi as a guidepost. Among individual medicinals for
conditions like this, we find *Wu Yao* (Linderae Radix), *Xiao Hui Xiang*
(Foeniculi Fructus), and *Ju He* (Citri Reticulatae Semen); among formulas we
find *Ju He Wan* (Tangerine Pip Pill).

The kidney

The fact that the kidney plays a role in the normal physiology of men will come as no surprise to all practitioners and students of Chinese medicine. In fact, one may argue that at times it is overemphasized. When this occurs it degrades our understanding of the physiological roles of the other viscera-bowels and ignores the pathological importance of repletion conditions such as depressions, binds, and evils in men's diseases. Such unexamined assumptions represent an oversimplification of male physiology and pathology and at times lead to inappropriate supplementation of repletion. For example, many modern Chinese books and articles stress the importance of repletion pathomechanisms such as damp-heat, phlegm, and blood stasis—in fact usually in combination with or rooted in spleen-kidney vacuity—in male illnesses such as acute and chronic prostatitis (Tan and Tao, 1999).

However, even in light of the above, there is no defensible reason to ignore the often pivotal role of the kidney in male physiology. The premodern references below will showcase a few important aspects of kidney physiology and will show their importance to male function.

Premodern references

Zhen Jiu Jia Yi Jing states: "The kidney stores essence and essence houses the will. Its breath is yawning and its humor is spittle."

Zhong Zang Jing (*The Central Treasury Canon*)[14] states: "The kidney houses the essence-spirit, is the root of life, and connects outward through the ears. In men, it blocks [*i.e.*, restrains] essence. In women, it envelops [*i.e.*, contains blood]. It stands in interior-exterior relationship with the bladder and the foot lesser yin and greater yang are their [corresponding] channels."

Chapter 9 of *Su Wen* states: "The kidney governs hibernation, is the root of sealing and storage, and is the dwelling place of essence. Its bloom is in the hair, and its fullness is in the bones. It is the yin within lesser yin and it flows to the qi of winter."

Chapter 1 of *Su Wen* states: "[When a] male is eight years old, his kidney qi is replete and his teeth are fully developed. At 16 years old, his kidney qi is exuberant, his heavenly tenth (*tian gui*) arrives, his essential qi flows, his yin and yang are harmonious, and he is able to produce a child."

Explanation

In order to comprehend the meaning of the premodern statements above, we must clarify two meanings for the term "essence" (*jing*); both will shed light on the role of the kidney in male physiology. In the first and broad meaning of

---

[14] *Zhong Zang Jing* is attributed to Hua To who lived in the 2nd century CE, during the Eastern Han dynasty.

essence, it is the fundamental substrate from which all other essential elements—namely qi, blood, and fluids—derive. As such, essence is raw material which must be in abundance so that a man's viscera-bowels, bodily orifices, etc., are sufficiently nourished.[15] Only when a man's body is adequately nourished can it function optimally. In the second and more specific meaning of essence as "reproductive essence," it stands for reproductive essence in a genetic-like sense[16] and also specifically refers to semen. From this statement and others like it, we are reminded of the importance of the kidney in all male reproductive and sexual functions.

The second and third passages above, point out the role of the kidney in restraining essence (semen) and in this respect, liken kidney qi to the natural phenomena of winter and hibernation. In terms of andrology, the sealing and storing nature of kidney qi is necessary for normal ejaculation.

In the well-known passage from chapter 1 of *Su Wen* above, we see that the concept of heavenly tenth (*tian gui*) applies not only to women, but also to men. The arrival of heavenly tenth—in men and women—represents the attainment of sexual and reproductive maturity and is immediately dependent on an exuberance of "kidney qi," which here stands for kidney essence. Because of the previously mentioned mutually-reinforcing relationship between early heaven essence (*xian tian zhi jing*) and later heaven essence (*hou tian zhi jing*), however, the arrival of heavenly tenth is also indirectly dependent on investment from later heaven (the spleen and stomach). As a child ages, his physiologically vacuous spleen and stomach matures to the point of being able to engender and then store a surplus of liver blood in the kidneys as kidney essence. Gradually then, kidney essence—otherwise known in such discussions as kidney "essential qi"—builds up in direct proportion to the amount of this stored surplus liver blood. By the time a boy turns 16, his kidney qi is exuberant enough to overflow in the form of heavenly tenth, and he reaches puberty.[17]

Pathology

If, owing to either natural endowment insufficiency or insufficient investment from later heaven, kidney essence is vacuous, then a boy can experience delayed onset of puberty and secondary sexual characteristics. Moreover, according to Chinese andrology, this can result in small genitals, genital retraction, and infertility.

[15] It is revealing to note that the Chinese character for essence (*jing*) contains the rice or grain (*mi*) radical (#119). Considering the traditional grain-based (*i.e.*, rice, millet, wheat, sorghum) diet of broad regions of China, one may draw analogy between grain—the root of survival and avoidance of starvation—and essence as a basic staple of life.

[16] Here I mean "genetic-like" as a deliberate reference to the Western medical model in which genetic material from both the male and female combine at the moment of conception. I also think that the Chinese medical concept of essence resembles the modern Western understanding of stem cells—undifferentiated raw substance (cells) from which any other substance (or cells) can be derived.

[17] See also Book 1, Chapter 1 on the history of andrology in Chinese medicine.

If there is kidney qi vacuity and a failure of sealing and storage, then male sexual dysfunctions such as premature ejaculation and seminal efflux may occur.

The six bowels

Although the five viscera are much more important in andrology, for the sake of completion, I do wish to explore a few aspects of the bowels (*fu*) in relation to male function. There is also an another theme that serves as the backdrop for this discussion—that the bowels are subject in general to diseases of repletion and obstruction. This is expressed quite eloquently in chapter 11 of *Su Wen* which states:

> "The stomach, large intestine, small intestine, triple burner, [and] the bladder—these five—are engendered from heaven qi; [as such] they are manifestations of heaven. Thus, they drain but do not store. They receive turbid qi from the five viscera and are [therefore] called conveying and transforming bowels. [Within these bowels] there cannot be long-term abiding, [but only] transporting and draining."

The gallbladder

Premodern references

Pi Wei Lun states: "The gallbladder is the lesser yang upbearing qi of spring. [When] spring qi upbears, the ten thousand transformations are quiet. If gallbladder qi-spring upbears, the rest of the viscera follow."

Chapter 8 of *Su Wen* states: "The gallbladder holds the office of justice; whence decision emanates."

There is a widely held axiom in Chinese medicine which states: "When the gallbladder is vacuous, then the spirit is spontaneously timid."

Explanation

In the quote from the *Pi Wei Lun* above, Li Dong-Yuan points out the role of the gallbladder in maintaining the normalcy of the qi dynamic (upbearing, downbearing, exit, and entry) among the viscera and bowels. As such, we find that the gallbladder and the liver function in concert, that their channels net together and thus they form an interior-exterior pair. Moreover, they both belong to wood which has the nature of free coursing, and thus they mutually govern free coursing. It is true that in terms of free coursing, gallbladder function overlaps with that of the liver, and in Chinese herbal medicine is usually treated through the liver. In acumoxa therapy however, the gallbladder channel (and other channels which net with it) are essential therapeutic options for encouraging liver and gallbladder free coursing.

Further, I submit that we should not jettison whole segments of Chinese visceral manifestation theory without careful consideration of the ramifications of doing so. In this case, I argue that by preserving a clear understanding of the gallbladder as it is described in premodern literature, we maintain the conceptual link to certain gallbladder pathomechanisms. As a result we bring existing gallbladder treatment strategies into sharper focus and provide fuel which may power new insights for gallbladder-based treatments. When we sever such links, we lose a cognitive key to learning, teaching, and applying Chinese medicine.

The last two statements above reveal the role of the gallbladder in emotional life and also reflect gallbladder physiology in relation to that of the liver and heart. Premodern sources often contain references to this aspect of gallbladder function and assert that the gallbladder endows humans with courage and "decision-making." Wang (2001) explains these psychological attributes of the gallbladder in terms of relationships between the gallbladder, liver, and heart and not as independent features of the gallbladder alone. For our purposes in this study of andrology, considering the gallbladder in this light presents diagnostic and therapeutic options for treating men with anxiety related to sexual dysfunction and andropause. These options can supplement those which emphasize liver and heart physiology and pathomechanisms for such conditions.

Pathology

When liver and gallbladder free coursing and upbearing become depressed, various andrological conditions may arise. These include yang wilt, mounting qi, scrotal pain, and inability to ejaculate. Also, damp-heat may pour downward from the center burner and into the liver and gallbladder channels. This pathomechanism can lead to conditions such as rigid yang, acute and chronic prostatitis, inability to ejaculate, and hematospermia.

In pathology, the connection between the gallbladder and emotional life is most clearly seen in patterns such as gallbladder-heart timidity[18] and gallbladder depression with phlegm-fire harassing the heart. These patterns can play a role in male sexual dysfunctions including yang wilt, premature ejaculation, and andropause.

The stomach

Premodern references

Jing Yue Quan Shu states: "The stomach governs intake and the spleen governs movement and transformation. One takes in and the other moves; together they engender and transform essential qi."

---

[18] There are several names for this pattern in the Chinese medical literature including gallbladder-heart qi vacuity, gallbladder qi vacuity, and gallbladder vacuity-cold. It is clear that in Chinese herbal medicine, treatment of this pattern and its complications usually requires a combination of treatment strategies including but not limited to supplementing spleen and heart qi, nourishing blood, transforming phlegm, and resolving depression. Consider representative formulas for these patterns such as *Shi Yi Wei Wen Dan Tang* (Eleven Ingredients Gallbladder-Warming Decoction) and *Ding Zhi Wan* (Mind-Stabilizing Pill).

Chapter 29 of *Su Wen* states: "The four limbs could not be endowed with qi from the stomach if it were not for the spleen endowing [the stomach with qi]; [without this coordination, qi] cannot reach the channels."

Jing Yue Quan Shu states: "All those who wish to examine diseases must first examine the stomach qi. All those who wish to treat diseases, must—on principle—look after stomach qi. If the stomach qi-origin is damaged, no one can be free from worry."

Explanation

While I explore the centrality of normal spleen function to the health of men above, here I would like to draw attention to the important contribution the stomach makes to the engenderment of qi, blood, essence, and fluids. While modern Western authorities on Chinese medicine typically emphasize the spleen's role in the formation of these essential elements of the human body—sometimes to the detriment of showing the importance of the stomach—premodern Chinese sources do not. As we can see from Zhang Jing-Yue's proclamation above, perhaps we should reexamine our assumptions that the stomach is not as important as the spleen in Chinese visceral manifestation theory.

The stomach is responsible for the intake and decomposition of water and grain. If the stomach does not decompose water and grain, then the spleen is unable to move and transform their essence. So, we can see that although one's spleen may be functioning normally, if one's stomach is not, there can still be negative implications for one's ability to engender qi, blood, essence, and fluids. In point of fact, in clinical practice we most often see diseases of the spleen and stomach presenting together; this reflects the reality that the spleen and stomach are fully integrated in both their physiology and pathology. If we do not retain the role of the stomach itself in this physiology and pathology, however, we may lose cognitive links which—in certain clinical circumstances—guide us to stomach channel points (in addition to points on the spleen channel) and to medicinals which specifically treat the stomach (as distinct from, and in addition to, those that treat the spleen). I believe a clear example of the latter lies in our clinical mandate to select medicinals and formulas for abducting and transforming food when treating the pattern "food stagnation in the stomach duct."

Pathology

In light of the above, the stomach plays an important role in a man's physiology because the health of the anterior yin is in direct proportion to the health of the stomach. All the later heaven nourishment required by the penis, scrotum, testes, bladder, etc., ultimately originate in the stomach. The stomach therefore may play an indirect role in the development of almost any andrological condition. Some more commonly-encountered conditions include yang wilt, infertility, dribbling urinary block, and chronic prostatitis.

Whether due to repletion, vacuity, or both, stomach diseases can affect a man's health. For example, if there is turbid dampness obstructing the spleen and stomach, yang wilt may occur. This pathomechanism is revealed when we see that a spleen-stomach supplementing formula such as *Liu Jun Zi Tang* (Six Gentlemen Decoction) is a useful formula to treat certain cases of yang wilt.[19] For a further exploration of this idea from the perspective of the stomach channel, see Book 1, Chapter 3 on the channels and network vessels.

The small intestine

Premodern references

Lei Jing states: "The small intestine is located below the stomach. It receives water and grain from the stomach and separates the clear and the turbid; as a result, fluid percolates [downward] and exits from the anterior [yin] and [solid] waste exits from the posterior [yin]. Spleen qi transforms and upbears [and the] small intestine transforms and downbears. So, [the small intestine is called the place] whence the transformation of things emanates."

Zhu Bing Yuan Hou Lun (*On the Origin and Indicators of Disease*)[20] states: "The bladder and the kidney stand in exterior-interior relationship; together they govern water. When water enters the small intestine, it flows downward to the bladder, travels to the [anterior] yin, and becomes urine."

Explanation

The first statement above clarifies the role of the small intestine in both digestion and urination and suggests a close link between the spleen and the small intestine. In fact, we usually see small intestinal function described as one aspect of splenic function, and this is reflected in the fact that most modern discussions of the physiology of the small intestine in the Chinese literature amalgamate the small intestine with the spleen. As such, the role of the small intestine in digestion is included in the discussions of the spleen and it is generally assumed that splenic movement and transformation of water and grain occurs at least in part through small intestinal separation of the clear and the turbid. Zhang Jing-Yue, by succinctly saying "[The] spleen qi transforms and upbears [and the] small intestine transforms and downbears," also hints at such a close link. This connection is also clear in herbal medicine in that supplementing the small intestine requires fortifying the spleen and draining dampness; there are no medicinals that supplement the small intestine without also supplementing the spleen.

---

[19] The specific textual basis for the connection between yang wilt and stomach vacuity was first suggested to me by my colleague Fan Jian-Min (personal communication, 2001) who directed me to chapter 44 of *Su Wen* which states: "When yang brightness is vacuous, there is slackness of the ancestral sinew (*i.e.*, the penis)." This shows the connection between yang brightness vacuity (in this case yang brightness-stomach vacuity) and yang wilt. I have since noted in clinical practice that men will also experience positive effects on their sexual function from spleen-supplementing formulas. This pathomechanism is explored in greater detail in Book 1, Chapter 5.

[20] *Zhu Bing Yuan Hou Lun* was written by Chao Yuan-Fang and published in 610 CE, during the Sui dynasty.

Although I agree that the relationship between the spleen and the small intestine is extremely close, I also feel that understanding the specific role of the small intestine in the formation of stool and urine clarifies aspects of physiology and pathomechanisms—and by extension of treatment—which are difficult to grasp without this understanding in place. Simply stated, when the small intestine "separates the clear and the turbid," it: 1) transforms the "clear" essence of water and grain and sends the "turbid" dregs further downward to the large intestine where it is "mutated" by the large intestine into stool and is then subjected to large intestinal conduction and conveyance; it is thereby expelled through the anus and; 2) separates "clear" or liquid from the "turbid" or solid dregs. It sends the liquid to the bladder for excretion and the solid to the large intestine.

Pathology

Once we understand the physiological functions of the small intestine, we can progress to comprehending its pathomechanisms and we can see their significance to the practice of andrology. While a more detailed discussion of these pathomechanisms is presented in their corresponding chapter, a brief mention here is essential to understanding small intestinal physiology in the context of andrology. If the small intestine fails to separate the clear and the turbid properly in either of the two ways expressed above, then two issues arise. First, this means that there is splenic movement and transformation failure and therefore water and grain essence and water-damp are not being transformed. (See the spleen section above for a discussion of the pathological implications of this.) Secondly, bladder qi transformation and its role in the formation and excretion of urine will be adversely affected. We usually label this as either spleen and small intestinal vacuity and/or obstruction, or as heart and small intestinal heat (a.k.a. small intestinal repletion heat and heart fire conducting into the small intestine). As a result of either of these pathomechanisms, a myriad of andrological complaints may arise including yang wilt, dribbling urinary block, strangury, prostatic hyperplasia, and hematospermia.

The large intestine

Premodern references

Chapter 8 of *Su Wen* states: "The large intestine holds the office of conveyance, whence mutation emanates."

Explanation

The large intestine conducts and conveys out stool. Its role of "mutation" is taken to mean that it receives the dregs left over from splenic movement and transformation and from the small intestine's function of separating the clear and the turbid, and then mutates these dregs into a formed stool which it conveys outward through the anus. So the large intestine plays an important role in the formation and ejection of turbid waste and helps to prevent any accumulation or stagnation from forming in the lower burner and in the anterior yin region. This role is also understood in light of the fact that the large intestine is the largest bowel in the lower body; hence, free flow within it encourages free flow to all the other organs in the lower burner, and the anterior yin region, including the penis, the testes, and the scrotum.

Pathology

If the large intestine fails in its functions of conduction and conveyance and mutation and either diarrhea or bound stool results, then male physiology can be adversely affected. For example, if there is persistent diarrhea (and this invariably means that there is also disease of both the spleen and small intestine), then there will be a loss of luxuriance and containment (as a result of qi and blood vacuity) for the male anterior yin region and yang wilt, premature ejaculation, infertility, and seminal efflux can occur. On the contrary, if stool becomes bound within the large intestine so as to form a substantial accumulation and thus a blockage to the free flow of qi and blood to the penis and testes, the same diseases can result but due to repletion pathomechanisms rather than to those of vacuity. In such cases, attacking and precipitating methods as embodied within formulas such as *Da Cheng Qi Tang* (Major Qi-Infusing Decoction) and its variants can be applied.

Since the large intestine and the lung stand in interior-exterior relationship, any vacuity or repletion of the large intestine can affect the lung and prevent the lung from functioning normally. The lung functions most likely to be adversely affected by large intestinal pathology in andrological diseases would be its ability to serve as the upper source of water, its depurative downbearing, and its function of regulating the waterways (triple burner). If these functions fail, then dribbling urinary block and strangury occur because lung qi fails to transform fluids and to power triple burner, kidney, and bladder qi transformation. In the case of infertility, the lung would be unable to send enriching nourishment to the anterior yin region thus denying yin-fluids to serve as the partial material basis for semen.

The bladder

Premodern references

Chapter 8 of *Su Wen* states: "The bladder holds the office of the river island; it stores fluids. Qi transformation enables [the bladder] to outthrust [fluid]."

Xue Zheng Lun (*On Blood Pathoconditions*)[21] states: "The *Inner Canon* says [the bladder] holds the office of the river island, [that it] stores fluids, [and that] qi transformation enables it to outthrust. This refers to outthrust of sweat and urine."

Xue Zheng Lun (*On Blood Pathoconditions*) explains: "Although urine is outthrust from the bladder, [this outthrust] is actually dependent on [the fact that the] lung is the upper source of water; [when] the upper source [is] clear, [the]

---

[21] *Xue Zheng Lun* was written by Tang Rong-Chuan in 1884, during the Qing dynasty.

lower source is free [and] clear. [The] spleen is the dike, when the dike is uninhibited, the waterways are uninhibited."

Explanation

The most significant contribution of these three premodern statements about the bladder is their emphasis on the fact that it is bladder qi transformation which outthrusts urine from the bladder. Qi transformation (*qi hua*)—one of the five basic physiological functions of qi—describes the role of the bladder in outthrusting both urine (from the bladder bowel itself) and sweat (from the interstices, which are also under the influence and regulation of the foot greater yang channel). Of these two aspects of bladder qi transformation, however, the former is most pertinent to andrology.

In the human body, qi is the motile and active force which must be in sufficient supply and must not become depressed. The force exerted by qi as it is expressed through the viscera and bowels and the free flow of qi throughout the body are essential to normal functioning. Qi therefore drives all the physiological processes of each viscera and bowel. Hence, the bladder's ability to excrete urine smoothly, completely, and efficiently is in direct proportion to bladder qi power and free flow. Bladder qi power and free flow in turn depends on the power and free flow of lung qi, spleen qi, small intestinal qi, liver qi, kidney qi, and—by extension—triple burner qi.

Pathology

When bladder qi transformation is either underpowered due to lung, spleen or kidney qi vacuity, or depressed due to externally-contracted wind evil or liver depression, micturition is adversely affected. These bladder pathomechanisms then are important factors in the development of andrological conditions such as acute and chronic prostatitis, benign prostatic hyperplasia, prostate cancer, strangury, and dribbling urinary block.

The triple burner

Premodern references

Difficulty 31 of the *Nan Jing* states: "The triple burner is the path of water and grain, [and is the] place from which qi begins and [at which it] ends."

Difficulty 38 of the *Nan Jing* states: "So, there are six bowels [and the sixth] is called the triple burner; it is the special courier of original qi; it governs and maintains all the various [forms of] qi."

Difficulty 66 of the *Nan Jing* states: "The triple burner—the special courier of original qi—governs the free movement of all three qi, and passes through the five viscera and six bowels."

Chapter 8 of the *Su Wen* states: "The triple burner holds the office of the sluices; it manifests as the waterways."

Explanation

For the purposes of brevity, here we must place aside the longer review of the historical debate about the triple burner within Chinese medicine. Of course, the main point of disagreement has always been centered on whether or not the triple burner has its own individual morphological structure or whether its functions are an amalgamation of the structures and functions of other viscera and bowels. When modern Chinese doctors attempt to correlate the traditional functional concept of the triple burner to known anatomical structures in the human body, they usually suggest that the triple burner includes the lymphatic system, connective tissue, the nervous system, the digestive system, the urinary system, and the circulatory system (Wang, 2001).

In any case, while premodern literate physicians have disagreed about the anatomy of the triple burner, modern Chinese doctors generally agree that the triple burner is functionally concerned with: 1) the movement and transformation of water and grain; 2) the movement and distribution of original qi (*yuan qi*) and; 3) the metabolism of fluids. Thus, the conceptual umbrella of "triple burner" includes the functions of all the other viscera and bowels in these specific three aspects, and not only helps to explain physiology and pathology, but also serves as an important cognitive tie to the triple burner channel and its network connections as clinical treatment options. For example, without an understanding of triple burner physiology, one lacks the theoretical rationale for grasping the use of *Zhi Gou* (SJ-6) for helping to move stool, *Tian Jing* (SJ-10) for downbearing counterflow qi and transforming phlegm, and *San Jiao Shu* (BL-22) for disinhibiting urine and draining dampness (Deadman and Khafagi, 1998).

Pathology

Considering the three aforementioned physiological functions of the triple burner, and the relationships among the triple burner and the other viscera and bowels, let us clarify certain aspects of triple burner pathology and treatment. Firstly, as triple burner physiology is largely subsumed within the physiology of other viscera, bowels, and tissues, most modern Chinese herbalists generally treat and positively affect the triple burner indirectly by treating its associated viscera and bowels. As an added clinical bonus, however, acumoxa therapists who accept Chinese channel and network vessel theory have the triple burner channel and its networks available as therapeutic options.

If the triple burner fails in its role of movement and transformation of water and grain, we usually see this as a disorder of the spleen, stomach, and intestines, and we treat it as such. When water and grain is not transformed, the anterior yin is denied nourishment; this leads to andrological conditions such as infertility, yang wilt, dribbling urinary block, and premature ejaculation.

When the triple burner does not function as the "special courier of original qi," the natural outcome is either qi vacuity, qi depression, or both. Once again, Chinese herbalists generally would identify the other viscera and bowels involved—which are usually the spleen, stomach, liver, bladder, kidney, or lung—and treat accordingly. Under this heading, we find conditions such as yang wilt, dribbling urinary block, urinary incontinence, inability to ejaculate, and mounting qi.

Finally, when the triple burner as "the waterways" is either underpowered or depressed, water-damp collects and phlegm-rheum arises. Medicinal treatment is generally aimed at the lung, spleen, liver, kidneys, and urinary bladder. Clinical manifestations include yin stem phlegm node, scrotal node, water mounting, benign prostatic hyperplasia, and dribbling urinary block.

Disease Causes and Pathomechanisms in Andrology

One of the key distinguishing features of any medicine is its understanding of the causes and progression of illness. For Chinese medicine, this data lies under the heading "disease causes and pathomechanisms" (*bing yin bing ji*). Theoretically, a licensed practitioner of Chinese medicine should be thoroughly familiar with disease causes and pathomechanisms and should be able to apply them in clinical practice with ease and creativity. It is my experience, however, in over sixteen years of teaching and practicing Chinese medicine, that the overwhelming majority of Western students and practitioners of Chinese medicine have a very shaky understanding of Chinese medical theory, including disease causes and pathomechanisms. Hence, it is necessary here to take some time to cover these core concepts in some detail and with clarity of language and thought. Without the core cognitive structure of disease causes and pathomechanisms, our ability to apply Chinese medicine in the clinical practice of andrology is significantly stunted.

While a discussion of disease causes and pathomechanisms could be a very broad one (and indeed in a first-year theory course it should be), the focus of my attention here is on revealing disease causes and pathomechanisms that are specific to andrology. Thus, this chapter serves as the theoretical underpinning for the chapters on specific diseases in Book 2 of this text, which is a more clinically-organized presentation of the pathomechanisms of specific diseases. For more information regarding a Chinese disease category mentioned in this chapter but for which there is not a detailed individual chapter in Book 2, refer to Book 1, Chapter 6 on Chinese andrological disease categories, which gives a broad overview of Chinese andrological disease categories.

The Six Main Causes of Men's Diseases

Although these six disease causes are listed separately below for the purpose of efficient teaching and learning, experienced clinicians know that most patients develop illness due to a combination of two or more disease causes simultaneously. Further, according to the dictum from chapter 33 of *Su Wen* (*Plain*

Questions),[1] "for evil to encroach, qi must be vacuous," even diseases caused by repletion evils often occur because of the pathomechanism of "evil qi taking advantage of vacuity." So, in fact most diseases present with what eight-principle pattern discrimination describes as vacuity-repletion combination disease, namely vacuity of right qi (*zheng qi*) allowing for an evil to either invade from the exterior or to be engendered in the interior as a result of weakened viscera-bowel function. The six main causes of men's disease are:

1. The six excesses (especially cold, dampness, and heat)
2. Affect-mind damage
3. Dietary irregularities
4. Overtaxation
5. External injuries
6. Natural endowment insufficiency and Constitutional vacuity

The Six Excesses

Cold evil

Cold—being a yin evil—is fundamentally constricting, obstructing, binding, and congealing. It damages (*shang*)[2] yang qi in that it obstructs its free flow and its transforming power. According to chapter 66 of *Ling Shu* (*Magic Pivot*),[3] cold evil first invades through the feet and then travels upwards to the abdomen and umbilical region where it stagnates and congeals qi and blood. It may also directly strike the interior (the viscera and bowels, bones, or internal pathways of the channels and network vessels), or it may enter the body through excessive intake of cold food or fluid. Regardless of its route of entry or source of development, cold causes: 1) the functions of the viscera and bowels (being manifestations of yang qi transformation and qi dynamic) to become obstructed; 2) the free flow of qi and blood within the channels and network vessels to become slowed, bound, and congealed and; 3) the qi, blood, and fluids within the tissues of the bodily form to become bound. For the purposes of our discussion, cold binds within the male anterior yin region and is the cause of many diseases of men.

Pathomechanisms of cold

According to *Ling Shu*: "The foot reverting yin sinew…follows [its course] up the inner thigh and binds at the yin organ and connects with the [other] sinews [there].… damage by cold entering leads to yin [*i.e.*, genital] retraction."

As the *Ling Shu* reveals to us in this quote, cold evil tends to "bind" or become stagnated in the foot reverting yin liver channel. This has profound implications

---

[1] *Su Wen* is the first section of *Huang Di Nei Jing* (*The Yellow Emperor's Inner Canon*), which was written in the 1st century CE.

[2] It is important to note that the word damage (*shang*) sometimes means "to make vacuous" and sometimes "to obstruct or hinder normal function." In this case, the latter meaning is implied.

[3] *Ling Shu* is the second section of *Huang Di Nei Jing*, which was written in the 1st century CE.

for andrological diseases. For example, as yin-cold "damages" yang qi in the anterior yin region, symptoms such as cold mounting pain, lesser abdominal hypertonicity and pain, testicular pain, a cold sensation in the genitals, yang wilt, cold semen, and retracted genitals can develop. Further, if yin-cold accumulates and thus congeals fluids in the anterior yin region and causes the formation of cold-dampness, there may also be a sensation of cold and damp in the scrotum and inguinal area as well as water mounting, which includes the biomedically-defined condition scrotal hydrocele.

In my opinion, cold evil is a common cause of disease in men, even in 21st century North America where central heating is ubiquitous. In my own clinical experience, I have seen men with yang wilt, cold mounting, and acute and chronic prostatitis either caused by or exacerbated by exposure to cold evil. Although these men invariably live in heated homes and enjoy a comfortable Mediterranean climate (they live and work in southern California), they work in conditions of cold or engage in recreational activities such as swimming, boating, and surfing which involve significant exposure to cold. One such man with cold mounting is a butcher who has worked in a meat freezer his entire working life. In his medical history lie two examples of the effects of cold evil—hernia and hydrocele.

Dampness

Dampness—like cold—is a yin evil. Thus, its fundamental pathomechanisms relate to its ability to obstruct and inhibit qi dynamic. The heavy, sticky, and thus stagnating nature of dampness is especially troublesome for the male anterior yin region, as once dampness is formed, it has a tendency to "pour downward" (xia zhu), and to "brew and bind" (yun jie) in the lower burner and in the liver channel. These two tendencies of dampness are often lost in less-careful translations of Chinese medicine into English, yet are nonetheless essential for understanding the disease causes and pathomechanisms of dampness.

Dampness pours downward

If dampness "pours downward" into the lower burner and liver channel, logic dictates that it must originate in some superior (i.e., higher) location. In fact, it usually forms in the center burner as a natural and spontaneous outcome of splenic movement and transformation failure. It then pours downward into the lower burner, including into the anterior yin region. When spleen qi is markedly vacuous and center qi fall is present, the spleen then fails to raise the clear essence of water and grain, fails to move and transform water-damp, and fails in its management of the small intestine's qi-transforming function of separating the clear and turbid; as a result, turbid dampness pours downward into the lower burner. Once located in the lower burner, dampness tends to "brew" and "bind" there, and this directly reflects the obstructive and transformation-inhibiting nature of dampness. The usual outcome of brewing and binding of dampness is that heat will transform from damp depression and hence lead to damp-heat—the mutual binding of dampness and heat.

Dampness and kidney yang vacuity

Although dampness as a cause of male anterior yin disease usually derives from splenic movement and transformation failure, it often also results from kidney yang vacuity. Indeed, it is not uncommon to find that both spleen and kidney yang vacuity are present. When kidney yang is debilitated and life gate fire is waning, water-damp is not transformed and instead collects and congeals. Since the kidney governs the two lower yin (the anterior and posterior yin), accumulated water-damp that affects the kidneys will often lead to diseases of the anterior and posterior yin regions.

Signs and pathomechanisms of dampness

The signs of dampness in the male anterior yin region include water mounting, damp sensation of the genitals, yang wilt, infertility manifesting as decreased sperm motility and increased abnormal morphology, unctuous strangury (*gao lin*), dribbling urinary block (*long bi*), and damp skin lesions on and around the scrotum, penis, and inguinal area.

When there is brewing and binding of damp-heat (perhaps the more common scenario among Western males), symptoms reflect not only the obstructing nature of dampness but also the scorching nature of heat and include burning sensations in the genital and inguinal area, skin lesions with thick white or yellowish fluid, unctuous or heat strangury, dribbling urinary block with dark scanty urine and burning sensations in the urethra and bladder, yang wilt, infertility manifesting as decreased sperm motility, decreased seminal volume and increased seminal viscosity, and hot sweaty malodorous genitals.

If damp-heat becomes severely depressed and this depression transforms fire toxin, or if damp-heat fire toxin invades the anterior yin region directly from the exterior (as in the case of a sexually-transmitted organism or poor genital hygiene), fire rots the scrotal flesh and decocts blood to form blood stasis, and scrotal or testicular welling-abscess develops.

Some Chinese texts on andrology include a few other particularly severe anterior yin diseases in such discussions like scrotal wind (*yin nang feng*), sloughing scrotum (*tuo nang*), and lower body gan [sore] (*xia gan [chuang]*).

Wiseman and Feng (1998) define scrotal wind in the following passage and suggest that it might be reframed into Western medicine as either scrotal eczema, neurodermatitis, or riboflavin deficiency: "Dryness and itchiness of the scrotum relieved by bathing in hot water and in severe cases with red pimples the size of millet seeds that exude fluid when scratched, and are sometimes associated with scorching heat pain. Scrotal wind is caused by liver channel damp-heat and external invasion of wind" (p. 516).

Sloughing scrotum, Wiseman and Feng (1998) explain, is characterized by "Redness and swelling of the scrotum causing ulceration that in severe cases leaves the testes exposed. Sloughing scrotum is attributed to damp-heat fire toxin pouring downward into the liver channel" (p. 540). Although this definition offers no Western medical correlate for sloughing scrotum, severe inflammation or infection is likely.

The definition of lower body gan [sore]—which is also attributed to damp-heat and toxin, and in modern Chinese medicine is usually assumed to be caused by a sexually-transmitted agent such as herpes genitalia—includes "A sore of the penis, yin head (glans penis), or foreskin. ...that starts with a bean-like lump that is neither painful nor ruptures...or that starts as a small sore and gradually ruptures" (Wiseman and Feng, 1998, p. 368).

Heat

In basic contrast to cold and dampness, heat is a yang evil. As such, its nature is to flame upward, to scorch and consume fluids, and to damage qi. In Chinese andrology, heat is a frequent cause of disease because it readily affects the bladder, the essence chamber (including the prostate), the scrotum and testes, and the penis. In all cases and despite its location, the clinical characteristics of heat are heat sensations, redness, swelling, and pain (usually of a burning or stinging character), and if heat becomes depressed or is especially severe and accompanied by toxin, there will be pus.

Of course, there are many sources of heat, and we fundamentally categorize these sources under the headings of repletion heat and vacuity heat in terms of eight-principle pattern discrimination. Repletion heat comprises externally-contracted heat, damp-heat, phlegm-heat, heat toxin, and depressed heat. The term depressed heat in this context largely encompasses heat derived from the transformation of depressed liver qi and is an important cause of disease in men because the liver channel skirts the genitals. The main causes of vacuity heat in andrology are insufficiency of lung and/or kidney yin. Implicit in the discussions of heat pathomechanisms below is the assumption that the clinician must be clear about the origins of the heat that drives the specific pathomechanisms in any given case.

There are a number of common pathomechanisms of heat in Chinese andrology including: 1) heat distressing the bladder; 2) heat harassing the essence chamber; 3) heat scorching yin-fluids; 4) heat entering construction-blood and; 5) heat rotting healthy tissue leading to pus (as in scrotal or testicular welling-abscess).

Heat distressing the bladder

When heat distresses the bladder, it obstructs bladder qi transformation and scorches the urinary pathway. Hence, it produces signs including inhibited and burning urination, scanty reddish urine, scorching pain in the lesser abdomen, scorching or stinging sensation in the urethra, and urinary urgency. This pathomechanism is a common factor in andrological conditions such as acute and chronic prostatitis and interstitial cystitis when heat signs are clearly present. Clinicians should be careful here not to, in a "knee-jerk" fashion, equate any Western disease with the suffix "itis" with heat in Chinese medicine. The Chinese disease categories that most directly correlate with these Western diseases include dribbling urinary block (*long bi*) and strangury (*lin*). Within the context of these Chinese disease categories, the pathomechanism of heat distressing the bladder exists within the specific patterns of bloody strangury, heat strangury, and the heat patterns of dribbling urinary block.

Heat harassing the essence chamber

Heat harassing or scorching the essence chamber is a frequent culprit in male infertility, acute and chronic prostatitis, and hamatospermia. In the context of male infertility, heat from various sources (but most commonly from kidney yin vacuity and hyperactive ministerial fire and/or liver depression with depressed fire) harasses the essence chamber and thereby interferes with either the formation, quantity, morphology, or delivery of sperm and semen. For example, when heat decocts the seminal fluid (a manifestation of essence), it may increase its viscosity to the point of interfering with the ability of sperm to travel to and fertilize an ovum. If, when sperm are formed, they are subject to heat evil, their morphological structure (including their head, body, and tail) may form abnormally to the extent that they are either nonfunctional or lessfunctional and are thus unable to successfully reach and fertilize an ovum.

Acute, and especially chronic prostatitis often presents clinically with complicated vacuity-repletion complexes; among the more common combination of patterns in these diseases are spleen and kidney qi vacuity with depression of damp-heat in the liver channel. Hence, we often find the pathomechanism of heat harassing the essence chamber present.

Hematospermia is a reasonably common problem among middle-aged men; it is very often caused by kidney yin vacuity and hyperactive ministerial fire with or without depressed fire in the liver channel. In both cases, fire scorches the network vessels (*luo mai*) within the essence chamber and causes blood to move recklessly outside its normal pathway; thus, it becomes visible in the ejaculate.[4]

Heat scorching yin-fluids

Once heat is present in the anterior yin region—regardless of its origin—it frequently damages yin-fluids. The outcome of this pathomechanism is either scorching of fluids (which we usually describe as fluid damage or fluid depletion), or decoction of physiological yin-fluids into phlegm. In the case of the former, heat damages fluids and fluids become scant, as in the disease of scanty semen (including decreased seminal volume). In the latter, heat decocts fluids into phlegm which binds in the anterior yin region, as in the diseases testicular phlegm node (scrotal mass) and yin stalk phlegm node (Peyronie's disease).

---

[4] Although blood in the ejaculate (hematospermia) is a fairly common and usually benign sign from the perspective of Western urology, it may be a sign of a more serious disorder including prostate cancer. Thus, a thorough urological exam should be conducted in order to rule out a more sinister disease process when this sign presents in clinical practice (Fauci *et al.*, 1998). For more information, see Hematospermia: Book 2, Chapter 7.

Heat entering construction-blood

In terms of qualifying the pathomechanism of heat entering construction-blood, the main consideration is the presence of heat-induced bleeding. Any andrological disease which has heat-induced bleeding is in fact manifesting this pathomechanism. In a more specific sense, however, this pathomechanism refers to the entrance of a heat evil more deeply into the interior as in the course of an infectious disease such as acute bacterial prostatitis with prostatic abscess or as in scrotal abscess. In addition to the signs of prostatitis, the classic signs of heat entering construction-blood are generalized heat effusion that is worse at night, bleeding, absence of thirst, heart vexation and insomnia, clouded spirit and delirious speech, faint maculopapular eruptions (which are dark purple if the heat truly penetrates into the blood aspect), crimson red tongue without fur, and a fine rapid pulse.

Heat rotting healthy tissue

I find the Chinese medical description of the pathomechanisms of welling-abscess quite interesting. Inherent in all discussions of welling-abscess—both modern and premodern—are the themes of depressed heat engendering heat toxin, heat decocting blood and creating blood stasis, and heat rotting (*fu*) healthy tissue into pus. In Chinese medical logic, welling-abscesses are organized very broadly under the headings of external welling-abscess (*wai yong*) and internal welling-abscess (*nei yong*). As the penis, testes, and scrotum are part of the exterior of the body in the Chinese medical framework, Chinese andrology mainly deals with external welling-abscesses in the form of scrotal abscess, crotch-boring sore,[5] and testicular abscess.

Affect-mind damage

At the core of Chinese medicine lies the assumption that the mind and body are one. As physicians of Chinese medicine, we infer from this that when a man's emotional life is smooth and relatively untroubled by extremes of emotions such as fear, anxiety and preoccupation, resentment and indignation, depression, etc., his sexual, urinary, and reproductive functions will be normal. It follows logically then that emotional challenges can adversely affect a man's health. The most common affect-mind damage pathomechanisms presenting in men are: 1) binding depression of liver qi with qi depression transforming fire; 2) anxiety and preoccupation damaging the heart and spleen and; 3) fright and fear damaging the kidney and heart. As the interpretation of human emotional experience should be considered in the context of culture, we Western practitioners of Chinese medicine must reframe Chinese descriptions of emotional states in ways that speak to the reality of our patients' experience. I have attempted to do this in a simple and clinically-relevant way in my discussions below.

---

[5] For more details on crotch-boring sore, see Book 1, Chapter 6 on Chinese andrological disease categories as well as Book 2, Chapter 1 on prostatitis. In short, this Chinese disease category probably overlaps with the Western medical disease prostatic abscess.

Binding depression of liver qi

Binding depression of liver qi with qi depression transforming fire is an extremely common pathomechanism among men in our patient population. Although excessive anger is the most frequently mentioned emotion in connection with this pathomechanism in English language discussions, premodern and modern Chinese texts include more subtle descriptions that are definitely applicable to modern Western clinical practice. These include resentment, indignation, hatred, irascibility, regret, and unfulfilled desires. Strictly speaking, the last two usually present when there is binding depression of liver qi without heat from depression, and do not require heat-clearing, but only depression-resolving treatments. However, the balance of those listed above do all involve a greater or lesser degree of depressed heat, and so do require heat-clearing or fire-draining treatments in addition to depression-resolving treatments.

To understand how this basic pathomechanism leads to andrological diseases, the first fact we need in place in our cognitive map of Chinese medicine is that the liver channel skirts the anterior yin region. Secondly, we must fully understand that a man can only have and maintain an erection, or experience resolution of an erection when the qi and blood in his liver channel is smoothly flowing in and out of the penis. If we understand these facts, then we may grasp how this pathomechanism can cause either yang wilt, persistent erection, or yin protraction (*yin zong*). Further, when we know that depressed heat in the liver viscus conducts downward through the liver channel and into the anterior yin region, we can understand how this pathomechanism can lead to conditions such as hematuria, hematospermia, premature ejaculation or inability to ejaculate, and scorching sensation in the urethra. In essence, we are then observing the pathomechanisms of heat as I have described them above, but we have identified the source of the heat as liver depression, which is in turn caused by affect-mind damage.

In my experience, men who are subject to this pathomechanism often have a history of: 1) unresolved emotional conflicts from within their family of origin; 2) sexual, physical, or emotional abuse; 3) unresolved conflicts from current or past intimate romantic relationships or; 4) post-traumatic stress from wars, natural disasters, or other intense emotional trauma. Indeed, many of these men have experienced more than one of these.

Anxiety and preoccupation

If we wish to fully grasp the ramifications of these affects on male function we need only understand a few basic facts about the heart and spleen in Chinese physiology.[6] In short, the heart is the sovereign viscus and therefore directs the physiological activities of all of the other viscera and bowels, and it engenders blood and stores the spirit. The spleen governs the movement and transformation of water and grain essence which is one of the substantial requirements for

---

[6] For a detailed coverage of heart and spleen physiology as it pertains to normal male functioning, see Book 1, Chapter 4 on viscera-bowel physiology.

the formation of blood. The heart engenders blood which nourishes the spleen and the spleen provides the heart with nourishment in the form of water and grain essence. When they are both functioning normally, there is abundant qi and blood, and the spirit is calm. When a man's spirit is calm and nourished, his sexual, reproductive, and urinary functions are normal.

When a man has a tendency to worry and to be preoccupied with his work, relationships, and health (including his sexual and reproductive health), or when he simply uses his intellectual capacity to excess in his work, he runs the risk of damaging his spleen qi. When spleen qi is damaged and not replenished with proper diet, rest, and other nourishing life (*yang sheng*) methodologies, the source for the engenderment and transformation of qi and blood is depleted. Since the relationship between the heart and spleen is such a close one, and since the heart depends on the spleen for nourishment, we frequently see such men in clinic with a dual vacuity of the heart and spleen pattern. As a result, the anterior yin is underpowered and undernourished. This is a frequent cause of yang wilt, premature ejaculation, and infertility manifesting as decreased sperm concentration, abnormal morphology, and decreased motility. Further, dual vacuity of the heart and spleen is a common pattern in andropause.

Fright and fear

Strictly speaking, fright (*jing*) corresponds to the heart and fear (*kong*) corresponds to the kidneys. Fright damage usually refers to disease caused by a sudden and fearful event or sound, and fear damage pertains to disease caused by exposure to ongoing fearful conditions. Although these differences exist on paper, in real life, these two affects often occur together and do tend to mutually promote one another. Due to this fact and to the especially intimate physiological and pathological relationships between the heart and kidneys in Chinese medicine, fright and fear usually damage both of these viscera. In Chinese texts, the descriptions of emotional states caused by these affects include closing the door in fear as if someone were coming to seize or arrest one, general disquietude, and being easily flustered. When I reframe these descriptions in culturally-relevant ways, I conclude that my patients with general anxiety disorder, post-traumatic stress disorder, panic disorder, and paranoia (sometimes in response to the use of drugs such as cannabis or cocaine) exhibit this pathomechanism.

In terms of male sexual dysfunction, these affects are common causes of yang wilt (often caused by or complicated by performance anxiety) and premature ejaculation. More specifically, when fright and fear damage the heart and kidneys, a few scenarios are possible: 1) excessive fright and fear cause hyperactive sovereign fire (heart fire) which in turn inflames ministerial fire (kidney fire). As a result, kidney qi is unable to secure the essence gate, and leads to premature ejaculation; 2) excessive fright and fear cause hyperactive heart fire to inflame ministerial fire which then scorches kidney yin-essence; yang wilt results from undernourishment of the anterior yin and the yin stem (the penis) in particular or; 3) fright and fear damage heart and kidney qi and lead to an underpowered and undernourished yin stem and to insecurity of the essence gate. In this third scenario, yang wilt and premature ejaculation do not result from harassment by fire but are instead caused by lack of qi to activate and secure.

Dietary irregularities

Among the male patients I have seen in clinical practice who eat the typical American diet—high in saturated fats, processed foods, iced and heavily-sugared soft drinks, and very low in fiber and fresh vegetable intake—phlegm, dampness, and damp-heat are endemic. Some of these men under thirty years of age who are physically active and of muscular build seem to be able to tolerate such a diet without outward signs of dramatic weight gain. However, once they turn thirty (or even earlier in some cases), if they do not: 1) significantly alter their diets by reducing their intake of calories, saturated fats, and iced drinks, and by increasing their intake of fiber and; 2) maintain their activity levels, they invariably become significantly overweight. In my opinion, as these younger men age, their weakened center burner is less able to tolerate the unhealthful dietary practices of their youth. The inevitable result of such a profoundly center burner earth-challenging diet and lifestyle is phlegm, dampness, and damp-heat. These yin evils—as evils having form—constitute substantial impediments to the smooth flow of qi and blood through the channels and network vessels throughout the body and to the anterior yin. This process is encouraged by the fact that dampness tends to pour downward into the lower burner. Hence, by following along with the typical American fast-food and sedentary lifestyle, these men unknowingly set themselves up for yang wilt, infertility, prostatitis, and benign prostatic hyperplasia.

One of the not-so-subliminal messages delivered to the masses of American men via the fast-food and meat industries and via cultural biases in favor of high meat intake is some form of the assumption that "real men eat lots of meat," which associates male virility with high meat intake. Ironically, we know that high saturated fat intake is associated with hypercholesterolemia, coronary artery disease, and hypertension, and that these diseases are usually associated with erectile dysfunction.[7] To maintain male sexual and reproductive health, I recommend a combination of a modern Western understanding of healthful nutrition, a Chinese medical view, and an anthropologically-validated model of human nutrition. This includes a moderate intake of lean meats as part of a balanced diet including plenty of cooked fresh vegetables, legumes, some fruits, and whole grains (gluten-free grains for those with sensitivities). According to Chinese nourishing life traditions, a balanced diet combined with exercise, intake of supplementing medicinals when appropriate, and a balanced emotional life guarantees male sexual and reproductive function into old age.

On the other side of the coin, there is a population of men who in overcompensating for the ills of the typical American diet, have gone way too far in the

---

[7] For a comparative and provocative look at Western and Chinese diet, see Campbell, T.C. and Campbell, T.M. (2005).

opposite direction. Sometimes by rigidly adhering to a raw food vegan diet, these men weaken their spleen and stomach yang. Some simply cannot tolerate such a diet and wisely realize the need for change when they experience abdominal bloating, aversion to cold, and diarrhea after only a few weeks or months. Some others do seem able to tolerate the diet for longer periods of time even perhaps for years, but begin to experience the deleterious effects after their late twenties, when they begin to experience fatigue, aversion to cold, low libido, and yang wilt. In some cases, there is an obsession with cleansing the body in response to the onslaught of a vague sense of "toxins" from our modern and polluted environment. In fact, this obsession sometimes goes so far as to form what I believe is a subclinical and undiagnosed eating disorder along with an anxiety disorder. In clinical practice, it is a challenging issue and requires much patient education and demands that the practitioner patiently and slowly help the patient to alter his attitudes towards food and health. I find this set of circumstances fairly common among young men who are members of the alternative medicine community. In Chinese medical terms, in these cases there is not only dietary irregularity operating as a disease cause, but also anxiety and preoccupation. These men are often preoccupied with cleansing and with adhering to the diet to which they have a philosophical (bordering on religious) commitment, yet the purported benefits are not validated by my clinical experience or by historical or anthropological data.

There is another aspect of diet that connects with culture and emotional well-being that is not usually discussed in a straightforward Chinese text on andrology, but I believe is worth mentioning here. Shared meals can be vehicles for emotional support. In traditional cultures all over the world such as Chinese and European cultures, meals are not only times for obtaining physical sustenance, but also represent opportunities for family and friends to connect emotionally. In the fast-food and overworked culture of American society, our male patients have fewer chances to bond with friends and family. In my experience, this serves to amplify the negative effects of stress on their health.[8]

Overtaxation

The two main forms of overtaxation that affect men are overwork and sexual taxation (excessive sexual activity).

I. Overwork and dietary irregularities

For men in our modern Western patient population, overwork is endemic. It is common for men we see in our practice to be working full-time in demanding careers, and to be taking work home in the evenings and on weekends. Further, they may have domestic responsibilities to maintain their homes and to be actively involved in raising their children should they have any. What often comes along with such a busy life is an erratic eating schedule in which one: 1) foregoes a nourishing but time-consuming breakfast in favor of grabbing a coffee and pastry on the way to the office and; 2) skips lunch or grabs

---

[8] For a fascinating look at food and meals in American culture, see Pollan, M. (2006).

a sandwich in order to catch up on e-mails and phone messages. The combination of overwork and "grab and go" erratic eating schedules lead to tired anxious men who have decreased libidos and fertility, and yang wilt.

From the perspective of Chinese medicine, overtaxation damages and consumes qi and blood, and debilitates liver blood, spleen qi, kidney qi, and kidney essence.[9] Conditions for which overtaxation is cited as a disease cause include but are not limited to yang wilt, seminal efflux, infertility, foxy mounting[10], dribbling urinary block, taxation strangury, essence turbidity, turbid urine, and andropause.

Specific pathomechanisms of overtaxation

When overtaxation damages liver blood, there is insufficient blood to fill the penis and yang wilt occurs. When overtaxation damages kidney qi and leads to insecurity of the essence gate, seminal efflux and premature ejaculation occurs. If overtaxation leads to debility of kidney essence, there is no substantial foundation for the production and activity of sperm and male infertility results. Overtaxation that damages the spleen and kidney qi and leads to depressed cold evil in the liver channel and the lesser abdomen may cause foxy mounting. When overtaxation damages the spleen and kidney qi and causes splenic movement and transformation failure as well as kidney, bladder, and triple burner qi transformation failure, this leads to taxation strangury and/or dribbling urinary block. If taxation damages the spleen and kidney qi, it may cause wasted essence to form in the essence chamber and to flow downward to the penis causing essence turbidity, which is characterized by rice water-like penile discharge and is a possible signs of prostatitis. Overtaxation that causes splenic movement and transformation failure and kidney, bladder, and triple burner qi transformation failure results in the formation of dampness that pours downward into the lower burner and causes turbid urine.

2. Sexual taxation

Whenever we bring up the topic of sexual taxation, a number of questions invariably follow such as: 1) How much sex is too much? 2) Is masturbation more damaging than sex with a partner? 3) Is it wise to practice seminal retention because any loss of semen damages kidney essence and therefore should be avoided? 4) Is male homosexual sex somehow inherently imbalanced in terms of yin and yang and therefore inherently harmful?

If one wishes to answer these questions along traditional Chinese lines, it is best to consult the nourishing life (*yang sheng*) literature which focuses on the regulation of sexual life, and on the use of sexual activity to cultivate and

---

[9] In point of fact, the stress that invariably accompanies the overtaxed life also leads to binding depression of liver qi and depressed heat.

[10] This is a condition in which the small intestine periodically protrudes into the scrotum and retracts back upwards in a stealthy "fox-like" manner. For more information, see Book 1, Chapter 6 on Chinese andrological disease categories.

maintain essence. There has been an explosion of popular literature on these subjects in recent years, not all of which have been responsibly researched; hence we should be discriminating about the sources we select and regard as definitive.[11] Even among definitive sources, however, there exist a wide variety of opinions on how frequently men may ejaculate before suffering damage to kidney essence. My approach here is very pragmatic. So, instead of attempting to take a very traditional stance on these issues that might not be culturally applicable to our patient population, I prefer to deal with them in the same way that I deal with them with my patients.

I think it is important to state some facts about the men we see in our practices. They are 21st century Western men who grew up under the influence of the sexual revolution. Generally speaking, they are more comfortable with exerting their sexuality than their grandfathers were, but they may be more subject to performance anxiety. And they live in a world where sexually-transmitted diseases such as AIDS, hepatitis B, and Chlamydia are endemic.

Frequency of sex

When a male patient asks me how frequently he can have sex, my response is based on the consideration of a few factors, namely, the strength of his constitution, his age, and the season of the year. Based on my understanding of these factors, my response is usually in the range of one to five times per week. My advice is to use a basic number like this as a guide but to pay attention to one's body, regarding signs such as fatigue, weakness of the back and knees, decreased frequency of morning erections, decreased firmness of erections, and decreased orgasmic intensity as barometers for detecting weakened kidney qi and for the need to reduce sexual frequency. Paying attention to seasonal fluctuations and linking our sexuality to it, winter is a time to conserve essence and slightly reduce our sexual activity, and spring and summer are seasons in which to become more active and increase our sexual activity.

Masturbation

When a man asks me whether I think masturbation is more damaging to essence than sex with a partner, I keep in mind that for a healthy man, sexual frustration and infrequency can themselves lead to liver depression, stagnation of qi, and stasis of blood, and that if he does not use masturbation as a release he might be more likely to seek casual sex and thus be exposed to a sexually-transmitted disease, engage in risky casual "cruising" encounters, or be party to an unwanted pregnancy. Further, deep-seated guilt about masturbation among young sexually vigorous men who do not have partners might be more damaging than any alleged damage caused by masturbation. With these considerations in mind, and having no moral bias against it, I usually say that it is fine for him to masturbate at a similar frequency at which he should have sex with a partner, to feel good about pleasing himself, but to avoid excessive masturbation just as he should avoid excessive sexual activity of any kind.

---

[11] For a responsibly and accurately translated selection of Daoist sexual texts, see Wile (1992).

Some Chinese doctors' advice to avoid masturbation completely is not based on a moral stance against it, but on the belief that it does damage essence more than sex with a partner does. My personal opinion on this issue attempts to balance traditional views on masturbation with modern realities. I do feel, however, that excessive masturbation—just as excessive sexual activity of any kind—damages kidney essence.

Seminal retention practices

As any reader who is familiar with Chinese nourishing life practices will recall, there is a tradition of avoiding or limiting the frequency of ejaculation because loss of semen is regarded as loss of essence, and should therefore be limited or avoided. This is based on three treasures theory in which essence, qi, and spirit comprise the three fundamental aspects of the human body, and in which essence is the fundamental substrate from which qi and spirit derive. Debilitation of essence then leads to vacuity of qi and insufficient spirit. Because of this, there are many systems of *qi gong* and behaviors to adopt while having sex which have as their goal controlling ejaculation and avoiding seminal loss. While delaying ejaculation for a reasonable period of time as a means of increasing one's own and one's partner's sexual satisfaction is universally accepted by modern Chinese practitioners of andrology, complete seminal retention and avoidance of ejaculation is generally not. The main objection exerted by modern Chinese authorities is that seminal retention can cause qi stagnation and blood stasis to become depressed in the essence chamber and other parts of the anterior yin, and is a potential cause of prostatic hyperplasia, prostatitis, and prostate cancer, as well as other anterior yin diseases. I personally allow for the possibility of being able to properly and beneficially practice such techniques. However, I doubt they can be learned from a book or video tape. On the contrary, they require careful mentorship with an experienced and authentic teacher. Authentic seminal retention practices usually include a means of dissipating and even harnessing the qi generated by orgasm or near-orgasm, thus theoretically preventing the formation of depression of qi and blood.

Some men who are trying to practice seminal retention become very anxious and concerned about the slightest loss of semen during sex or sleep. I have personally seen young male patients in my practice who were *qi gong* or martial arts students, were attempting to practice seminal retention (usually from having read about it in a book), and who had a great deal of anxiety about how much irreparable damage their kidney essence would suffer as a result of an occasional wet dream. Needless to say, their young and active ministerial fire was finding a way to break through their attempts to harness it. Other than making them anxious, however, I cannot say whether they had as yet suffered any other damage, nor have I seen a significant number of older men who had practiced seminal retention for many years. Hence, I cannot speak authoritatively about their experience. Presumably, Chinese doctors have seen many more of these men, and have formed their opinions against seminal retention based on clinical observations.

Homosexuality

With respect to homosexual sex, I think any opinion that out-of-hand dismisses male homosexual sex as inherently imbalanced in terms of yin and yang is a moral/religious assertion and not a secular/medical one. In addition to being blatantly discriminatory, this attitude is based on the rigid assumption that men are yang and women are yin, and that sexual intercourse between a man and woman is the only possible way to experience a harmonious yin-yang exchange during sex. I feel this represents a naive understanding of yin and yang as it relates to gender and is a remnant of traditional antihomosexual biases in Chinese and Western culture that we should dispense with as inaccurate and discriminatory.

It is my observation that rather than conforming to a rigid male-female dichotomy, the yin-yang nature of any person *vis-à-vis* their gender is a manifestation of their place on a continuum of yin-femaleness and yang-maleness, and is therefore not a black and white matter. For example, I personally know many women who are inherently more yang-male than many men, and know many men who are inherently more yin-female than many women. Further, sexual orientation is arguably an inherent trait and not a learned behavior or a disease. Hence, I strenuously assert that we should not see male homosexual sex as inherently imbalanced or damaging within the scope of Chinese andrology. I should reinforce here, however, that anal intercourse, more common among homosexual men, does pose a greater risk (especially for the recipient) for the transmission of blood-borne infectious agents such as AIDS and various blood-borne varieties of the Hepatitis viruses, and any oral-anal contact ("rimming") exposes the "doer" to infectious agents such as *E Coli* as well as Hepatitis.

Finally, I have certainly seen many homosexual men who have "come out of the closet" who report a long history of emotional damage from the liver depression and depressed heat caused by having repressed their innate homosexuality for fear of being rejected by their friends and families. In such cases, the repression is clearly a manifestation of affect-mind damage as discussed previously.

External injuries

Any injury to the anterior yin region as a result of experiencing trauma during sports activities, car accidents, slips and falls, and surgery would directly damage the channels and network vessels and cause blood from within the network vessels to leave and leak into the surrounding bodily spaces. Any such "blood that has left the vessels" that has remained within the anterior yin region comprises "static blood," and is a substantial obstruction to local qi and blood flow. Blood stasis—from trauma or other causes—is responsible for many problems in andrology, as it represents an obstruction having "form" (*xing*), and thus is a significant cause of failed anterior yin functions when qi and blood flow to the essence chamber, penis, testes, and scrotum is compromised as a result of its presence. If an injury to the anterior yin region severs the network vessels more severely and causes copious bleeding, then blood will be more significantly damaged. This can be a cause of blood vacuity-related male diseases. In light of these pathomechanisms, trauma to the anterior yin region may be a factor in pain anywhere in the anterior yin region, and in other andrological conditions such as yin stem phlegm node (Peyronie's disease), blood mounting, hematuria, yang wilt, dribbling urinary block, and urinary incontinence.

Natural endowment insufficiency and constitutional vacuity

1. Natural endowment insufficiency

There is a commonly held misconception among students of Chinese medicine—and even among some practitioners—that one must be old (*i.e.*, over 40 years old) in order to have kidney vacuity. And this error seems amplified in the case of kidney essence vacuity. While it is true that one of the main causes of kidney essence vacuity is aging, it is not the only cause of it. To assume that kidney essence vacuity can only be acquired with age or through overtaxation (*i.e.*, sexual taxation) is to ignore that one can inherit it from one's parents or be subjected to essence-damaging conditions during gestation.[12] This comprises the Chinese medical understanding of the role of genetics in the inheritance of disease tendencies, as well as the role of factors affecting the parents at the time of conception, and the mother and fetus during gestation. These disease causes and pathomechanisms are embodied within the concept of natural endowment insufficiency.

To illustrate the manifestations of natural endowment insufficiency, we can look at problems that occur in early infancy and childhood such as the five slownesses (*wu chi*),[13] and the five limpnesses (*wu ruan*).[14] These are manifestations of natural endowment insufficiency of essence as the substantial material from which all other aspects of the bodily form and functional activity derive. These show that one may suffer an inborn vacuity of kidney essence that may in turn adversely affect the development of the entire body. In terms of male sexual and reproductive issues that develop later in life, natural endowment insufficiency can lead to problems such as delayed onset of puberty, abnormally-small genitalia, infertility, yang wilt, and premature ejaculation. The common pathomechanism among these various problems is fundamentally identical to that of the five slownesses and five limpnesses—insufficient material substance. In the case of older boys and men, however, there is insufficient substance to: 1) engender and nourish the bodily form (including the penis, testes, and scrotum); 2) engender reproductive substance in the form of semen and sperm and; 3) provide the substantial yin basis for yang functions

---

[12] This is the Chinese medical explanation why infants born to mothers who smoked during their pregnancy have low birth weight.

[13] The five slownesses (*wu chi*) are slowness to stand, slowness to walk, slowness to grow hair, slowness to teethe, and slowness to speak.

[14] The five limpnesses (*wu ruan*) are softness of the head, limpness of the neck, limpness of the hands and feet, and limpness of the mouth.

such as getting and maintaining an erection, making sperm motile, and to either appropriately discharge from or secure essence within the essence chamber.

2. Constitutional vacuity

Many Chinese texts use the term constitutional vacuity—in the sense of later heaven or acquired constitution—to mean causes of disease that occur after birth. These include serious illnesses that so damage the body that from that point forward one is prone to certain pathologies; one then has a constitutional tendency to develop certain diseases. For example, a serious infectious diarrhea that occurred in early childhood can damage the spleen and stomach—the later heaven source of essence—so significantly that kidney essence is not replenished at a normal rate.[15] The natural result of this process in the affected boy is delayed onset of puberty and slower growth patterns. The pathomechanisms for natural endowment insufficiency and constitutional vacuity are essentially the same in that they both involve a lack of nourishment and inadequate source of substance to bring luxuriance to the bodily form, the viscera and bowels, the channels and network vessels, and the orifices. The difference is essentially one of timing—natural endowment insufficiency is present at birth (and perhaps even in the uterus), and acquired constitutional vacuity develops after birth.

---

[15] Here I allude to the fact that later heaven essence enriches and engenders early heaven essence. That is, under healthy conditions, any surplus water and grain essence absorbed by the spleen can be stored in the kidneys as essence. For further discussion, see the kidney and spleen sections in Book 1, Chapter 4 on the viscera and bowels.

Chinese Andrological Disease Categories: Definitions and Definitive Signs

What are Chinese Andrological Disease Categories?

The diagnostics of Chinese medicine consist of many different methods and means of categorizing and making sense of patients' complaints. Among all of the available diagnostic methods, the method of discrimination of patterns (*bian zheng*) is probably the best-known one in the West, and for good reason. Most practitioners of Chinese medicine ultimately determine treatment by discriminating from among several possible patterns and they design their treatment strategy accordingly. And while this is an effective means of diagnosis, there is yet another overarching structure that is very helpful—disease discrimination (*bian bing*)—which many Western practitioners have overlooked because the secondary Western-Chinese medical literature has not generally been explicit in pointing it out.[1]

Since we most often treat our patients according to pattern discrimination, I am often asked why we should bother discriminating Chinese disease categories at all. My response is that generally, the Chinese disease discrimination model provides an additional layer of clinical organization that actually brings pattern discrimination into sharper cognitive focus in a very practical way. As the saying goes: "same pattern, different disease, different treatment." This means that the same pattern—take kidney yang vacuity as an example—may manifest in different diseases, and each of those diseases requires a different treatment.

Looking at Chinese andrology in terms of Chinese disease categories, dribbling urinary block, urinary incontinence, and yang wilt can all present clinically as a kidney yang vacuity pattern. While the core treatment for all three of these diseases would essentially be the same (warming and supplementing kidney yang), they each require an

---

[1] Of notable exception here is the work of Bob Flaws who has taken great pains to clarify the diagnostic methodology of Chinese medicine. I also offer my own work here as in Damone (2002).

additional nuance added to that common core that makes the treatment even more accurate and effective. So, in addition to warming and supplementing kidney yang, dribbling urinary block also requires disinhibiting dampness and freeing urination, urinary incontinence requires restraining urine, and yang wilt requires treatments that have the specific effect of stimulating the rising of the penis. In my own clinical experience, it is often these nuanced treatments that yield quicker and better clinical outcomes than general treatments do.

Further, the Chinese medical literature is mostly organized under a disease-based rubric and not according to pattern-based logic, so that when doctors of Chinese medicine wish to research the Chinese literature—premodern and modern alike—for the treatment of any specific patient, we mainly access texts with disease categories as the chapter headings. Once we go to any specific disease chapter, we then encounter coverage of the common patterns encountered for that disease. Andrological disease categories are the Chinese medical disease categories under which men's diseases are organized and accessed in the Chinese literature.

Reframing Chinese Andrological Disease Categories Into Western Disease Categories

Before going into defining some of the more common Chinese andrological disease categories and providing the main signs and patterns they manifest with, we have to deal with another matter: How do we reframe Chinese medical disease categories into their constituent Western disease categories?

At this point the reader should take note that this text is organized by Western disease categories; hence, the specific disease chapters in Book 2 are titled accordingly. For example, see Chapters 1 and 2 devoted to benign prostatic hyperplasia (BPH) and prostatitis respectively. One of the first sections of each of these chapters is devoted to reframing these Western-defined diseases into their constituent Chinese diseases. We do this by comparing the history, signs and symptoms, and prognosis of the Western and Chinese diseases, but the most important ground for comparison is the signs and symptoms. Once we understand and become adept at the reframing process and we have a sophisticated understanding of both Chinese and Western andrology, we can accurately reframe in either direction.

In Book 2 of this text, which is devoted to specific diseases and their treatments, I have chosen to use Western disease categories as the organizing principle and then reframe them into Chinese disease categories. I have done this in part to make the text accessible for use in the clinic, and in part because Chinese andrological texts are often organized this way.[2] In this chapter,

---

[2] See Book 1, Chapter 1 on the history of Chinese andrology for a detailed explanation of why this is so. In short, modern Chinese andrology is a manifestation of what is known as "Integrated Chinese-Western Medicine" (*zhong xi yi jie he*).

however, I mainly define Chinese andrological diseases, but to some extent also reframe in the opposite direction both to introduce a broader range of Chinese andrological diseases and to model the reframing process from Chinese diseases to their Western counterparts.

There are many more Chinese andrological disease categories than (for practical reasons) I can cover in detail in this text. A comprehensive coverage of all andrological diseases—including an exhaustive search of the premodern literature, specific patterns and their treatments, and modern research—would make for a much longer book and would require much more research. As a means of balancing the lack of detailed information for some Chinese andrological diseases, in this chapter I provide brief descriptions and definitive signs for a broad spectrum of Chinese andrological diseases, many of which are not specifically covered in Book 2 of this text. In doing so, I strive to give readers a broader cross-sectional view of the andrology literature. Further, by including examples of premodern references that exhibit some important, unique, and at times challenging perspectives, I hope to alert readers to the unplumbed depths of Chinese andrology (and indeed Chinese medicine in general) and to thereby provoke further research into these topics.

Chinese Andrological Disease Categories

Diseases of the penis

1. Yang wilt (*yang wei*)

Main signs, causes, and patterns

Refers to a condition in which the penis does not rise up or become hard enough to enable penetration of a responsive partner. This disease is most often seen in aging men, and is commonly caused by sexual overtaxation and/or waning of life gate fire from aging, but may additionally result from thought and fright damaging the heart and spleen, liver depression, liver channel damp-heat, yin phlegm-dampness obstructing yang qi, and blood stasis.

In vacuity patterns, the pathomechanism is that the penis lacks warmth, power, or nourishment for erection. In repletion patterns, there may be sufficient warmth and power, but qi stagnation and/or substantial evils obstruct the free flow of qi and blood to the penis and hence interfere with normal erectile response.

Note: Yang wilt is also called yin wilt (*yin wei*) in some sources.

Noteworthy premodern references

Of special interest is the relationship of yin wilt to the heart described in *Bian Zheng Lu* (*Pattern Discrimination Record*).[3] The pathomechanism is related to insufficiency of heart qi and a resulting inability of sovereign fire (physiological

---

[3] *Bian Zheng Lu*, a fourteen-volume medical collection, was compiled by Chen Shi-Feng in 1687, during the Qing dynasty.

fire of the heart) to lead and govern the ministerial fire (physiological fire of the kidneys).

Lin Pei-Qin, in *Lei Zheng Zhi Cai (Systematized Patterns with Clear-Cut Treatments)*[4] describes the role of the stomach in the pathomechanisms of yang wilt as follows: "In those with stomach vacuity and scanty food [intake], water and grain lack fullness and [as a result] essence-marrow loses its effulgence."

Western medical correlates and associated conditions

Erectile dysfunction; benign prostatic hyperplasia (BPH); chronic prostatitis; depression; post-traumatic stress disorder (PTSD); diabetes; peripheral vascular disease; heart disease

2. Rigid yang (*yang qiang*)
Main signs, causes, and patterns

This disease category refers to a condition in which the penis becomes erect and does not become flaccid for a long time, and in which there is an inability to ejaculate. This is later followed by spontaneous discharge of semen. Less commonly, this term refers to a condition in which, after having intercourse, a man has unretractable protrusion of the tongue. In modern andrology, this disease category is most often used to describe the former condition, and is usually attributed to yin vacuity with hyperactive ministerial fire, upward harassment of vacuity fire and inability of lung-metal to move downward,[5] exuberant fire-toxin, liver channel damp-heat, liver channel blood stasis, or to liver depression and depressed heat in the liver channel.

Note: Rigid yang is also called rigid center (*qiang zhong*), yin protrusion (*yin ting*), genital protraction (*yin zong*), and rigidity of the penis (*jing qiang*).

Noteworthy premodern references

A less severe manifestation of this condition is embodied under the heading of readily-obtained erections (*yang wu yi ju*), and is generally attributed to similar causes, though according to *Yan Fang Xin Bian (New Compilation of Empirical Formulas)*,[6] it is sometimes attributed to frenetic stirring of ministerial fire agitating the heart.

---

[4] *Lei Zheng Zhi Cai* was published in 1839, during the Qing dynasty.

[5] This pattern is described in *Shen Xian Ji Shi Liang Fang (Spirit Immortal World Salvation Good Remedies)*. The text goes on to say that this is lung-metal failing to perform depurative downbearing to enrich and nourish kidney yin in order to naturally (*i.e.*, physiologically) drain hyperactive kidney fire.

[6] *Yan Fang Xin Bian* was published in 1846, during the Qing dynasty. It was originally an eight-volume compilation of empirical formulas from many specialties in Chinese medicine, but grew into 24 volumes in later publications either by rearrangements of the original chapters or by the addition of new content.

Mei Shi Yan Fang Xin Bian (*Mei's New Compilation of Empirical Formulas*)[7] relates this condition to "kidney stagnation leaking disorder (*shen zhi lou ji*)" and recommends blood-quickening and qi-rectifying medicinals to treat it.

Western medical correlates and associated conditions

Priapism; sexual addiction disorder

3. Pain in the penis (*jing zhong tong*)

Main signs, causes, and patterns

As the name implies, this disease refers to a condition in which there is pain within the penis. The most common patterns cited include liver channel qi depression, liver channel blood stasis, hyperactive heart fire conducting into the small intestine (also known as small intestinal repletion heat), kidney vacuity, invasion of cold evil, and spleen and lung qi vacuity. At times, this condition is associated with itching (from wind and/or damp-heat), and with swelling (from heat and/or dampness).

Since the penis is the ancestral sinew and all sinews are ascribed to the liver, and the liver channel encircles the genitals, depressed liver qi leads to qi depression and sometimes also to blood stasis within the penis. Where there is a lack of free flow of qi or blood, there is pain. So, pain within the penis develops. If depressed heat is present, there may be stinging or burning pain.

When heart fire is hyperactive, it may flame downward and conduct into the small intestine. Fire then conducts into the bladder and its urinary pathway, which extends through the penis. Hence, stinging and burning pain occurs along with frequent but inhibited urination.

The kidneys govern growth and reproduction and are responsible for nourishing and powering the anterior yin region,[8] including the penis. If the penis is undernourished or underpowered, free flow of qi, blood, and essence within it may be compromised; this lack of free flow may lead to pain.

Cold—as a yin evil—is constricting and congealing. If it enters the liver channel and the penis, it obstructs qi and congeals blood and causes pain.

In the case of lung and spleen qi vacuity, lack of lung qi to power the waterways and to perform depurative downbearing to the bladder, kidney, and penis may lead to depression of qi within the penis, and therefore to pain.

---

[7] *Mei Shi Yan Fang Xin Bian* was published in 1878 by Mei Qi-Zhao, during the Qing dynasty. It represents eight volumes of additional material that was at first added to the previously published *Yan Fang Xin Bian* (*New Compilation of Empirical Formulas*) but later published independently. See note 6 above.

[8] The kidneys govern "the two yin," which means the anterior and posterior yin regions.

If spleen and lung qi are vacuous they fail to power the small intestine in its role of separating the clear and the turbid, which is in part responsible for smooth, efficient, and therefore pain-free urination. Typically, this will be dull pain within the penis which is worse with exertion and better with rest.

Noteworthy premodern references

I found a useful passage from the Qing dynasty text *Qian Zhai Yi Hua* (*Medical Discussion from the Hidden Room*),[9] where it states: "In old age, [when there is] frequent urination at night, it is efficacious to eat glutinous rice cakes at night. Men who have pain within the penis during urination, and [who still have] frequent urination but the urine is not reddish, [should] boil and drink one *liang* of *Sheng Huang Qi* (Astragali Radix Cruda) and two *qian* of *Gan Cao* (Glycyrrhizae Radix). Those with a severe case [should] take it twice a day and it will be cured."

In *Zhu Bing Yuan Hou Lun* (*On the Origin and Indicators of Disease*),[10] pain in the penis is associated with vacuity taxation disease (*xu lao*) as revealed in the following passage: "[In] kidney qi vacuity detriment, wind evil invades.[11] [Evil] qi flows into the kidney channel and yin and qi attack each other; the true and evil mutually contend, and as a result there is pain within the penis. However, those with cold only have pain; [those who] have accompanying heat, also have swelling."

Western medical correlates and associated conditions

Urethritis; acute and chronic prostatitis; acute cystitis; chronic interstitial cystitis

4. Small penis (*yin jing duan xiao*)
Main signs, causes, and patterns

This Chinese disease category applies to men who have abnormally-small penises, either as a result of early or later heaven insufficiency.

Men who have early heaven insufficiency (which are generally not considered treatable), are also referred to as "heavenly eunuchs (*tian yan*)" in premodern literature. Early heaven natural endowment vacuity of kidney essence results in underdevelopment of the penis, scrotum, and testes.

If there is later heaven insufficiency—meaning in this case spleen-stomach vacuity leading to kidney essence vacuity—which results in a lack of replenishment

---

[9] *Qian Zhai Yi Hua* was compiled by Wang Shi-Xiong and published in 1853 as a compilation of empirical medical experiences in over forty categories of medicine.

[10] *Zhu Bing Yuan Hou Lun* was written by Chao Yuan-Fang and published in 610 CE, during the Sui dynasty. A very influential text, it gives the disease causes, signs, and pathomechanisms of hundreds of diseases.

[11] This is usually described in premodern literature as "wind evil taking advantage of vacuity."

of kidney essence through the mutual transformation of liver blood and kidney essence, the penis may either not develop at puberty or may shrink in size later in life. In this latter example, supplementing later heaven can maximize each man's potential penis size by optimizing the nourishment it receives either at puberty or in middle age or older age.

Noteworthy premodern references

In *Dan Fang Jing Hua* (*The Quintessence of Dan-[Xi's] Formulas*),[12] we find the following case report on a case of small penis: "A certain gentleman of about twenty years of age [came for treatment], with a constitutionally weak body and genitals that looked just like those of a young child. They were especially tiny and had not yet matured, so that he looked just like a heavenly eunuch. [We] used ground pig's penis washed in vintage grain liquor until clean and stewed it on a civil flame to a fatty [consistency]. [He] took it consistently for about five or six years [and his penis] became like that of an adult."

Western medical correlates and associated conditions

Hypogonadism

5. Other diseases of the penis

Yang retraction (*yang suo*);[13] swelling of the penis (*jing zhong*); cold in the penis (*yin han*)[14] and; cold-tipped penis (*yin tou han*).

Most of these additional diseases of the penis have overlapping signs and pathomechanisms with some of the other diseases I do cover either in this chapter or in Book 2. As such, they do not warrant individual coverage. Further, once we master the underlying principles of andrology, we should be able to reason through the diagnosis and treatment of various penile diseases and reframe them into Chinese medical logic even when we cannot find specific references to them in textbooks and clinical manuals such as this one.

Seminal diseases

1. Premature ejaculation (*zao xie*)

Main signs, causes, and patterns

This disease category refers to a condition in which a man ejaculates very quickly after the initiation of intercourse, or in severe cases, ejaculates even before intromission occurs. It is commonly attributed to kidney yin vacuity and hyperactive ministerial fire, dual vacuity of kidney yin and yang, noninteraction of the heart and kidney, liver channel damp-heat, and liver depression with depressed fire. It is often associated with other andrological diseases such

---

[12] Publication date unavailable.
[13] See retracted genitals (*yin suo*).
[14] See cold genitals (*yin han*).

as yang wilt, seminal emission, and easy erection and occasionally with hematospermia. In fact, premodern sources generally discuss this condition together with seminal emission and relatively rarely list it as a separate disease.

In cases of heat (either vacuity or repletion), the essence gate is overly excited due to hyperactivity of ministerial fire, and in cases of yang qi vacuity, insecurity of the essence gate causes premature release of semen. When there is also hematospermia, hyperactive ministerial fire scorches the essence chamber and causes frenetic movement of blood within its network vessels. As a result, blood leaks into the seminal fluid and is discharged along with the semen during ejaculation.

Noteworthy premodern references

Of note is a reference to the treatment of premature ejaculation in *Yan Fang Xin Bian* (*New Compilation of Empirical Formulas*).[15] For men with those conditions who have tried "one hundred treatments without result," the author recommends the use of ten earthworms, washed clean in water and pounded together with the juice of *Jiu Cai Zi* (Allii tuberosi Semen), which should be boiled with wine and taken drenched daily for several days. The cited predicted outcome is the ability to last a long time during intercourse and a good chance of engendering a child. In some premodern texts, this condition is called chicken essence (*ji jing*).

Western medical correlates and associated conditions

Premature ejaculation; benign prostatic hyperplasia; chronic prostatitis; anxiety disorders; depression

2. Seminal emission (*yi jing*)
Main signs, causes, and patterns

This disease category refers to involuntary loss of semen that is not associated with conscious sexual activity. When it occurs during sleep and with dreams of engaging in sexual acts, it is called dream emission (*meng er yi jing*), dreaming of intercourse (*meng jiao*), seminal loss while dreaming (*meng shi jing*), or dream ejaculation (*meng xie*). When not associated with dreaming, it is called seminal efflux (*hua jing*).

Essence is stored in the kidneys and governed by the heart. Therefore, seminal emission is often caused by detriment and damage to the heart and kidneys caused by excessive thought and preoccupation as well by taxation from excessive vexation and sexual intemperance. It is important to note that these heart-kidney patterns can be either heart-kidney yin vacuity patterns or heart-kidney yang vacuity patterns. In the case of yin vacuity, insufficiency of kidney yin-essence makes the ministerial and sovereign fire hyperactive and causes them to harass the essence gate. In yang vacuity, the essence-governing power

---

[15] See note 6 in this chapter.

of the heart and the essence storage-power of the kidneys lacks warmth and power; as a result, the essence gate becomes insecure.

Other causes include spleen-stomach damp-heat, spleen qi vacuity, and hyperactive liver yang from insufficiency of liver yin-blood.

Excessive consumption of rich, thick-flavored foods, and alcohol leads to the formation of damp-heat in the center burner, which pours downward into the essence chamber. Once there, depressed heat and phlegm form and obstruct the physiological essence-storing function of the essence chamber.

Enduring damp-heat in the center burner and excessive thought and preoccupation weaken the spleen. When spleen qi is vacuous, it fails to move and transform the essence of water and grain and to play its role in engendering qi and blood. As a result, qi loses its restraining power and blood is not engendered sufficiently; hence, the essence gate becomes insecure and the anterior yin region loses its nourishment.

If liver yin-blood is vacuous, ministerial fire within the liver becomes hyperactive and harasses the heart and kidneys; this leads to insecurity of the essence gate as described under the heart and kidney patterns above.

Note: Seminal emission is also called seminal emission (*yi xie*),[16] seminal loss (*shi jing*), and essence desertion (*tuo jing*).

Noteworthy premodern references

There is an especially rich record of discussions of seminal emission in the premodern literature. I have chosen just a few that exhibit some interesting and clinically relevant ideas.

One of the earliest references to seminal emission occurs in Zhang Zhong-Jing's famous text, *Jin Gui Yao Lue Fang Lun* (*Essential Prescriptions of the Golden Coffer*),[17] in which he associates seminal loss with stringlike tension in the lesser abdomen, dizzy eyes, hair loss, a cold-tipped penis and an extremely vacuous scallion-stalk pulse that is also slow. His recommended formula is *Gui Zhi Jia Long Gu Mu Li Tang* (Cinnamon Twig Decoction Plus Dragon Bone and Oyster Shell).

On the subject of dream emissions, *Bian Que Xin Shu* (*Bian Que's Heart Text*),[18] states: "When a man dreams of intercourse and does not ejaculate, his

---

[16] In this case, the English language translation is the same, but the second character in the Chinese word *yi xie* is different. *Xie* means "to discharge."

[17] *Jin Gui Yao Lue Fang Lun* was originally published during the Eastern Han dynasty, and was part of the same text as *Shang Han Lun* (*On Cold Damage*). The original title of the text (*Shang Han Lun* and *Jin Gui Yao Lue Fang Lun* combined) was *Shang Han Za Bing Lun* (*On Cold Damage and Miscellaneous Diseases*).

[18] *Bian Que Xin Shu* was published in 1146, during the Song dynasty.

heart and kidney qi are replete; when [such] dreams result in [seminal] emission, his heart and kidney are vacuous."

In *Dan-Xi Xin Fa (Dan-Xi's Heart Approach)*,[19] Zhu Dan-Xi (Zhu Zhen-Heng) comments that the treatment for essence desertion is the same as that of abnormal vaginal discharge, and proceeds to describe damp-heat patterns, qi and blood vacuity patterns, and heart and kidney patterns.

In *Pu Ji Fang (Universal Salvation Formulary)*,[20] we find the following interesting quote: "There are also those who are young with exuberance of qi and celibate Daoist men who are compelled to control their sexual desire, [and who] as a result of [stirring] of [their sexual] desire have [seminal] emission; no medicine can prevent and contain this."

In *Bian Zheng Lu (Pattern Discrimination Record)*,[21] there is a noteworthy description of how liver blood vacuity leads to dream emission. The explanation revolves around the fact that when liver blood is vacuous and then liver-wood is dry, the fire within the liver becomes hyperactive and harasses the heart and kidneys.

Western medical correlates and associated conditions

Chronic prostatitis; anxiety disorders

3. Essence turbidity (*jing zhuo*)

Main signs, causes, and patterns

This disease category refers to a condition in which there is clear urine, but during urination there is a turbid and pasty substance collecting at the opening of the urinary meatus. There may also be pain and itching of the penis. If the turbid and pasty discharge is white, the disease is more specifically called white turbidity (*bai zhuo*); if it is red, it is called red turbidity (*chi zhuo*).

Causes include: 1) excessive consumption of alcohol which leads to vanquished essence[22] and stasis-obstruction; 2) detriment and damage to kidney yin-essence leading to frenetic movement of ministerial fire which harasses vanquished essence and causes it to be expelled and; 3) damp-heat pouring downward into the essence chamber. In enduring cases, even when the root was one of repletion, there is usually also tip vacuity in the form of kidney yin and/or yang vacuity, as well as spleen vacuity patterns.

---

[19] *Dan Xi Xin Fa* was published in 1481, during the Yuan dynasty.
[20] *Pu Ji Fang* was edited by Teng Hong and published in 1406, during the Ming dynasty.
[21] See note 3 in this chapter.
[22] Vanquished essence (*bai jing*) refers to semen that has been despoiled by evil qi.

Noteworthy premodern references

Zheng Zhi Hui Bu (Supplemental Essays on Patterns and Treatments)[23] clarifies that essence turbidity is "caused by vanquished essence flowing into the urinary orifice, which [becomes] stagnated and difficult to expel." The passage goes on to say that fire within the heart and kidney channels causes essence to flow out with the urine.

Western medical correlates and associated conditions

Acute and chronic prostatitis; urethritis; sexually-transmitted infectious diseases; male infertility

4. Hematospermia (*xue jing*)
Main signs, causes, and patterns

This disease category applies when there is blood mixed with semen. It is commonly caused by either damp-heat harassing the essence chamber, static blood obstructing the essence pathway, yin vacuity with hyperactive ministerial fire, and dual vacuity of spleen and kidney qi.

In the case of damp-heat, the main disease cause is usually excessive intake of greasy-fried, sweet foods, and dairy products which lead to splenic movement and transformation failure. As a result, dampness collects in the center burner and pours downward to the essence chamber and becomes depressed there. Depressed dampness engenders heat and combines with dampness. Then damp-heat harasses the network vessels within the essence chamber and causes frenetic movement of blood into the semen. Additionally, however, damp-heat toxin may directly enter the penis and essence chamber by having unhygienic sex.

Blood stasis results from either external injury to the anterior yin region or from internal damage by the seven affects; in either case, qi depression and blood stasis accumulate in the essence chamber. During sexual activity, when the movement of qi caused by the stirring of sexual desire, and ejaculation encounters the blocked static blood, the network vessels are damaged and blood leaks into the semen.

Further, especially vigorous or forceful sexual acts can directly traumatize the essence chamber.

Insufficiency of kidney essence comes from: 1) natural endowment insufficiency; 2) sexual intemperance; 3) excessive intake of warm and dry yang-assisting medicinals or; 3) enduring depressed heat scorching yin and leading to hyperactive ministerial fire. This vacuity fire enters the essence chamber, scorches the network vessels, and leads to frenetic movement of blood into the semen.

---

[23] *Zheng Zhi Hui Bu* was written by Li Yong-Cui and published in 1687, during the Qing dynasty.

In the pattern of dual vacuity of the spleen and kidneys, taxation-fatigue or dietary irregularities damage the spleen qi—which is the source of engendering and transformation of qi and blood—and lead to vacuity of both qi and blood. Since blood is the mother of qi, qi is the commander of blood, and essence and blood share the same source, blood vacuity leads to yin-essence insufficiency. The kidneys lose their nourishment and their sealing and storage capacity (due to insecurity of kidney qi), and spleen qi is unable to restrain blood; this leads to blood in the semen.

Note: We should differentiate this condition from two other Chinese disease categories: blood strangury (*xue lin*) and hematuria (*xue niao*). Blood strangury applies when there is blood in the urine and there is also rough, painful, and inhibited urination. We use the term hematuria for those with blood in the urine without pain.

Noteworthy premodern references

In the section on vacuity taxation emission of blood and semen, *Zhu Bing Yuan Hou Lun (On the Origin and Indicators of Disease)*[24] we find the earliest mention of this disease. It states: "This is caused by taxation damage to kidney qi. The kidneys store essence and essence is formed from blood. Vacuity taxation causes the seven damages and the six extremes,[25] and [brings] detriment to both qi and blood. When the kidneys tend to vacuity, [they are] unable to store essence, so that essence and blood are emitted together."

Western medical correlates and associated conditions

Hematospermia; prostate cancer; acute and chronic prostatitis; epididymitis

Testicular and scrotal diseases

1. Mounting qi (*shan qi*)

Main signs, causes, and patterns

This disease was first described in chapter 55 of *Su Wen (Plain Questions)*. It has many other names including mounting pathocondition (*shan zheng*), mounting (*shan*), bladder and small intestinal qi, small intestinal qi pain, bladder qi, and running piglet qi (*ben tun*). This is probably due to the fact that the disease category of mounting qi in ancient times was used very broadly to describe many different diseases.

In the premodern literature, we find two common schema for differentiating mounting into either five or seven patterns. The five-pattern schema appeared

---

[24] See note 10 in this chapter.

[25] The six extremes (*liu ji*) refers to six types of relatively serious vacuity detriment diseases: qi extreme; blood extreme; sinew extreme; flesh extreme; bone extreme and; essence extreme. This comprises the list as it appeared in Zhang Zhong-Jing's *Jin Gui Yao Lue Fang Lun (Essentials of Prescriptions from the Golden Coffer)*, though later authors changed it slightly.

in *Zhu Bing Yuan Hou Lun* (*On the Origin and Indicators of Disease*),[26] and the seven-pattern schema first appeared in *Su Wen* (*Plain Questions*). In general, however, this disease is caused by some form of evil qi accumulating in the yin aspect of the body, and the common denominator among all its various patterns is that this disease is located in the liver channel. So, there is a dictum in Chinese medicine: "all mounting is ascribed to the liver."

Very broadly, the disease category of mounting qi has two main uses in andrology. It defines a condition in which there is either: 1) something protruding from inside of the body cavity accompanied by qi pain, and/or sudden and intense abdominal pain accompanied by unsmooth urination or bowel movements or; 2) a disease located in the genitals, the testicles, or the scrotum characterized by either swelling, ulceration, or pus, by the emission of vanquished essence and turbid substance from the urethra,[27] by testicular or scrotal swelling and pain, or by other, generally painful, symptoms in the abdomen.

As mentioned above, there have been many mounting patterns described in different premodern texts. Not all of these has survived the test of time, so that many of them are not used in contemporary clinical practice. Although the subject of mounting qi could require an extremely long discussion, it is useful to have a basic understanding of these conditions in premodern terms, because such an understanding is helpful for reframing certain Western-defined diseases (as listed below) into Chinese medicine. Rather than taking on the daunting task of defining every pattern that ever appeared under the heading of mounting, in accordance with Tan (1999), I am limiting my discussion to the four types of mounting considered most relevant to contemporary clinical practice—foxy mounting (*hu shan*), water mounting (*shui shan*), blood mounting (*xue shan*), and prominent mounting (*tui shan*).

• Foxy mounting (*hu shan*)
According to Wiseman and Feng (1995), foxy mounting refers to the "[p]rotrusion of the small intestine into the scrotum. The intestine retracts periodically of its own accord, and can be drawn back in by the patient himself in lying posture." The name derives from the stealthy and fox-like way in which the intestine slides in and out of the scrotum, which is likened to a fox lair. The main patterns discriminated for this disease are liver depression and qi stagnation, internal collection of cold-dampness, and center qi fall.

Noteworthy premodern references
Shou Shi Bao Yuan (*Prolonging Life and Preserving the Origin*)[28] states: "In those with foxy mounting, qi exits and the scrotum becomes enlarged and swollen, and causes the man to be unable to endure it. At night, qi enters, the swelling and dis-

---

[26] See note 10 in this chapter.
[27] See also essence turbidity (*jing zhuo*) in this chapter.
[28] *Shou Shi Bao Yuan* was written by Gong Ting-Xian, and published during the Ming dynasty.

tention completely disappear, and there is slight relief from the suffering. A concealed fox is an animal. During the day, it leaves its hole to urinate, and at night it returns to its hole and does not urinate. [In the same way,] the symptoms [of this disease] disappear at night and this is why it is called foxy mounting."

Western medical correlates and associated conditions

Inguinal hernia; umbilical hernia; scrotal hernia

• Water mounting (shui shan)

This type of mounting is distinguished either by the presence of sweating and dampness of the scrotum with leakage of yellowish fluid or by a swollen, enlarged, and translucent scrotum. It is generally attributed to kidney vacuity and water collection, liver channel damp-heat, blood stasis obstructing the network vessels, and internal collection of cold-dampness. When this condition occurs in young infants, it is called early heaven water mounting and when it occurs in adults, it is called secondary water mounting.

Noteworthy premodern references

In *Bian Zheng Lu (Pattern Discrimination Record)*,[29] it states: "[When a] man has bladder block and dribbling, urine is inhibited, and there is pulling pain in the testicles accompanied by a sagging [sensation] and pain within the small intestine. Who would know this is due to binding of heat in the bladder? The bladder is the [bowel] which transforms water. When there is cold in the bladder, water is not transformed, and heat is also not transformed; [thus] water is not transformed and heat binds within the bladder, so that water is separated [out to] the channels and networks. Water [then] enters the testicles."

According to *Song Ya Zun Sheng Quan Shu (Life-Respecting Compendium [from the] Precipice of Song [Mountain])*,[30] "[In] water mounting, the scrotum is swollen and enlarged, and as clear as water. There is extreme sweating of the genitals and possibly itching of the genitals with leakage of yellowish fluid when scratched, or watery sounds in the abdomen when it is pressed, or possibly one testicle becomes enlarged and the other becomes smaller. The smaller one can disappear to the degree [that it is as if the man has] only one testicle, [because it is so] deeply pulled into the lesser abdomen and painful."

Western medical correlates and associated conditions

Scrotal hydrocele

• Blood mounting (xue shan)

Blood mounting refers to an accumulation of blood within the scrotum that either results from traumatic injury or after surgery. In both cases, blood spills out of the vessels and gathers within the scrotum. The main signs are signifi-

---

[29] See note 3 in this chapter.
[30] *Song Ya Zun Sheng Quan Shu* was compiled by Jing Dong-Yang and published in 1696, during the Qing dynasty.

cant scrotal swelling and distention, with pain and a heavy drooping sensation, and stasis macules on the scrotal skin. Blood stasis obstructed within the scrotal network vessels is the main pattern.

Noteworthy premodern references

According to *Jing-Yue Quan Shu* (*Jing-Yue's Complete Compendium*),[31] when "blood binds within the lesser abdomen, it is called blood mounting. However, [when one] inspects it, it is neither qi nor food, and the small intestine is hard and has form, the stools are bound and black, and the urine is uninhibited. It must be blood accumulation and it belongs to blood mounting."

Western medical correlates and associated conditions

Hernia; scrotal hematoma

• Prominent mounting (*tui shan*)

Prominent mounting results when there is chronic retention of lymphatic fluid within the scrotum which leads to chronic scrotal edema and the formation of fibrous tissue within the scrotum. The most prominent clinical signs are gradual thickening and hardening of the scrotal skin, and the absence of pain or itching.

Noteworthy premodern references

Yi Zong Bi Du (*Indispensable Medical Readings*),[32] states: "[In] prominent mounting, the scrotum is swollen and enlarged, [and weighs] from one *sheng* to one *dou*;[33] when severe, it can be as large as a wicker basket."

Song Ya Zun Sheng Quan Shu (*Life-Respecting Compendium [from the] Precipice of Song [Mountain]*)[34] states: "Prominent mounting is also called stubborn mounting (*wan shan*); the testicles [weigh] as much as one *sheng* or one *dou*, and there is neither pain nor itching. This is always ascribed to damp qi [accumulating] suddenly."

Western medical correlates and associated conditions

Elephantiasis of the scrotum; filariasis

2. Testicular phlegm (*zi tan*)
Main signs, causes, and patterns

Testicular phlegm is the premodern Chinese medical disease category that covers chronic ulcerative tuberculin infection of the testicles, epididymis, and spermatic cord. The main features of this condition include testicular swelling and

---

[31] *Jing-Yue Quan Shu* was written by Zhang Jing-Yue and published in 1624, during the Ming dynasty. It is one of the most celebrated works in Chinese medicine.
[32] *Yi Zong Bi Du* was written bu Li Zhong-Zi in 1637, during the Ming dynasty.
[33] These are premodern measurements equivalent to about one liter and ten liters in modern volume respectively.
[34] See note 30 above.

lumps, local sores, flowing thin watery pus containing a rotted thready substance, the opening of the sore is pitted, and eventually fistulas form. This is, by definition, a complicated, chronic and stubborn condition.

The pathomechanisms usually involve detriment and damage to the liver and kidneys which leaves the channels and networks open and vacuous so that cold dampness and turbid phlegm take advantage of the vacuity and flow downward into the lower burner and accumulate in the anterior yin region. Then, enduring cold dampness becomes depressed and transforms heat, which rots the flesh and creates pus. As the pus continuously flows over time, it creates a pathway out to the exterior of the body (a fistula). As a complication of the heat transforming from turbid phlegm depression, yin is damaged; this engenders interior heat from yin vacuity. Over time, yin vacuity affects the yang and leads to kidney yang vacuity. In summary, this condition is characterized by root vacuity and tip repletion. There is detriment and damage to the liver and kidneys at the root, combined with congelation and accumulation of turbid phlegm at the tip.

Noteworthy premodern references

In *Wai Ke Qi Xuan* (*Mysterious Inspiration of External Medicine*),[35] this condition is covered under the heading of scrotal cracking fistula (*yin nang po lie lou chuang*): "The exterior of the scrotum bursts and fishy-smelling water leaks out. [Even] after long-term treatment, it is not cured. This engenders a bayberry sore,[36] with toxin bound within it."

Other sources refer to this condition under different headings, including testicular leak (*shen lou*). For example, *Zheng Zhi Zhun Sheng* (*The Level-Line of Pattern Identification and Treatment*)[37] states: "*Shi Hui San* (Ten Cinders Powder) treats testicular leak, after yellow water has burst out and the sore looks like a fish's mouth; it extends life."

Western medical correlates and associated conditions

Tuberculosis of the testicles, tuberculosis of the epididymis; tuberculosis of the spermatic cord

3. Testicular welling-abscess (*zi yong*)
Main signs, causes, and patterns

This disease category refers to an abscess of the testicle, and is divided into acute and chronic types. In acute cases, the culprit is usually damp-heat pouring downward from the center burner leading to qi stagnation and blood sta-

---

[35] *Wai Ke Qi Xuan* was written by Shen Dou-Yuan and published in 1604, during the Ming dynasty. The first three chapters within this twelve-chapter text are devoted to the diagnosis and treatment of sores.

[36] Bayberry sore (*mei chuang*) is generally attributed to primary syphilis.

[37] *Zheng Zhi Zhun Sheng* was written by Wang Ken-Tang and published in 1602, during the Ming dynasty.

sis, as well as heat toxin and pus. Other causes include external contraction of cold damp or damp-heat evils (during unhygienic sexual activity) that become depressed in the lower burner and transform heat, external injury causing blood stasis that becomes depressed and transforms heat, and heat transformation from depression of vanquished essence caused by holding back ejaculation during sexual activity. The main signs include swelling and hardness of the affected testicle, intense pain, a local scorching sensation, and tense and shiny scrotal skin. In chronic cases, there is usually binding depression of liver qi from enduring anger and resentment and vacuity-detriment of the liver and kidneys which allows for an accumulation and congelation of phlegm-dampness. In such cases, the disease course is prolonged, and the affected testicle is enlarged and hard, but is not significantly painful and the scrotum is not red or hot (unless complicated by depressed heat). After several months or years, there will be watery pus, and a fistula may form. This condition is considered difficult to cure.

Noteworthy premodern references

Xuan Lu Yan Fang Xin Bian (Selected Writings from a New Compilation of Empirical Formulas)[38] states: "[When] the testicle is painful and on its exterior it is red and not rising upward, this is called testicular abscess. Gradually, pus forms. When it ulcerates, life is extended." This reference shows that in the course of abscess, it is a favorable event when pus is expelled. And the presence of unexpelled pus is associated with a poor clinical outcome.

Western medical correlates and associated conditions

Testicular abscess; epididymitis with abscess

4. Scrotal welling-abscess (*nang yong*)

This disease category applies when there is acute swelling, pain, and heat sensation of the scrotum that do not affect the testicles. Other important signs include reduction of pain and swelling after the expulsion of pus, generalized heat effusion, reddish hot urine, and dry mouth with a desire to drink cold fluids. In premodern sources, however, this distinction is far from clear, and we see many descriptions of this disease in the literature that list signs on the penis, testicles, and on the anterior yin region in general, along with those on the scrotum.

Main signs, causes, and patterns

The main causes are liver channel damp-heat pouring downward and brewing in the scrotum, prolonged sitting in damp clothes or in a damp location leading to damp depression and damp-heat toxin, repeatedly scratching the scrotum and breaking the skin allowing damp-cold or damp-heat toxin to enter

---

[38] I am not completely certain, but the title of this book suggests that it is selected writings from *Yan Fang Xin Bian*, which was published in 1846, during the Qing dynasty. See note 6 in this chapter for further explanation.

the channels, and overindulgence in greasy-fried, fatty and spicy-hot foods leading to damp-heat in the center burner that pours downward into the scrotum. Also, some authors attribute this condition to kidney yin vacuity with damp-heat pouring downward. In this case, damp-heat evil takes advantage of vacuity and becomes depressed in the scrotum.

In all of these cases, depressed evils in the scrotum transform heat, and engender heat toxin and pus.

Note: Scrotal welling-abscess is also called testicular sac welling-abscess (*shen nang yong*) and external kidneys welling-abscess (*wai shen yong*).

Western medical correlates and associated conditions

Scrotal abscess; filariasis

5. Kidney sac [*i.e.,* scrotal] wind (*shen nang feng*)
Main signs, causes, and patterns

This disease category applies when there are sores and rashes in the scrotal region. It begins with dryness and itching in the scrotal region and progresses to the formation of papules and vesicles which ooze an oily fluid when scratched. A damp ulceration forms which eventually scabs over. When this condition persists for a long period of time, the scrotal skin becomes scaly and intensely itchy. The main pattern is damp-heat pouring downward into the anterior yin region and engendering wind. Also called scrotal wind (*nang feng*) and bobble[39] wind (*xiu qiu feng*).

Noteworthy premodern references

Wai Ke Da Cheng (*The Great Compendium of External Medicine*),[40] states: "[In] kidney sac wind, there is itching, lumps, and stubborn numbness, breaking [of the skin] and flow of thick fluid. It is caused by liver channel wind dampness and requires *Long Dan Xie Gan Tang* (Gentian Liver-Draining Decoction) or *Chai Hu Sheng Shi Tang* (Bupleurum Dampness-Overcoming Decoction)."

In *Wai Ke Zhen Quan* (*True Interpretation of External Medicine*),[41] we find the following detailed description of kidney sac wind: "Kidney sac wind, also called bobble wind, begins with extreme dryness and itching, and a liking for bathing in hot water. In severe cases, lumps arise that have the shape of red millets, there is numbness and itching, [and after] scratching there is oozing of oily fluid. [Further,] the skin is painful and as hot as if being burned. It is ascribed to repletion heat and requires internal administration of *Jia Jian* [*Long Dan*] *Xie*

---

[39] According to the *Oxford American Dictionary*, a bobble is "a small ball made of strands of wool used as a decoration on a hat or on furnishings."
[40] *Wai Ke Da Cheng* was written by Qi Kun and published in 1665, during the Qing dynasty.
[41] *Wai Ke Zhen Quan* was written by Zou Yue and published in 1838, during the Qing dynasty.

Gan Tang ([Gentian] Liver-Draining Decoction with Modifications) and external use of *She Chuang Zi Tang* (Cnidium Decoction) as a steam wash."

Western medical correlates and associated conditions

Scrotal eczema; neurogenic dermatitis of the scrotum

6. Genital itching (*yin yang*)
Main signs, causes, and patterns

This disease category is mainly characterized by itching of the genitals. In severe cases, the itching is unbearable, and the patient cannot sit comfortably. It is commonly attributed to liver depression transforming heat, spleen vacuity with accumulation of dampness, and brewing and binding of damp-heat pouring downward, to lack of cleanliness of the external genitalia and sitting for long periods of time in damp areas. This exposes the genital region to damp evil. Those with preexisting vacuity are more susceptible to such an invasion as the evil takes advantage of the vacuity. An additional cause is yin vacuity and blood dryness failing to nourish and enrich the anterior yin region and engendering wind.

Noteworthy premodern references

Zhang Shi Yi Tong (*Zhang's Clear View of Medicine*)[42] states: "[For] itching in the [anterior] yin [due to] liver patients' damp-heat, [use] *Xiao Chai Hu Tang* (Minor Bupleurum Decoction) or *Zi Shen Wan* (Kidney-Enriching Pill). Itching and dryness in thin people is ascribed to yin vacuity. [Use] three *qian* of *Liu Wei Di Huang Wan* (Six-Ingredient Rehmannia Pill) taken together with one *qian* of *Zi Shen Wan* (Kidney-Enriching Pill). Externally, use a wash of *She Chuang Zi* (Cnidii Fructus)."

Western medical correlates and associated conditions

Scrotal fungal infection; "jock itch"; scrotal pruritis

7. Suspended welling-abscess (*xuan yong*)
Main signs, causes, and patterns

Refers to a welling-abscess in the perineal region, having all the usual features of abscess including redness, swelling, hardness, pain, pus, and heat sensation.

Note: Suspended welling-abscess is also called seabed leaking (*hai di lou*) and crotch-boring welling-abscess (*chuan dang yong*).

Noteworthy premodern references

Wai Ke Zhen Quan (*True Interpretation of External Medicine*)[43] states: "Suspended welling-abscess is also called seabed leaking [*hai di lou*]. It appears behind the scrotum and in front of the anus, on the point *Hui Yin* (CV-1). It is

---

[42] *Zhang Shi Yi Tong* was written by Zhang Lu and published in 1695, during the Qing dynasty.
[43] See note 41 in this chapter.

caused by detriment and damage to the three yin and congestion and stagnation of damp-heat. At the onset, there is redness and scorching hot pain; such cases are ascribed to yang and are easily cured. If it is clear, cold, and hard, and there are no discolorations of the skin, it is ascribed to yin and is difficult to treat."

In another section of the same text, we find the following: "Crotch-boring welling-abscess appears in front of the *Hui Yin* point and behind the scrotum. Follow the treatment methods for suspended welling-abscess. However, this [abscess] is tied to the skin at the hollow of the scrotum. It is an extremely critical [case] if toxin is engendered and it ulcerates abnormally quickly, if the root is deep and ulceration is delayed, if the rotting damages the urinary tube, or if there is leaking of urine and inability to retain [urine]."

Western medical correlates and associated conditions

Prostatic abscess; perineal abscess; prostate cancer; urethral fistula

8. Retracted genitals (*yin suo*)
Main signs, causes, and patterns

First mentioned in the *Ling Shu* (*Magic Pivot*), this disease category is used when the tissues of the anterior yin region retract inward and upward. In males, this includes the penis, the scrotum, and testes. The main cause is cold invading the foot reverting yin liver channel, though heat patterns are described in some sources.

The liver channel encircles the genitals. When cold evil invades the liver channel, the tissues of the anterior yin region contract and retract upward toward the abdominal cavity. As cold—a yin evil—obstructs yang qi and congeals blood, there is usually also pain in the genitals and hypertonicity and pain of the lesser abdomen.

Another cause is outward desertion of yang qi caused either by direct strike of cold into the lesser yin or by severe vomiting or diarrhea. In cases of yang brightness heat falling inward into the reverting yin channel, there is also abdominal fullness and bound stool, vexation and heat with thirst, and a replete forceful pulse. When there is liver-gallbladder heat, there is scrotal distention and penile retraction, abdominal pain, red eyes and dry lips, and a stringlike, tight pulse.

Note: This condition overlaps with scrotal retraction (*nang suo*), yang retraction (*yang suo*), and penile retraction (*jing suo*).

Noteworthy premodern references

Gu Jin Yi Tong Da Quan (*The Complete Compendium of Medical Works, Ancient and Modern*),[44] in its chapter on genital retraction and genital protraction has the following explanation this condition: "Genital retraction is due to the

---

[44] *Gu Jin Yi Tong Da Quan* was compiled by Xu Chun-Fu, and published in 1556, during the Ming dynasty.

genitals receiving cold and retracting up into the abdomen. Genital protraction[45] is caused by the genitals [*i.e.*, the penis] receiving heat and staying erect and long without receding. The *Ling Shu* states: "[When] the foot reverting yin is damaged by cold, there is genital retraction; [when] it is damaged by heat, it is protracted and erect without receding."

Bing Ji Sha Zhuan (*The Sand Seal of Pathomechanisms*)[46] relates the channels to this disease in the following passage: "The governing vessel, the liver channel, and the conception vessel all are channels that pass through the anterior yin [region]. And the greater yin and yang brightness unite there. All [of these channels] accumulate at the genitals. These [channels] have a major influence on a man's penis and a woman's jade gate [*i.e.*, vaginal meatus]. Cold causes the sinews to retract upward into the abdomen; this is a critical indication. [*Rou*] *Gui* [Cinnamomi Cortex], *Fu* [*Zi*] [Aconiti Radix preparata], *Chai* [*Hu*] [Bupleuri Radix], [*Bai*] *Shao* [Paeoniae Radix Alba], *Dang* [*Gui*] [Angelicae Sinensis Radix], and [*Fu*] *Ling* [Poria] are suitable."

Western medical correlates and associated conditions

Unknown

Infertility

Main signs, causes, and patterns

This disease category applies to men who have been having unprotected intercourse with a known fertile female for at least two years without impregnating her. Common causes include vacuity patterns such as spleen qi vacuity, kidney yin, yang, and essence vacuity, and repletion patterns such as binding depression of liver qi, damp-heat, phlegm, and blood stasis.

In the case of spleen qi vacuity, later heaven fails to engender early heaven. In other words, the basic pathomechanisms is that a vacuous spleen fails to move and transform the essence of water and grain, which results in qi and blood vacuity that eventually affects liver blood and kidney essence.

When there is kidney yin vacuity, vacuity fire scorches the essence chamber and damages semen, and kidney yin-essence fails to nourish and engender semen. In the case of kidney yang vacuity, debilitated life gate fire fails to warm and power the transformation of kidney essence to kidney qi and the transformation of kidney essence into semen. If kidney essence is insufficient, there is a lack of substantial raw material for the engenderment of liver blood and semen.

As for repletion patterns, the main pathomechanism is one of obstruction. This is true for liver depression, dampness, phlegm, and blood stasis, which all have

---

[45] See the discussion of rigid yang in this chapter.
[46] *Bing Ji Sha Zhuan* was written by Li Zhong-Zi, and published in 1667, during the Ming dynasty.

the ability to obstruct the essence chamber and to therefore impair male fertility by interfering with the normal formation or distribution of semen and sperm. Finally, repletion heat (either from liver depression transforming heat or from damp-heat) scorches the essence chamber and damages semen and sperm.

Noteworthy premodern references

Most early premodern sources stressed vacuity as the main cause of male infertility as we find in the following passages below. Later, during the latter Qing dynasty, and then especially during the modern era, doctors began discussing the role of repletion patterns such as blood stasis and damp-heat in male infertility. See Chapter 8 on infertility in Book 2 of this text for a fuller view.

Chapter 1 of the *Su Wen* (*Plain Questions*) states: "The kidneys govern water; they receive essence from the five viscera and six bowels and store it. So, when the five viscera are exuberant, [a man] can ejaculate. If the five viscera are all debilitated and the sinews and bones separate and fall, and [further] heavenly tenth has ceased, the beard becomes white, the body is heavy, and [one] cannot walk straight, [one] can no [longer] have children."

In *Zhu Bing Yuan Hou Lun* (*On the Origin and Indicators of Disease*),[47] we find the following interesting discussion of male infertility: "Men who have no children, [may have] semen as clear as water and as cold as frozen iron; these are indicators that they are unable to have children. Further, [there are] other men who are unable to have children who have seminal emission or inability to discharge semen [which] instead accumulates in the penis head. If they don't have these indicators, then they are able to have children. [One] should have intercourse at a yang time. Yang time is from midnight until the third watch [*i.e.*, 3–5 a.m.]. Having a child [*i.e.*, conceiving] at this time [will always result in having] an intelligent child who has a long life. Do not have a child at a yin time. Yin time is from noon until the twelfth watch [*i.e.*, 9–11 p.m.]. A child conceived during these times will always be stupid and will have a dark and short life. All should carefully follow this in detail. All women should wait one to three days from when their moon time arrives, when the child gate is open. If they have intercourse at this time, they will have a child. If they [let] four days pass, then [the child gate] is blocked and they cannot have a child.[48] Men whose pulse feels minute weak and rough cannot have children; their essential qi [*i.e.*, semen] is clear and cold."

Western medical correlates and associated conditions

Male factor infertility

---

[47] See note 10 in this chapter.
[48] This advice is clearly incorrect according to our modern understanding of female hormonal and ovulatory cycles.

Urinary diseases

1. Dribbling urinary block (*long bi*)

Main signs, causes, and patterns

This disease category is characterized by partially or completely blocked urinary flow. Originally two separate diseases, *long* referred to partial blockage of urinary flow with dribbling, and *bi* referred to complete blockage of urinary flow. Nowadays, the two disease categories are combined together into one condition called dribbling urinary block (*long bi*).

Causes include lung heat and qi congestion, binding of heat in the bladder, liver depression, vanquished essence and blood stasis obstructing the bladder, insufficiency of fluids, qi vacuity, and kidney yang vacuity.

In the case of lung heat and qi congestion, heat congests the lungs (the upper source of water) and disables lung depurative downbearing and waterway-regulation and results in urinary dribbling or block. When there is binding of heat in the bladder, bladder qi transformation becomes obstructed resulting in an inability to expel urine.

The liver channel encircles the genitals and liver and free-coursing helps to regulate the formation and excretion of urine. If liver qi is depressed, dribbling urinary block may result. Vanquished essence and blood stasis cause dribbling urinary block by blocking the waterways and obstructing urine flow. When there is insufficient fluid, there is no water to transform into urine, so this leads to dribbling urinary block. If there is lung, spleen, or kidney qi vacuity, the three sources of water and the triple burner lack power for regulating the waterways; this leads to dribbling urinary block. Finally, when there is kidney yang vacuity, there is no warmth and power for kidney and bladder qi transformation; hence, the waterways become obstructed and dribbling urinary block result.

Noteworthy premodern references

In *Jing-Yue Quan Shu* (*Jing-Yue's Complete Compendium*),[49] Zhang elaborated on the pathomechanisms of qi vacuity and blockage in dribbling urinary block as follows: "In humans, urine enters the bladder and the bladder bowel stores it. It is [by the action of] qi that urine is transformed; therefore, if there is qi, then there is urine. The exit of water depends on water and the reach of qi, so water is the beginning of urine and constant qi transformation enables it to exit! Because of transformation, there can be entry and exit. Without transformation and exit, there can be no transformation and entry." He emphasized the importance of supplementing and moving qi in order to treat dribbling urinary block by activating the bladder and kidney qi transformation of water.

---

[49] See note 31 in this chapter.

In an influential passage from *Zheng Zhi Hui Bu* (*Supplemental Essays on Patterns and Treatments*),[50] Li Yong-Cui offers the following discussion of dribbling urinary block: "There is binding of heat in the lower burner, bladder congestion and roughness, stagnation of the qi pathway, deep-lying heat in the lung with inability to both engender water and to carry out qi transformation, enduring disease with desiccated fluid and humor, liver channel indignation and qi block and stoppage, and spleen vacuity and qi weakness with loss of free flow, regulation, and diffusion." He offers further observations on the treatment of dribbling urinary block via the lungs as follows: "The entire body's qi is related to the lung. When the lung is clear, qi moves; [when] it is turbid, qi congests. Therefore, urinary stoppage is mostly due to the inability of lung qi to diffuse and spread. Diffusing and clearing metal along with downbearing qi governs its treatment." This insight remains a mainstay in the treatment of dribbling urinary block in modern clinical practice.

Western medical correlates and associated conditions

Acute and chronic prostatitis; benign prostatic hyperplasia (BPH); prostate cancer

2. Strangury (*lin zheng*)

Main signs, causes, and patterns

The main features of strangury are short rough painful urination, urinary urgency, and urinary incontinence. There have been several different patterns (from 5–8) for strangury described in different texts throughout Chinese medical history. In the modern clinical practice of andrology, we discriminate the following patterns: heat strangury; stone strangury; unctuous strangury; blood strangury; taxation strangury; and qi strangury.

The pathomechanisms of the various stranguries can be summarized under the headings of bladder damp-heat, spleen and kidney depletion and detriment, and binding depression of liver qi.

Bladder damp-heat is characterized by scorching heat and stabbing pain in the penis. If enduring damp-heat brews and accumulates in the bladder and decocts the urine, substances within the urine will eventually bind to form sand; this leads to stone strangury. When damp-heat congests and binds in the bladder, qi transformation is inhibited and unable to separate the clear and turbid; as a result, fatty humor exits along with urine, the urine becomes oily and unctuous, and unctuous strangury develops. When exuberant heat within the bladder scorches the bladder network vessels and makes blood move frenetically, there will be hematuria—the chief sign of blood strangury.

Spleen qi vacuity leads to center qi fall, while kidney vacuity leads to insecurity of the lower origin. Together, these conditions cause taxation strangury. When center qi fall leads to strangury symptoms, we refer to it as the vacuity type of

---

[50] See note 23 in this chapter.

qi strangury. Depletion and vacuity of kidney qi and insecurity of the lower origin result in an inability to process humor (*ye*), which drains downward and mixes with urine and makes it murky and turbid. This is characteristic of unctuous strangury. When depletion and vacuity of kidney yin results in vacuity fire which scorches the bladder network vessels and makes the blood move frenetically, this is referred to as yin vacuity fire blood strangury.

Anger and indignation damage the liver and cause stagnation and nondiffusion of qi. Qi depression transforms fire and depressed fire harasses the bladder and interferes with bladder qi transformation. The result is lesser abdominal distention and pain with difficult, rough, dripping, incomplete, and painful urination. This is characteristic of the repletion pattern of qi strangury.

Noteworthy premodern references

Zhu Bing Yuan Hou Lun (*On the Origin and Indicators of Disease*)[51] has an excellent passage on strangury: "The various stranguries are caused by kidney vacuity and bladder heat...kidney vacuity will cause frequent urination, bladder heat will cause rough downbearing of water. The characteristics of strangury are frequency and nondiffusion. In heat strangury there is heat in the triple burner, qi struggles within the kidney, flows into the bladder, and produces strangury. In stone strangury [there is] dripping and expulsion of stones. Kidney rules water; [when] water is bound, stones are produced; thus, sand and stones are the guests of the kidney. [There is] kidney vacuity, so heat proliferates. Heat causes the disease of strangury. [During] urination, there is pain in the penis, incomplete excretion of urine, pain referring to the lesser abdomen, tenseness within the bladder, [and] expulsion of sand and stones from the urethra. In extreme [cases], the blockage and pain is so severe that it completely seals off the [outflow of urine]. In unctuous strangury, there is dripping and also fatty and greasy [urethral discharge]. This is why it is called unctuous strangury and flesh strangury. It [is caused by] the kidney's inability to process fatty humor, which then is excreted along with the urine."

Western medical correlates and associated conditions

Acute and chronic prostatitis; benign prostatic hyperplasia; cystitis; proteinuria; chronic nephritis

---

[51] See note 10 in this chapter.

General Treatment Principles in Chinese Andrology

In this chapter, I present the general treatment principles used in Chinese andrology and correlate them with common Chinese medicinal formulas and channels and acu-moxa points. Within the process of determining treatment based on pattern discrimination, identifying a treatment principle or strategy is of primary importance. Once one has discriminated the disease and pattern, establishing the treatment principle guides the direction of one's treatment. On a cognitive level, there is a direct and logical link between the pattern diagnosis, the treatment principle, and the selection of treatment modality. For example, once one knows that clearing heat and disinhibiting dampness is the dominant treatment strategy, certain empirically-effective medicinal formulas and acumoxa channels and points come into sharper focus and become more available to the clinician.

The standard treatment principle and corresponding treatments establish a starting point by getting one "in the ballpark." It is apparent to me, however, from practicing Chinese medicine for nearly twenty years, from having studied in China, from working side-by-side in clinical settings with Chinese colleagues, and from reading a fair amount of clinical literature in Chinese, that advanced clinicians are not overly bound by these protocols. Rather, they see such standard formulas and combinations as available templates which help focus their clinical efforts by providing a cognitive structure, while they do not feel beholden to them in any rigid way.

Successful clinical practice requires other skills and actions including intuition, experience, research, and a genuine sense of caring and compassion; indeed each patient needs a different mix of these factors to come together in their doctor, whose job sometimes requires being a "shape-shifter." In a clinical setting, the structure of treatment principles and standard treatments focus the clinician's mind on how to reach specific clinical goals and thus also provide a way for practitioners to share their clinical experiences with each other in verifiable and repeatable ways.

As we study these treatment principles, we must realize that the patterns which they are designed to treat combine in unique and challenging ways in every individual patient. Hence, the treatment for any given case would typically combine three or more of them in the same treatment. For example, it is quite common for men with chronic prostatitis to concurrently have kidney yang vacuity, damp-heat harassing the essence chamber, and blood stasis in the essence chamber. It follows logically then that the treatment for such men requires warming and supplementing kidney yang, clearing heat and disinhibiting dampness, and quickening blood and transforming stasis.

For detailed discussion of the disease causes and pathomechanisms that lead to the patterns these treatment principles correlate with, see the corresponding chapter on the disease causes and pathomechanisms in andrology. For treatment of the specific conditions mentioned in this section, see the second section of the text in which specific diseases are covered.

Clear Heat and Disinhibit Dampness

Damp-heat is a very common evil encountered in the clinical practice of Chinese andrology. The main pathomechanism is one of obstruction of kidney, bladder, and triple burner qi transformation. Common diseases associated with damp-heat include all of the following: dribbling urinary block, essence turbidity, infertility, turbid urine, urinary frequency, urinary urgency, and painful urination.

Chinese medicinals

For damp-heat pouring downward into the liver channel, use *Long Dan Xie Gan Tang* (Gentian Liver-Draining Decoction)

Long Dan Xie Gan Tang (Gentian Liver-Draining Decoction)
Long Dan Cao (Gentian Radix)
Huang Qin (Scutellariae Radix)
Shan Zhi Zi (Gardenia Fructus)
Mu Tong (Akebiae Caulis)
Ze Xie (Alismatis Rhizoma)
Che Qian Zi (Plantaginis Semen)
Dang Gui (Angelicae Sinensis Radix)
Sheng Di Huang (Rehmanniae Radix)
Chai Hu (Bupleuri Radix)
Gan Cao (Glycyrrhizae Radix)

For damp-heat in the kidney and bladder, use *Ba Zheng San* (Eight Corrections Powder) and/or *Bi Xie Fen Qing Yin* (Fish Poison Yam Clear-Turbid Separation Beverage)

Ba Zheng San (Eight Corrections Powder)
Che Qian Zi (Plantaginis Semen)
Qu Mai (Dianthi Herba)
Bian Xu (Polygoni Avicularis Herba)
Hua Shi (Talcum)
Shan Zhi Zi (Gardeniae Fructus)
Gan Cao (Glycyrrhizae Radix)

Mu Tong (Akebiae Caulis)
Da Huang (Rhei Radix et Rhizoma)

Bi Xie Fen Qing Yin (Fish Poison Yam Clear-Turbid Separation Beverage)[1]
Bi Xie (Dioscoreae Hypoglaucae Rhizoma)
Huang Bai (Phellodendri Cortex)
Shi Chang Pu (Acori Tartarinowii Rhizoma)
Fu Ling (Poria)
Bai Zhu (Atractylodis Macrocephalae Rhizoma)
Lian Zi Xin (Nelumbinis Plumula)
Dan Shen (Salvia Miltiorrhizae Radix)
Che Qian Zi (Plataginis Semen)

When damp-heat brews in the essence chamber, in the testes and scrotum, and in the bladder for long periods of time, depressed heat transforms heat toxin and decocts blood to form stasis, and also scorches the blood and rots the flesh. This explains the development of welling-abscesses (*yong*) in the anterior yin region such as testicular welling-abscess and scrotal welling-abscess. In such cases, the following medicinals may be added to clear heat and resolve toxicity and to quicken the blood and expel pus:

Pu Gong Ying (Taraxaci Herba)
Zi Hua Di Ding (Violae Herba)
Bai Jiang Cao (Patrinia Herba)
Hu Zhang (Polygoni Cuspidati Rhizoma)
Chi Shao (Paeoniae Radix Rubra)
Zao Jiao Ci (Gleditisiae Spina)
Sheng Huang Qi (Astragali Radix Recens)

Enduring damp-heat in the bladder and kidney will consume kidney yin, or vacuity fire from kidney yin vacuity decocts humor and leads to damp-heat. In either case, there is damp-heat in the kidney and bladder with liver and kidney yin vacuity concurrently. Use *Zhi Bai Di Huang Wan* (Anemarrhena, Phellodendron, and Rehmannia Pill) or *Zi Yin Chu Shi Tang* (Yin-Enriching Dampness-Eliminating Decoction) as the guiding formula.

Zhi Bai Di Huang Wan (Anemarrhena, Phellodendron, and Rehmannia Pill)
Zhi Mu (Anemarrhena Rhizoma)
Huang Bai (Phellodendri Cortex)
Sheng Di Huang (Rehmanniae Radix)
Shan Yao (Dioscoreae Rhizoma)
Shan Zhu Yu (Cornii Fructus)
Fu Ling (Poria)
Ze Xie (Alismatis Rhizoma)
Mu Dan Pi (Moutan Cortex)

---

[1] Note that this version of the formula derives from *Yi Xue Xin Wu* (*Medical Insights*), written by Cheng Guo-Peng in 1732, during the Qing dynasty.

Zi Yin Chu Shi Tang (Yin-Enriching Dampness-Eliminating Decoction)[2]
Chuan Xiong (Chuanxiong Rhizoma)
Dang Gui (Angelicae Sinensis Radix)
Bai Shao (Paeoniae Radix Alba)
Shu Di Huang (Rehmanniae Radix preparata)
Chai Hu (Bupleuri Radix)
Huang Qin (Scutellariae Radix)
Chen Pi (Citri Reticulatae Pericarpium)
Zhi Mu (Anemarrhenae Rhizoma)
Bei Mu (Fritillariae Bulbus)
Ze Xie (Alismatis Rhizoma)
Di Gu Pi (Lycii Cortex)
Gan Cao (Glycyrrhizae Radix)
Sheng Jiang (Zingiberis Rhizoma Recens)

Acumoxa therapy

To meet this treatment principle with acumoxa therapy usually involves choosing points from the kidney channel, the bladder channel, the liver channel, the gallbladder channel, the triple burner channel, the conception vessel, and the governing vessel depending on the location of the damp-heat and the therapeutic strategy of the practitioner.

Yin Gu (KI-10), *Jiao Xin* (KI-8), *Gan Shu* (BL-18), *San Jiao Shu* (BL-22), *Shen Shu* (BL-23), *Xiao Chang Shu* (BL-27), *Pang Guang Shu* (BL-28), *Wei Yang* (BL-39), *Li Gou* (LV-5), *Qu Quan* (LV-8), *Zhi Gou* (SJ-6), *Hui Yin* (CV-1), *Zhong Ji* (CV-3), *Guan Yuan* (CV-4), *Shi Men* (CV-5), *Zhong Wan* (CV-12), *Chang Qiang* (GV-1), *Yao Yang Guan* (GV-3), *Zhi Yang* (GV-9)

Course the Liver and Rectify the Qi

As binding depression of liver qi is a common cause of male sexual and reproductive diseases, this treatment principle is essential to daily clinical practice. Coursing the liver and rectifying qi means to course and free the qi dynamic and open depression, to smooth and quicken qi and blood, and to regulate the activity of the affect-mind (emotions). This treatment principle is used for treating yang wilt, premature ejaculation, inhibited urination, qi mounting, and for andropause.

Chinese medicinals

Chai Hu Shu Gan San (Bupleurum Liver-Coursing Powder) and *Xiao Yao San* (Free Wanderer Powder) are the guiding formulas.

Chai Hu Shu Gan San (Bupleurum Liver-Coursing Powder)
Chai Hu (Bupleurum Radix)

---

[2] This formula derives from *Wai Ke Zheng Zong* (*Orthodox Manual of External Medicine*), written by Chen Shi-Gong in 1617, during the Qing dynasty.

Bai Shao (Paeoniae Radix Alba)
Zhi Ke (Aurantii Fructus)
Chen Pi (Citri Reticulatae Pericarpium)
Chuan Xiong (Chuanxiong Rhizoma)
Xiang Fu (Cyperi Rhizoma)
Gan Cao (Glycyrrhizae Radix)

Xiao Yao San (Free Wanderer Powder)
Chai Hu (Bupleuri Radix)
Bo He (Mentha Herba)
Dang Gui (Angelicae Sinensis Radix)
Bai Shao (Paeoniae Radix Alba)
Bai Zhu (Atractylodis Macrocephalae Rhizoma)
Fu Ling (Poria)
Sheng Jiang (Zingiberis Rhizoma Recens)
Gan Cao (Glycyrrhizae Radix)

If enduring or severe liver depression transforms heat, use *Jia Wei Xiao Yao San* (Supplemented Free Wanderer Powder) or *Xiao Chai Hu Tang* (Minor Bupleurum Decoction). The former is used when there is liver depression, spleen vacuity and blood vacuity with either depressed heat or heat from blood vacuity. The latter is used when there is liver depression, spleen vacuity, and damp-heat.

Jia Wei Xiao Yao San (Supplemented Free Wanderer Powder)
Chai Hu (Bupleuri Radix)
Bo He (Mentha Herba)
Dang Gui (Angelicae Sinensis Radix)
Bai Shao (Paeoniae Radix Alba)
Bai Zhu (Atractylodis Macrocephalae Rhizoma)
Fu Ling (Poria)
Sheng Jiang (Zingiberis Rhizoma Recens)
Mu Dan Pi (Moutan Radix)
Shan Zhi Zi (Gardeniae Fructus)
Gan Cao (Glycyrrhizae Radix)

Xiao Chai Hu Tang (Minor Bupleurum Decoction)
Chai Hui (Bupleuri Radix)
Huang Qin (Scutellariae Radix)
Ren Shen (Ginseng Radix)
Ban Xia (Pinelliae Rhizoma)
Sheng Jiang (Zingiberis Rhizoma Recens)
Da Zao (Jujubae Fructus)
Gan Cao (Glycyrrhizae Radix)

If there is enduring liver channel qi depression with cold-dampness and blood stasis in the liver channel leading to testicular distention, pain, and swelling, *Ju He Tang* (Tangerine Pip Decoction) is the guiding formula.

Ju He Tang (Tangerine Pip Decoction)
Ju He (Citri Reticulatae Semen)
Hai Zao (Sargassum)
Kun Bu (Eckloniae Thallus)
Hai Dai (Laminariae Thallus)
Chuan Lian Zi (Toosendan Fructus)
Tao Ren (Persicae Semen)
Hou Po (Magnoliae Officinalis Cortex)
Mu Tong (Akebiae Caulis)
Zhi Shi (Aurantii Fructus Immaturis)
Yan Hu Suo (Corydalis Rhizoma)
Rou Gui (Cinnamomi Cortex)
Mu Xiang (Aucklandiae Radix)

Acumoxa therapy

In andrology, when using acumoxa therapy for coursing the liver and rectifying qi, we choose points from the liver and gallbladder channels, the bladder channel, the large intestine channel, the spleen channel, the conception vessel, and the governing vessel.

Tai Chong (LV-3), *Xing Jian* (LV-2), *Qu Quan* (LV-8), *Yang Ling Quan* (GB-34), *Gan Shu* (BL-18), *Dan Shu* (BL-19), *He Gu* (LI-4), *San Yin Jiao* (SP-6), *Hui Yin* (CV-1), *Zhong Ji* (CV-3)

Warm the Liver and Dissipate Cold

Warming the liver and dissipating cold means to dissipate cold evil from the liver channel and to warm and promote the orderly reaching and free coursing of yang qi within the liver channel and viscera. The natural outcome of this treatment principle is that qi and blood flows smoothly through the male anterior yin region.

Cold stagnating in the liver channel is an important pattern to be aware of as a cause of andrological conditions which exhibit signs such as lesser abdominal hypertonicity and pain, testicular pain and distention, internal retraction of the penis and genitals, cold genitals, and cold mounting.

Chinese medicinals

Very commonly, cold evil lodges in the liver channel when it takes advantage of liver blood or liver yang vacuity. The guiding formula for warming the liver channel, supplementing the liver and kidneys, and moving qi and stopping pain is *Nuan Gan Jian* (Liver-Warming Brew).

Nuan Gan Jian (Liver-Warming Brew)
Dang Gui (Angelicae Sinensis Radix)
Gou Qi Zi (Lycii Fructus)
Xiao Hui Xiang (Foeniculi Fructus)

Rou Gui (Cinnamomi Cortex)
Wu Yao (Linderae Radix)
Chen Xiang (Acquilariae Lignum)
Fu Ling (Poria)

Acumoxa therapy

When using acumoxa therapy for warming the liver and dissipating cold, we usually select points from the liver channel, the kidney channel, the spleen channel, the bladder channel, the governing vessel, and the conception vessel.

Da Dun (LV-1), *Tai Chong* (LV-3), *Qu Quan* (LV-8), *Li Gou* (LV-5), *Tai Xi* (KI-3), *Fu Liu* (KI-7), *San Yin Jiao* (SP-6), *Gan Shu* (BL-18), *Ming Men* (GV-4), *Hui Yin* (CV-1), *Zhong Ji* (CV-3), *Guan Yuan* (CV-4)

Quicken the Blood and Transform Stasis

To quicken the blood and transform stasis is to resolve and dissipate static blood; hence, by applying this treatment method, we aim to remove static blood from within the channels and network vessels, the viscera and bowels, and from anywhere else within the bodily form. In andrological diseases, static blood is usually caused by one or more of the following factors: 1) lodged damp-heat; 2) traumatic injury or; 3) enduring unresolved diseases in which there is heat, qi vacuity, or blood vacuity. The signs of stoppage and abiding of static blood include scrotal swelling, roughness and pain within the penis, swelling and hardness of the testes, enlargement of the prostate, yang wilt, infertility, and rigid center.

Chinese medicinals

Commonly used formulas include *Tao Hong Si Wu Tang* (Peach Kernel and Carthamus Four Agents Decoction), *Xue Fu Zhu Yu Tang* (House of Blood Stasis-Expelling Decoction), and *Di Dang Tang* (Dead-On Decoction).

Tao Hong Si Wu Tang (Peach Kernel and Carthamus Four Agents Decoction)
Tao Ren (Persicae Semen)
Hong Hua (Carthami Flos)
Dang Gui (Angelicae Sinensis Radix)
Chuan Xiong (Chuanxiong Rhizoma)
Chi Shao (Paeoniae Radix Rubra)
Sheng Di Huang (Rehmanniae Radix)

Xue Fu Zhu Yu Tang (House of Blood Stasis-Expelling Decoction)
Tao Ren (Persicae Semen)
Hong Hua (Carthami Flos)
Dang Gui (Angelicae Sinensis Radix)
Chuan Xiong (Chuanxiong Rhizoma)
Chi Shao (Paeoniae Radix Rubra)
Sheng Di Huang (Rehmanniae Radix)

Niu Xi (Achyranthis Bidentatae Radix)
Jie Geng (Platycodi Radix)
Chai Hu (Bupleuri Radix)
Zhi Ke (Aurantii Fructus)
Gan Cao (Glycyrrhizae Radix)

Di Dang Tang (Dead-On Decoction)
Shui Zhi (Hirudo)
Meng Chong (Tabanus)
Tao Ren (Persicae Semen)
Da Huang (Rhei Radix et Rhizoma)

In andrology—and indeed in general practice as well—static blood is usually the result of some combination of qi stagnation, damp-heat, qi vacuity, and/or cold congelation. Therefore, in many cases of blood stasis, in addition to directly quickening the blood and transforming stasis, we use the treatment principles of rectifying qi, clearing heat and disinhibiting dampness, supplementing the spleen and kidney qi, freeing the network vessels and warming the liver channel and dissipating cold to improve clinical results. Many of the formulas we use for treating blood stasis already embody some of these other treatment principles in the form of one or two medicinals. For more complex cases, however, it is usually necessary to modify the guiding formulas by adding medicinals aimed at these other treatment goals.

Acumoxa therapy

For quickening blood and transforming stasis in andrology, we usually select points from the spleen channel, the stomach channel, the bladder channel, and the conception vessel.

San Yin Jiao (SP-6), *Di Ji* (SP-8), *Shang Ju Xu* (ST-37), *Xia Ju Xu* (ST-39), *Da Zhu* (BL-11),[3] *Ge Shu* (BL-17), *Hui Yin* (CV-1), *Zhong Ji* (CV-3), *Guan Yuan* (CV-4)

Transform Phlegm and Soften Hardness

When we transform phlegm and soften hardness, we free the qi dynamic,[4] fortify the spleen in its movement and transformation of water-damp, and dissipate swellings and lumps. When there are conditions such as testicular phlegm node (scrotal mass), yin stem phlegm node (Peyronie's disease), scrotal swelling, prostatic hyperplasia, and lumps and swellings anywhere else in the male anterior yin region, this treatment principle can be used.

---

[3] ST-37, ST-39, and BL-11 are points ascribed to the sea of blood; hence they may be used for all disorders of the blood.

[4] Pertains to any of four aspects of the normal movement of qi—upbearing, downbearing, exit, and entry.

Depending on the particular case, this treatment principle takes on the more specific forms of warming and dissipating cold and transforming phlegm, clearing heat and transforming phlegm, and softening hardness and dissipating binds. Commonly, enduring spleen vacuity and splenic movement and transformation failure has led to the collection of water-damp and to the mutual binding of turbid phlegm and qi. In such cases, we must additionally supplement the spleen and move qi to transform phlegm.

Chinese medicinals

Commonly used guiding formulas include *Er Chen Tang* (Two Matured Ingredients Decoction), *Xiao Luo Wan* (Scrofula-Dispersing Pill), and *Yang He Tang* (Harmonious Yang Decoction). *Er Chen Tang* is of course the quintessential formula for transforming turbid phlegm and comprises the base formula for many other phlegm-transforming formulas. *Xiao Luo Wan* embodies the principle of softening hardness and as such is a good model for practitioners to keep in mind when needing to use this method. When combined with other phlegm-transforming formulas, *Yang He Tang* is used when there is phlegm due to cold congelation due to cold evil taking advantage of yang debility and blood vacuity.

Er Chen Tang (Two Matured Ingredients Decoction)
   Ban Xia (Pinelliae Rhizoma)
   Ju Hong (Citri Reticulatae Exocarpium Rubrum)
   Fu Ling (Poria)
   Gan Cao (Glycyrrhizae Radix)

Xiao Luo Wan (Scrofula-Dispersing Pill)
   Xuan Shen (Scrophulariae Radix)
   Mu Li (Ostreae Concha)
   Bei Mu (Fritillariae Bulbus)

Yang He Tang (Harmonious Yang Decoction)
   Shu Di Huang (Rehmanniae Radix preparata)
   Rou Gui (Cinnamomi Cortex)
   Ma Huang (Ephedrae Herba)
   Lu Jiao Jiao (Cervi Cornus Gelatinum)
   Bai Jie Zi (Sinapis Semen)
   Jiang Tan (Zingiberis Rhizoma Carbonisatus)
   Gan Cao (Glycyrrhizae Radix)

Acumoxa therapy

To transform phlegm and soften hardness for andrological diseases, we select points from the spleen channel, the stomach channel, the triple burner channel, the liver channel, and the bladder channel.

Tai Bai (SP-3), *Feng Long* (ST-40), *Tian Jing* (TB-10), *Tai Chong* (LV-3), *Qu Quan* (LV-8), *San Jiao Shu* (BL-22), *Pi Shu* (BL-20), *Wei Yang* (BL-39)

Supplementing the Spleen and Boosting Qi

The spleen is the later heaven source of qi, blood, and fluids and later heaven and early heaven have a mutually transforming relationship. Because of the pivotal role of the spleen in providing the source for nourishing the entire body, supplementing the spleen and boosting qi has far-reaching implications for normal male functioning. One of the central aspects of this is that when splenic movement and transformation of water and grain essence is functioning at an optimal level, there is more essence available for the kidneys to store because more blood is stored in the liver. Since the liver and kidneys share the same source—meaning in part that liver blood can be stored as kidney essence—the more blood that is created the more kidney essence there will be. The kidney stores essence and governs growth and reproduction and kidney qi transformation governs water metabolism. Kidney essence serves as the early heaven source for engendering qi, blood, and fluids. In short, when we supplement the spleen, we also indirectly supplement the kidneys and encourage them to function better both in terms of storing essence and in governing water metabolism.

The spleen is the later heaven source for engendering blood and blood nourishes the heart and enables it to govern the spirit. Considering the importance of heart blood in normal male emotional life and the role of spirit (*shen*)[5] in the normal physiological functions of a man's anterior yin region, in this context the spleen is yet again revealed as a very important viscus because it provides later heaven essence. This essence is one of the most important substantial foundations for engendering blood. When seen from the perspective of the practitioner of Chinese andrology, when the spleen fails to provide essence of water and grain, the heart-spirit lacks nourishment and the male anterior yin region suffers from a lack of luxuriance (*rong*). So, the treatment principle of supplementing the spleen and boosting qi can be used for conditions such as yang wilt, infertility, chronic prostatitis, andropause, and premature ejaculation.

We have already seen that spleen vacuity and a failure to move and transform water-damp is one of the major causes of turbid dampness and phlegm. Thus, the methods of supplementing the spleen and transforming dampness and phlegm are commonly used in the clinic. This means to provide more power to splenic movement and transformation and to eliminate any turbid dampness and phlegm that has accumulated as a result of this failed function. For a list of conditions this method is used for, look under the heading Transform Phlegm and Softening Hardness (p. 130).

Chinese medicinals

Commonly used formulas for spleen qi vacuity and nonluxuriance are *Gui Pi Tang* (Spleen-Returning Decoction) and *Ren Shen Yang Rong Tang* (Ginseng Construction-Nourishing Decoction). In such cases, we usually add medicinals

---

[5] For further discussion of the context in which I use the term spirit (*shen*) here, see the heart section of Book 1, Chapter 4 on the viscera and bowels (p. 58).

to either warm and supplement kidney yang, enrich and nourish kidney yin, or to nourish and enrich kidney essence as necessary.

Gui Pi Tang (Spleen-Returning Decoction)
Ren Shen (Ginseng Radix)
Huang Qi (Astragali Radix)
Bai Zhu (Atractylodis Macrocephalae Rhizoma)
Dang Gui (Angelicae Sinensis Radix)
Suan Zao Ren (Ziziphi Spinosae Semen)
Long Yan Rou (Longan Arillus)
Yuan Zhi (Polygalae Radix)
Fu Ling (Poria)
Mu Xiang (Aucklandiae Radix)
Gan Cao (Glycyrrhizae Radix)

Ren Shen Yang Rong Tang (Ginseng Construction-Nourishing Decoction)
Ren Shen (Ginseng Radix)
Huang Qi (Astragali Radix)
Bai Zhu (Atractylodis Macrocephalae Rhizoma)
Dang Gui (Angelicae Sinensis Radix)
Bai Shao (Paeoniae Radix Alba)
Shu Di Huang (Rehmanniae Radix preparata)
Rou Gui (Cinnamomi Cortex)
Fu Ling (Poria)
Ju Pi (Citri Reticulatae Pericarpium)
Wu Wei Zi (Schisandrae Fructus)
Yuan Zhi (Polygalae Radix)
Gan Cao (Glycyrrhizae Radix)

We use formulas such as *Liu Jun Zi Tang* (Six-Gentlemen Decoction), *Xiang Sha Liu Jun Zi Tang* (Costusroot and Amomi Six Gentlemen Decoction), and *Shen Ling Bai Zhu San* (Ginseng, Poria, and Atractylodis Powder) as guiding formulas when splenic movement and transformation failure leads to phlegm and turbid dampness. When treating these cases, we also warm and supplement kidney yang, transform bladder qi, and disinhibit water as necessary.

Liu Jun Zi Tang (Six Gentlemen Decoction)
Ren Shen (Ginseng Radix)
Bai Zhu (Atractylodis Macrocephalae Rhizoma)
Fu Ling (Poria)
Ban Xia (Pinelliae Rhizoma)
Chen Pi (Citri Reticulatae Pericarpium)
Gan Cao (Glycyrrhizae Radix)

Xiang Sha Liu Jun Zi Tang (Costusroot and Amomi Six Gentlemen Decoction) is *Liu Jun Zi Tang* (Six Gentlemen Decoction) with the addition of:
Mu Xiang (Aucklandiae Radix)
Sha Ren (Amomi Fructus)

Shen Ling Bai Zhu San (Ginseng, Poria, and Atractylodis Powder)
Ren Shen (Ginseng Radix)
Bai Zhu (Atractylodis Macrocephalae Rhizoma)
Fu Ling (Poria)
Shan Yao (Dioscoreae Rhizoma)
Lian Zi (Nelumbinis Semen)
Sha Ren (Amomi Fructus)
Jie Geng (Platycodi Radix)
Bai Bian Dou (Dolichoris Semen)
Gan Cao (Glcyrrhizae Radix)

When the spleen is vacuous and center qi falls, the clear essence of water and grain is not borne upward to the lung and heart and water-damp seeps downward into the anterior yin region. This is a complication of spleen qi vacuity and when it develops, we use the treatment principle of boosting qi and upbearing the clear in addition to that of supplementing the spleen and boosting qi. Commonly used medicinals are:
Chai Hu (Bupleuri Radix)
Sheng Ma (Cimicifugae Rhizoma)
Ge Gen (Puerariae Radix)
He Ye (Nelumbinis Folium)

Acumoxa therapy

To supplement the spleen and boost qi, we select points from the spleen channel, the stomach channel, the liver channel, the bladder channel, and the conception vessel.

Tai Bai (SP-3), *San Yin Jiao* (SP-6), *Zu San Li* (ST-36), *Zhang Men* (LV-13), *Pi Shu* (BL-20), *Wei Shu* (BL-21), *Xiao Chang Shu* (BL-27), *Qi Hai* (CV-6), *Zhong Wan* (CV-12), *Shan Zhong* (CV-17)

Astringe Essence and Restrain Urine

When there is insecurity of kidney qi, the essence gate fails to contain essence within the essence chamber, and insecurity of the bladder results in an inability to properly contain urine. This leads to conditions such as seminal emission, seminal efflux, premature ejaculation, nocturia, enuresis, and urinary incontinence. When used along with the appropriate kidney-supplementing medicinals, astringing essence and restraining urine further secures the root by helping kidney qi to perform its containment function in the anterior yin region. In clinical practice, medicinals having this action are usually used together with warming and supplementing kidney yang, enriching and nourishing kidney yin, and nourishing kidney essence.

When treating any kidney disease pattern, we should also keep in mind that the spleen (later heaven) and the kidneys (early heaven) mutually transform. So, when we supplement the spleen, we indirectly supplement the kidneys and vice versa. And since the spleen is the later heaven source for the engenderment of qi, and one of the five physiological functions of qi is containment, also supplementing the spleen in cases where there is efflux and drainage is a sound strategy. Therefore, in clinical practice, astringing essence and restraining urine is often also combined with that of supplementing the spleen and boosting qi.

Chinese medicinals

Commonly used formulas include *Jin Suo Gu Jing Wan* (Golden Lock Essence-Securing Pill), *Gui Zhi Jia Long Gu Mu Li Tang* (Cinnamon Twig Decoction Plus Dragon Bone and Oyster Shell), and *Sang Piao Xiao San* (Mantis Egg-Case Powder). *Jin Suo Gu Jing Wan* is primarily used for astringing essence and is usually combined with other formulas that mainly supplement kidney qi. *Gui Zhi Jia Long Gu Mu Li Tang*, which is also mostly used for astringing essence, was designed by Zhang Zhong-Jing and appeared for the first time in the *Jin Gui Yao Lue Fang Lun* (*Essential Prescriptions of the Golden Coffer*).[6] While its action and composition may not seem directly targeted at supplementing the kidneys and astringing essence, if we are able to see its base formula—*Gui Zhi Tang* (Cinnamon Twig Decoction)—as a supplementing formula, then its applicability here comes into clearer view. Most modern andrology practitioners combine it with kidney-supplementing formulas and medicinals when using it in clinical practice. A distinguishing feature of *Sang Piao Xiao San* is that it not only supplements the kidneys, astringes essence, and restrains urine, but also supplements the heart and promotes interaction between the heart and kidneys. Among these three formulas, it is generally the most frequently used for restraining urine.

Jin Suo Gu Jing Wan (Golden Lock Essence-Securing Pill)
Sha Yuan Ji Li (Astragali Complanati Semen)
Qian Shi (Euryales Semen)
Lian Xu (Nelumbinis Stamen)
Long Gu (Fossilia Ossis Mastodi)
Mu Li (Ostreae Concha)

Gui Zhi Jia Long Gu Mu Li Tang (Cinnamon Twig Decoction Plus Dragon Bone and Oyster Shell)
Gui Zhi (Cinnamomi Ramulus)
Bai Shao (Paeoniae Radix Alba)
Long Gu (Fossilia Ossis Mastodi)
Mu Li (Ostreae Concha)
Sheng Jiang (Zingiberis Rhizoma Recens)
Da Zao (Jujubae Fructus)
Gan Cao (Glcyrrhizae Radix)

Sang Piao Xiao San (Mantis Egg-Case Powder)
Sang Piao Xiao (Mantidis Ootheca)
Yuan Zhi (Polygalae Radix)

---

[6] *Jin Gui Yao Lue Fang Lun* was published during the Eastern Han dynasty.

Shi Chang Pu (Acori tatarinowii Rhizoma)
Long Gu (Fossilia Ossis Mastodi)
Ren Shen (Ginseng Radix)
Fu Shen (Poria Sclerotium Pararadicis)
Dang Gui (Angelicae Sinensis Radix)
Gui Ban (Testudinis Plastrum)

Acumoxa therapy

For astringing essence and restraining urine in andrology, we select points from the kidney channel, the spleen channel, the bladder channel, the conception vessel, and the governing vessel.

Tai Xi (KI-3), *Fu Liu* (KI-7), *San Yin Jiao* (SP-6), *Shen Shu* (BL-23), *Zhi Shi* (BL-52), *Pang Guang Shu* (BL-28), *Zhong Ji* (CV-3), *Guan Yuan* (CV-4), *Yao Yang Guang* (GV-3), *Ming Men* (GV-4)

Warm and Supplement Kidney Qi and Kidney Yang

Debilitated life gate fire is a common cause of male dysfunction. This is because when kidney life gate fire is waning, then the anterior yin cannot be warmed and nourished; under such conditions, male sexual-reproductive and urinary functions are compromised. When there is yang vacuity, cold spontaneously is engendered in the interior, or cold evil can take advantage of vacuity by invading from the exterior.

Warming and supplementing kidney yang can also be described as warming and supplementing the true fire of the lower origin. In this context, the "lower origin" points to the kidneys as the source of all yang qi and therefore all the physiological warming and steaming actions within the entire body. In this light, there are usually systemic signs of kidney yang vacuity, but signs specific to andrology include yang wilt, retracted genitals, cold genitals, withered and retracted testes, small penis, infertility, nocturia, cold-damp scrotum, and urinary frequency.

When warming the yang, we should take care to observe Zhang Jing-Yue's advice when he said: "[To] effectively supplement yin, [one] must seek yin within yang; [to] effectively supplement yang, [one] must seek yang within yin."[7] According to Wang (2003), overly emphasizing warm supplementation when treating kidney yang vacuity can damage yin and cause fire to upbear; this may lead to throat swelling, dryness, and pain, exacerbation of hypertension, burning urination, and hematospermia. Further, since we usually see kidney yang vacuity together with some degree of insufficiency of kidney essence and spleen yang vacuity, we usually add some medicinals to enrich and engender kidney essence and to warm and supplement spleen yang.

---

[7] This idea is found in *Jing-Yue Quan Shu* (*Jing-Yue's Complete Compendium*), published in 1624, during the Ming dynasty.

Chinese medicinals

In the clinical practice of Chinese andrology, because of the close interrelationships among the various physiological aspects of the kidneys, whenever there is kidney vacuity, multiple facets of this problem occur together. For example when there is kidney yang vacuity, there is often also insecurity of kidney qi, collection of evil water, and kidney essence vacuity; when there is kidney yin vacuity, there is often also kidney essence vacuity, etc. The question becomes not whether or not one aspect of kidney vacuity will occur with another aspect, but more which aspects are occurring together. And following logically from this, the clinician's job becomes matching treatments with the unique combination of these factors for each specific case. I believe this also accounts for some of the overlap in strategy among different kidney supplementing formulas—explaining why for example interior-warming, essence-enriching, damp-draining, and essence-securing medicinals are often used together in a given kidney-supplementing formula.

Jin Gui Shen Qi Wan (Golden Coffer Kidney Qi Pill) warms and supplements kidney yang and frees water, *You Gui Wan* (Right-Restoring [Life Gate] Pill) warms and supplements kidney yang and enriches essence-blood, *Wu Zi Yan Zong Wan* (Five-Seed Progeny Pill) supplements and disinhibits kidney qi and enriches essence-blood, and *Gui Lu Er Xian Gao* (Immortal Tortoise Shell and Deerhorn Glue Paste) supplements and boosts kidney qi and strengthens yang, and enriches yin and essence.

Jin Gui Shen Qi Wan (Golden Coffer Kidney Qi Pill)
Fu Zi (Aconiti Radix lateralis preparata)
Rou Gui (Cinnamomi Cortex)
Shu Di Huang (Rehmanniae Radix preparata)
Shan Yao (Dioscoreae Rhizoma)
Shan Zhu Yu (Corni Fructus)
Fu Ling (Poria)
Ze Xie (Alismatis Rhizoma)
Mu Dan Pi (Moutan Cortex)

You Gui Wan (Right-Restoring [Life Gate] Pill)
Shu Di Huang (Rehmanniae Radix preparata)
Shan Yao (Dioscoreae Rhizoma)
Shan Zhu Yu (Corni Fructus)
Gou Qi Zi (Lyci Fructus)
Tu Si Zi (Cuscutae Semen)
Lu Jiao Jiao (Cervi Cornu Gelatinum)
Du Zhong (Eucommiae Cortex)
Fu Zi (Aconiti Radix lateralis preparata)
Rou Gui (Cinnamomi Cortex)

Wu Zi Yan Zong Wan (Five-Seed Progeny Pill)
Gou Qi Zi (Lycii Fructus)
Tu Si Zi (Cuscutae Semen)

Wu Wei Zi (Schisandrae Fructus)
Fu Pen Zi (Rubi Fructus)
Che Qian Zi (Plantaginis Semen)

Gui Lu Er Xian Gao (Immortal Tortoise Shell and Deerhorn Glue Paste)
Lu Jiao (Cervi Cornu)
Gui Ban (Testudinis Plastrum)
Ren Shen (Ginseng Radix)
Gou Qi Zi (Lycii Fructus)

Acumoxa therapy

For warming and supplementing kidney qi and kidney yang, we select points from the kidney channel, the spleen channel, the bladder channel, the conception vessel, and the governing vessel.

Tai Xi (KI-3), *Fu Liu* (KI-7), *San Yin Jiao* (SP-6), *Shen Shu* (BL-23), *Zhi Shi* (BL-52), *Zhong Ji* (CV-3), *Guan Yuan* (CV-4), *Yao Yang Guang* (GV-3), *Ming Men* (GV-4)

Enrich and Supplement Kidney Yin

This method is used for depletion and vacuity of kidney yin and recovers the fundamental yin-humor. This makes the genitals get softened and nourished and supplements and makes semen full. It treats conditions such as scanty semen, inability to ejaculate, turbid semen, seminal dribbling, dream emission, andropause, and premature ejaculation.

Chinese medicinals

Commonly used formulas include *Liu Wei Di Huang Wan* (Six-Ingredient Rehmannia Pill), which supplements kidney yin, *Zuo Gui Wan* (Left-Restoring [Kidney Yin] Pill) which supplements kidney yin and enriches essence-blood, and *Da Bu Yuan Jian* (Major Origin-Supplementing Brew) which supplements kidney yin and additionally supplements kidney yang as well as qi and blood. Kidney yin vacuity is usually accompanied by hyperactive ministerial fire; when this occurs, we not only enrich yin but also clear heat and drain fire with formulas such as *Da Bu Yin Wan* (Major Yin Supplementation Pill) and *Zhi Bai Di Huang Wan* (Anemarrhena, Phellodendron, and Rehmannia Pill).

Yin supplementing medicinals are enriching and greasy and can therefore obstruct the movement and transformation of the spleen and stomach. When giving such medicinals—and especially when giving them over a long period of time, it is important to add medicinals that fortify the spleen, rectify qi, and transform food stagnation to the formula.

Liu Wei Di Huang Wan (Six-Ingredient Rehmannia Pill)
Shu Di Huang (Rehmanniae Radix preparata)
Shan Yao (Dioscoreae Rhizoma)

Shan Zhu Yu (Corni Fructus)
Fu Ling (Poria)
Ze Xie (Alismatis Rhizoma)
Mu Dan Pi (Moutan Cortex)

Zuo Gui Wan (Left-Restoring [Kidney Yin] Pill)
Shu Di Huang (Rehmmaniae Radix preparata)
Shan Yao (Dioscoreae Rhizoma)
Shan Zhu Yu (Corni Fructus)
Gou Qi Zi (Lycii Fructus)
Chuan Niu Xi (Cyathulae Radix)
Tu Si Zi (Cuscutae Semen)
Lu Jiao Jiao (Cervi Cornus Gelatinum)
Gui Ban Jiao (Testudinis Carapacis et Plastri Gelatinum)

Da Bu Yuan Jian (Major Origin-Supplementing Brew)
Ren Shen (Ginseng Radix)
Shan Yao (Dioscoreae Rhizoma)
Du Zhong (Eucommiae Cortex)
Shu Di Huang (Rehmmaniae Radix preparata)
Dang Gui (Angelicae Sinensis Radix)
Gou Qi Zi (Lycii Fructus)
Shan Zhu Yu (Corni Fructus)
Zhi Gan Cao (Glycyrrhizae Radix cum Liquido Fricta)

Da Bu Yin Wan (Major Yin Supplementation Pill)
Shu Di Huang (Rehmanniae Radix preparata)
Gui Ban (Testudinis Plastrum)
Zhi Mu (Anemarrhenae Rhizoma)
Huang Bai (Phellodendri Cortex)

Zhi Bai Di Huang Wan (Anemarrhena, Phellodendron, and Rehmannia Pill)
Zhi Mu (Anemarrhenae Rhizoma)
Huang Bai (Phellodendri Cortex)
Shu Di Huang (Rehmmaniae Radix preparata)
Shan Yao (Dioscoreae Rhizoma)
Shan Zhu Yu (Corni Fructus)
Fu Ling (Poria)
Ze Xie (Alismatis Rhizoma)
Mu Dan Pi (Moutan Cortex)

Acumoxa therapy

For enriching and nourishing kidney yin, we select points from the kidney channel, the spleen channel, the bladder channel, and the conception vessel.

Ran Gu (KI-2), Tai Xi (KI-3), Zhao Hai (KI-6), San Yin Jiao (SP-6), Shen Shu (BL-23), Zhi Shi (BL-52), Zhong Ji (CV-3), Guan Yuan (CV-4)

Enrich and Replenish Kidney Essence

In order to understand the use of this treatment principle, we have to compre-hend the meaning of kidney essence in this phrase. Consistent with three treas-ures (essence, qi, and spirit) theory, essence is the substantial foundation for all other physiological aspects of the body, and is especially associated with marrow as well as growth and reproduction. This we see reflected in statements of fact such as "the kidney stores essence," "essence engenders marrow and marrow fills the brain," and "the kidneys govern growth and reproduction." In androl-ogy, when we engender kidney essence, we are striving to directly add to the quantity of essence stored in the kidney in order to increase marrow, to encour-age growth and development (including the progression towards puberty), to fill the brain and strengthen weakened sense organs (which are manifestations of brain function in Chinese medicine),[8] to nourish and enrich the male anterior yin region, and to increase the quantity and quality of semen and sperm.

Chinese medicinals

In his much celebrated book *Lin Zheng Zhi Nan Yi An* (*A Clinical Guide with Case Histories*), written in 1766, during the Qing dynasty, Ye Tian-Shi states: "Essence and blood have form. [Therefore do not] use grasses and wood—sub-stances which lack feeling—in order to supplement and boost them; their qi does not correspond [to essence and blood]." This reflects an older idea within Chi-nese medicine—perhaps dating back to the *Nei Jing* (*Inner Canon*)—which as-sumes that in order to engender essence one must use "medicinals with affinity to flesh and blood" (*xue rou you qing zhi pin*). This usually means thick-flavored medicinals and specifically animal products such as *Gui Ban* (Testudinis Plas-trum), *Lu Rong* (Cervi Cornu Pantotrichum), and *E Jiao* (Asini Corii Colla) which have a "flesh and blood" quality. However, some doctors have suggested that this also applies to substances such as *Dong Chong Xia Cao* (Cordyceps) and *Feng Wang Jiang* (Royal Jelly) (Ni, Y.T., personal communication, 1991).

Although the general consensus seems to be that animal products are needed to enrich and replenish essence, we also use certain other thick-flavored plant-based medicinals like *Shu Di Huang* (Rehmanniae Radix preparata) and *Huang Jing* (Polygonati Rhizoma). Further, there is resonance between some seed medicinals (or at least those with the word *zi* in the Chinese name)[9] and essence. Of course, these are medicinals that are otherwise known to supple-

[8] If readers are tempted to judge this assertion as a manifestation of Western medicine and not a premodern notion, they should think again. For establishing a clear understanding of the connec-tion between the brain and the sense organs at the time of the *Nei Jing* (*Inner Canon*), consider chapter 28 of *Ling Shu* (Magic Pivot), which states: "If the upper body qi is insufficient, the brain will be unfilled and the ears will suffer ringing, the head will suffer emptiness, and the eyes will be dizzy," chapter 33 of *Ling Shu*, which states: "Insufficiency of the sea of marrow leads to tin-nitus," and chapter 80 of *Ling Shu* which states: "The essential qi of the five viscera and six bow-els all pour into the eyes and enable sight. [The eye] is joined with the essence of the tendons, bones, blood, and qi which [together] form a system that connects with the brain above."
[9] Many of these are not technically seeds in a modern Western botanical sense.

ment the kidneys and not just any seed. This explains why medicinals such as *Gou Qi Zi* (Lycii Fructus), *Nu Zhen Zi* (Ligustrum Lucidi Fructus), and *Tu Si Zi* (Cuscutae Semen) are used to engender kidney essence.

When there is kidney essence vacuity, there is always vacuity of at least one other major aspect of the kidneys (yin, yang, or qi), so engendering kidney essence is always used together with medicinals that warm and supplement kidney yang, secure and bind kidney qi, or enrich kidney yin as appropriate. *You Gui Wan* (Right-Restoring [Life Gate] Pill) warms and supplements kidney yang and enriches essence-blood, *Jin Suo Gu Jing Wan* (Golden Lock Essence-Securing Pill) secures kidney qi and engenders kidney essence, *Wu Zi Yan Zong Wan* (Five-Seed Progeny Pill) supplements and disinhibits kidney qi and enriches essence-blood, and *Gui Lu Er Xian Gao* (Immortal Tortoise Shell and Deerhorn Glue Paste) supplements and boosts kidney qi and strengthens yang, and enriches yin and essence. *Zuo Gui Wan* (Left-Restoring [Kidney Yin] Pill) supplements kidney yin and enriches essence-blood.

You Gui Wan (Right-Restoring [Life Gate] Pill)
Shu Di Huang (Rehmmaniae Radix preparata)
Shan Yao (Dioscoreae Rhizoma)
Shan Zhu Yu (Corni Fructus)
Gou Qi Zi (Lyci Fructus)
Tu Si Zi (Cuscutae Semen)
Lu Jiao Jiao (Cervi Cornu Gelatinum)
Du Zhong (Eucommiae Cortex)
Fu Zi (Aconiti Radix lateralis preparata)
Rou Gui (Cinnamomi Cortex)

Jin Suo Gu Jing Wan (Golden Lock Essence-Securing Pill)
Sha Yuan Ji Li (Astragali Complanati Semen)
Qian Shi (Euryales Semen)
Lian Xu (Nelumbinis Stamen)
Long Gu (Fossilia Ossis Mastodi)
Mu Li (Ostreae Concha)

Wu Zi Yan Zong Wan (Five-Seed Progeny Pill)
Gou Qi Zi (Lycii Fructus)
Tu Si Zi (Cuscutae Semen)
Wu Wei Zi (Schisandrae Fructus)
Fu Pen Zi (Rubi Fructus)
Che Qian Zi (Plantaginis Semen)

Gui Lu Er Xian Gao (Immortal Tortoise Shell and Deerhorn Glue Paste)
Lu Jiao (Cervi Cornu)
Gui Ban (Testudinis Plastrum)
Ren Shen (Ginseng Radix)

Zuo Gui Wan (Left-Restoring [Kidney Yin] Pill)
Shu Di Huang (Rehmmaniae Radix preparata)

Shan Yao (Dioscoreae Rhizoma)
Shan Zhu Yu (Corni Fructus)
Gou Qi Zi (Lycii Fructus)
Chuan Niu Xi (Cyathulae Radix)
Tu Si Zi (Cuscutae Semen)
Lu Jiao Jiao (Cervi Cornus Gelatinum)
Gui Ban Jiao (Testudinis Carapacis et Plastri Gelatinum)

Acumoxa therapy

For enriching and replenishing kidney essence, we select points from the kidney channel, the spleen channel, the bladder channel, the conception vessel, and the governing vessel.

Tai Xi (KI-3), *Fu Liu* (KI-7), *San Yin Jiao* (SP-6), *Shen Shu* (BL-23), *Zhi Shi* (BL-52), *Gao Huang Shu* (BL-43), *Zhong Ji* (CV-3), *Guan Yuan* (CV-4), *Yao Yang Guang* (GV-3), *Ming Men* (GV-4)

Nourish the Heart and Calm the Spirit

As many male andrological conditions (especially male sexual dysfunction, andropause, and infertility) have emotional causes and ramifications, nourishing the heart and calming the spirit is a very useful treatment principle in the andrology clinic.

For example, I have successfully treated a man with yang wilt from liver depression with depressed heat who also had hyperactive heart fire from depressed liver fire flaming upward and harassing the heart. So, in addition to having yang wilt and being angry and frustrated about it, he also experienced insomnia and had a red-tipped tongue. Although the root pattern was clearly the liver pattern, which called for coursing the liver, rectifying qi, and clearing heat, I also used the treatment principle of nourishing the heart and calming the spirit to good effect.

In cases of male infertility, there is invariably emotional conflict for the man and his partner. Such men often struggle with feelings of inadequacy and even shame about their infertility. These feelings invariably affect the heart and should be factored into a holistic treatment approach. There are many more examples of using the spirit-calming treatment principle in the Chinese andrology case literature.

When we recall that the heart stores the spirit and that spirit directs the physiological activities of the entire body—including a man's anterior yin region—treating the heart for andrological problems makes even more sense.[10] Nourishing the heart and calming the spirit is commonly used to treat either the root or tip pattern in conditions such as seminal efflux, premature ejaculation, yang wilt, andropause, and male infertility.

---

[10] For a further discussion of this perspective on the heart and its role in male physiology, see the heart section in Book 1, Chapter 4 (p. 58).

Chinese medicinals

Very often, we use the spirit-calming method when there is noninteraction of the heart and kidneys. This is because when hyperactive ministerial fire (kidney yin vacuity fire) flames upward it makes the sovereign fire (heart fire) hyperactive. *San Cai Feng Sui Dan Tang* (Heaven, Human, and Earth Marrow- Retaining Elixir) and *Gui Zhi Jia Long Gu Mu Li Tang* (Cinnamon Twig Decoction Plus Dragon Bone and Oyster Shell) are the guiding formulas to treat this pattern. When liver depression with depressed fire flames upward and harasses the heart-spirit, we use *Jia Wei Xiao Yao San* (Supplemented Free Wanderer Powder). And when the spirit is unquiet due to heart-spleen dual vacuity, we use *Gui Pi Tang* (Spleen-Returning Decoction) or *Ren Shen Yang Rong Tang* (Ginseng Construction-Nourishing Decoction).

In each of these scenarios we usually add medicinals to nourish the heart and calm the spirit along with medicinals to settle and calm the spirit if they are not already present in sufficient numbers or strength in the guiding formula. Common choices include:

> *Suan Zao Ren* (Ziziphi Spinosae Semen)
> *Bai Zi Ren* (Biotae Semen)
> *Ye Jiao Teng* (Polygoni multiflori Caulis)
> *Long Gu* (Fossilia Ossis Mastodi)
> *Mu Li* (Ostreae Concha)

When hyperactive heart fire and ministerial fire result in insecurity of the essence gate, securing and binding medicinals such as *Wu Wei Zi* (Schisandrae Fructus) are also added.

San Cai Feng Sui Dan (Heaven, Human, and Earth Marrow-Retaining Elixir)

> *Tian Men Dong* (Asparagi Radix)
> *Shu Di Huang* (Rehmanniae Radix preparata)
> *Ren Shen* (Ginseng Radix)
> *Huang Bai* (Phellodendri Cortex)
> *Sha Ren* (Amomi Fructus)
> *Zhi Gan Cao* (Glycyrrhizae Radix cum Liquido Fricta)

Gui Zhi Jia Long Gu Mu Li Tang (Cinnamon Twig Decoction Plus Dragon Bone and Oyster Shell)

> *Gui Zhi* (Cinnamomi Ramulus)
> *Bai Shao* (Paeoniae Radix Alba)
> *Long Gu* (Fossilia Ossis Mastodi)
> *Mu Li* (Ostreae Concha)
> *Sheng Jiang* (Zingiberis Rhizoma Recens)
> *Da Zao* (Jujubae Fructus)
> *Gan Cao* (Glcyrrhizae Radix)

Jia Wei Xiao Yao San (Supplemented Free Wanderer Powder)

> *Chai Hu* (Bupleuri Radix)

Bo He (Mentha Herba)
Dang Gui (Angelicae Sinensis Radix)
Bai Shao (Paeoniae Radix Alba)
Bai Zhu (Atractylodis Macrocephalae Rhizoma)
Fu Ling (Poria)
Sheng Jiang (Zingiberis Rhizoma Recens)
Mu Dan Pi (Moutan Radix)
Shan Zhi Zi (Gardeniae Fructus)
Gan Cao (Glycyrrhizae Radix)

Gui Pi Tang (Spleen-Returning Decoction)
Ren Shen (Ginseng Radix)
Huang Qi (Astragali Radix)
Bai Zhu (Atractylodis Macrocephalae Rhizoma)
Dang Gui (Angelicae Sinensis Radix)
Suan Zao Ren (Ziziphi Spinosae Semen)
Long Yan Rou (Longan Arillus)
Yuan Zhi (Polygalae Radix)
Fu Ling (Poria)
Mu Xiang (Aucklandiae Radix)
Gan Cao (Glycyrrhizae Radix)

Ren Shen Yang Rong Tang (Ginseng Construction-Nourishing Decoction)
Ren Shen (Ginseng Radix)
Huang Qi (Astragali Radix)
Bai Zhu (Atractylodis Macrocephalae Rhizoma)
Dang Gui (Angelicae Sinensis Radix)
Bai Shao (Paeoniae Radix Alba)
Shu Di Huang (Rehmanniae Radix preparata)
Rou Gui (Cinnamomi Cortex)
Fu Ling (Poria)
Ju Pi (Citri Reticulatae Pericarpium)

Acumoxa therapy

For nourishing the heart and calming the spirit in andrology, we choose points from the heart channel, the pericardium channel, the spleen channel, the stomach channel, the liver channel, the kidney channel, the bladder channel, the conception vessel, and the governing vessel.

Shen Men (HT-7), *Shao Hai* (HT-8), *Jian Shi* (PC-5), *Nei Guan* (PC-6), *Da Ling* (PC-7), *San Yin Jiao* (SP-6), *Feng Long* (ST-40), *Xing Jian* (LV-2), *Tai Chong* (LV-3), *Zhu Bin* (KI-9), *Jue Yin Shu* (BL-14), *Xin Shu* (BL-15), *Shen Mai* (BL-62), *Ju Que* (CV-14), *Jiu Wei* (CV-15), *Bai Hui* (GV-14)

Prostatitis

Western Medicine

The term prostatitis refers to various inflammatory conditions of the prostate including acute bacterial prostatitis, chronic bacterial prostatitis, and nonbacterial prostatitis. Acute bacterial prostatitis is suggested when there is abrupt emergence of symptoms accompanied by bacteriuria and/or pyuria. It is relatively easily diagnosed. Making a differential diagnosis for chronic prostatitis, however, is a bit more difficult and requires culture and analysis of specimens of the patient's midstream urine, his urine following prostatic massage, and his prostatic expressate. Based on the presence or absence of bacteria and on the number of leukocytes present, one makes the diagnosis of either chronic bacterial prostatitis, nonbacterial prostatitis, or chronic nonbacterial noninflammatory prostatitis (prostatodynia).

Acute bacterial prostatitis

Acute bacterial prostatitis is an acute infectious disease of the prostate which most often affects young men. However, it may occur at any age, and in older men it is especially prevalent among patients with an indwelling urethral catheter. The symptoms include abrupt onset of urinary urgency, burning and painful micturition, hematuria, fever, chills, perineal and back pain, lower abdominal fullness and pain, malaise, and body aches.

Diagnosis

Upon examination, the prostate gland is tender, edematous, focally or diffusely swollen and indurated, and warm (Beers *et al.*, 1999). The main laboratory findings include pyuria on urinalysis and positive urine culture. The offending pathogen is cultured either from expressed prostatic fluid (though prostate massage is not recommended in acute bacterial prostatitis) or from urine, and is reportedly usually a gram-negative enteric pathogen such as *E. Coli* or *Klebsiella*. According to Schlossberg (2001), acute bacterial prostatitis occurs when there is reflux of infected urine into the prostatic ducts and canaliculi. The possibility of sexual transmission of other agents is also reported. While prostatic massage in these cases usually does yield purulent secretions which can be cultured, it is not advised in acute bacterial prostatitis because it carries the risk of causing bacteremia.

Treatment

Generally, while physicians await for the culture and sensitivity results, they empirically treat with antimicrobial agents such as trimethoprim-sulfamethoxasole, ampicillin, or ciprofloxacin (Hoole *et al.*, 1999). Then they adjust their treatments accordingly when the test results arrive; apparently, this therapy is effective in a high percentage of cases if: 1) the offending organism is sensitive to the chosen drug(s) and; 2) the patient takes his medicine diligently; that is, he takes the proper dosage and completes the entire course of therapy. Fauci *et al.* (1998) posit that drugs such as these—which do not normally readily enter the prostate—are better absorbed by an acutely inflamed prostate and that this accounts for their rapid effectiveness in acute bacterial prostatitis. This fact also sheds light on the relatively disappointing results these drugs yield in chronic bacterial prostatitis. Prostatic abscess develops in some cases and usually requires hospitalization for more aggressive therapy, including but not limited to IV antibiotics and surgical drainage (Greene *et al.*, 1998). General supportive treatments for acute prostatitis include bed rest, hydration, analgesics, sexual activity to reduce prostatic congestion, and stool softeners if constipation or painful defecation develops (Hoole *et al.*, 1999). Of note is that some sources suggest insisting on a 4–6 week course of antimicrobial therapy to prevent the development of chronic bacterial prostatitis.[1]

Chronic bacterial prostatitis

Chronic bacterial prostatitis may be asymptomatic in a certain percentage of patients and thus may be accidentally diagnosed through routine urinalysis during physical examination or during a workup for male infertility. Physical examination of the prostate is normal, though Sobel (2000) reports that it might be indurated. When symptoms are present, they include enduring and recurrent pelvic and perineal distention and pain. Periodically, the infection may spread to the bladder and cause obstructive urinary symptoms including burning and/or urgent urination; hence, according to Fauci *et al.* (1998), chronic bacterial prostatitis should be considered in all middle-aged men with a history of recurrent cystitis.

Diagnosis

Diagnosis is established by culturing one of the same offending organisms that causes acute bacterial prostatitis (often *E. Coli* or *Klebsiella*) from prostatic expressate or from the urine after prostatic massage. The prostate expressate

---

[1] This raises some critical clinical and ethical questions for clinicians of Chinese medicine as well as for patients including: 1) Is the cost-benefit analysis in favor of antimicrobial therapy in acute bacterial prostatitis?; 2) How does the effectiveness of Chinese medicine for acute bacterial prostatitis compare with that of Western medicine? and; 3) Should Chinese medicine be considered a primary or complementary therapy for acute prostatitis?

usually also contains an elevated number of polymorphonuclear lymphocytes (PMNs) just as in chronic nonbacterial prostatitis.

Treatment

Treatment requires long-term administration (perhaps twelve weeks or longer) of the same antimicrobial agents used for acute bacterial prostatitis, though results are not always satisfactory and relapse is common. Nickel *et al.* suggest that prostatic massage used along with antimicrobial therapy improves clinical outcomes, though prostatic massage remains very controversial. Over-the-counter analgesics (NSAIDs) as well as the other comfort measures described for acute bacterial prostatitis (bed rest, warm sitz baths, stool softeners, and sexual activity) are also often recommended. Total prostatectomy is considered the cure for this condition, but due to the significant morbidity associated with it, is only used as a last resort.

Chronic nonbacterial prostatitis

The symptoms of chronic nonbacterial prostatitis are essentially the same as those of chronic bacterial prostatitis. However, while bacteria can be cultured from the prostatic expressate or urine of patients with chronic bacterial prostatitis, none is found in these patients.

Diagnosis

Chronic nonbacterial prostatitis should be considered in patients with chronic pelvic and perineal distention and pain, obstructive voiding, and possibly even sexual dysfunction, whose post-massage urine and prostatic expressate culture negative for bacteria yet contain ≥1000 leukocytes per microliter. There is in fact a specific increase of polymorphonuclear lymphocytes (PMNs) just as that which occurs with chronic bacterial prostatitis.

Treatment

The cause of chronic nonbacterial prostatitis is unknown and there is no generally accepted treatment. While the etiology and therapy for this condition are hotly debated, some authorities suspect an infectious agent (which might be sexually transmitted) and therefore advocate long-term antimicrobial therapy (Sobel, 2000). Comfort measures as listed for chronic bacterial prostatitis are also used.

Chronic nonbacterial noninflammatory prostatitis (prostatodynia)

Men who have prostatitis with chronic pelvic and perineal distention and pain, obstructive voiding, and possibly even sexual dysfunction, but who lack any objective evidence of either bacterial or inflammatory involvement have chronic nonbacte-rial noninflammatory prostatitis.

Diagnosis

The prostatic expressate and post-massage urine cultures negative and does not contain an elevated number of leukocytes.

Treatment

As the causative agent is unknown, and as there is neither infection nor inflammation, there is no specific therapy for chronic nonbacterial noninflammatory prostatitis. Comfort measures should be recommended as listed for the other types of prostatitis. Due to the chronic relapsing and therefore frustrating nature of this condition, some patients find solace in support groups and stress reduction therapies and use complementary medicine.

Western Complementary Medicine

Due to the questionable effectiveness of conventional treatments for chronic prostatitis, and to the frustrating nature of the symptoms, many patients seek complementary treatments. In addition to sitz baths (sometimes with herbs) and self-administered prostatic massage, some patients also take various vitamin and antioxidant supplements as well as phytotherapy products, avoid certain foods such as caffeine, alcohol, and spicy foods, receive acupuncture, and practice meditation in an attempt to relieve their symptoms. Recent studies suggest that doing pelvic floor strengthening exercises can reduce the symptoms of patients with chronic noninflammatory nonbacterial prostatitis by 50% (Potts and Fynn). Further, according to Shoskes *et al.* (1999), a proprietary brand of Quercitin (a bioflavonoid naturally occurring in red wine, onions, and green tea) taken at 500 mg/twice a day for one month was found to reduce the symptoms of chronic nonbacterial prostatitis by 25% in a statistically significant number of patients.

Chinese Medicine

Disease discrimination

When we deduce premodern Chinese disease categories from the signs and symptoms of prostatitis, we find the closest matches in strangury (*lin zheng*),[2] white turbidity (*bai zhuo*), essence-turbidity (*jing zhuo*), and dribbling urinary block (*long bi*).[3] The clinical features of the damp-heat patterns or "damp toxin" (*shi du*) patterns of these diseases correspond quite closely with the symptoms of acute bacterial prostatitis, and the taxation and qi vacuity patterns relate to the symptoms of chronic prostatitis. In a relatively small number of cases, the patterns of unctuous strangury (*gao lin*) and bloody strangury (*xue lin*) may also be useful.

---

[2] In Bensky and Gamble (1986), this disease category is translated as "painful urinary dysfunction." Maciocia (1994) utilizes the term "painful urination syndrome." We should be clear that this is an important clinical reference point for patients who suffer urinary discomfort and pain. The biomedical correlates of strangury include—but are not limited to—prostatitis, cystitis, urethritis, and nephritis.

[3] This Chinese disease category has received little attention in Western texts on Chinese internal medicine but appears in standard Chinese texts on the subject. Wu and Fischer (1997) do mention it, but the coverage is rather cursory.

These Chinese disease entities provide a conceptual and clinical structure around which to organize a Chinese medical approach to prostatitis. They apply not only to the diagnosis of prostatitis, but also to its pathomechanisms, treatment, and prognosis. Hence, it is within the premodern writings on these disease categories that we modern Chinese doctors find the empirical basis for our diagnosis and treatment of prostatitis, which we can apply and evaluate in the modern clinic and in research settings.

The earliest-known mention of strangury in premodern literature occurs in chapter 71 of *Su Wen* (*Plain Questions*);[4] in this passage, it is known as strangury stoppage (*lin bi*). In chapters 11 and 13 of *Jin Gui Yao Lue Fang Lun* (*Essential Prescriptions of the Golden Coffer*),[5] Zhang Zhong-Jing refers to it as strangury-tightness (*lin bi*) and as strangury (*lin*). The most commonly quoted passage occurs in chapter 13—which is devoted to the conditions of dispersion-thirst (*xiao ke*), inhibited urination (*xiao bian bu li*), and strangury (*lin*)—where it states: "[In the] disease of strangury, [one's] urine has the appearance of millet, the lesser abdomen is stringlike and tense, [and there is] pain and tautness within the navel." Hua To, in the *Zhong Zang Jing* (*The Central Treasury Canon*),[6] differentiated several patterns for strangury yet stated that all strangury is characterized by "lack of free flow among the five viscera, disharmony among the six bowels, and glomus (*pi*) and inhibition[7] within the triple burner," and that heat strangury is characterized by "rough voiding of urine which is as red as blood." Further, Chao Yuan-Fang's Sui dynasty classic—*Zhu Bing Yuan Hou Lun* (*On the Origin and Indicators of Disease*)[8]—relates strangury to "lack of free flow within the waterways (*shui dao bu tong*)." Taxation strangury provides a good model for chronic prostatitis. In *Zheng Zhi Hui Bu* (*Supplemental Essays on Patterns and Treatments*)[9] it states: "Taxation strangury occurs immediately after labor. [There is pain] referring to the qi thoroughfare. It is also called vacuity strangury." These premodern references demonstrate that the main clinical features of strangury are caused by stoppage, inhibition, and lack of free flow which leads to painful and inhibited micturition. Since these symptoms are often present in men with prostatitis, strangury serves as one of the clinical templates for its Chinese diagnosis and treatment.

---

[4] *Su Wen* is the first section of the *Huang Di Nei Jing* (*Yellow Emperor's Inner Canon*), which was published in the 1st century CE, during the Eastern Han dynasty.

[5] *Jin Gui Yao Lue Fang Lun* was written by Zhang Zhong-Jing and published during the Eastern Han dynasty.

[6] *Zhong Zang Jing* is attributed to Hua To and was published in the second century CE, during the Eastern Han dynasty.

[7] Some texts simply say urinary obstruction (*xiao bian bi sai*)

[8] *Zhu Bing Yuan Hou Lun* (*On the Origin and Indicators of Disease*) was written by Chao Yuan-Fang during the Sui dynasty around 610 C.E.

[9] *Zheng Zhi Hui Bu* (*Supplemental Essays on Patterns and Treatments*) was written by Li Yong-Cui and published in 1687, during the Qing dynasty.

In the process of looking for resonance between Western medicine and Chinese medicine for prostatitis, we must also investigate the disease categories of white turbidity (*bai zhuo*) and essence turbidity (*jing zhuo*) (Cheung, 1992 and 1994). According to Wiseman and Feng (1998), white turbidity is a condition characterized by "discharge of a murky white substance from the urethra, associated with inhibited urination with clear urine," and essence turbidity is characterized by "persistent discharge from the urethra like rice water or like flower and water paste"; additionally, there may be "pain like the cutting of a knife or like a burning fire." As prostatitis may present with these symptoms, we should not overlook these Chinese disease categories.

Dribbling urinary block (*long bi*) is actually an amalgam of what were originally two urinary diseases—dribbling (*long*) and block (*bi*). An early reference to these conditions is found in chapter 8 of the *Su Wen* (*Plain Questions*), which states: "[Concerning the] triple burner...repletion causes blockage and dribbling and vacuity causes enuresis. Enuresis requires supplementation; blockage and dribbling require drainage." *Zhu Bing Yuan Hou Lun* (*On the Origin and Indicators of Disease*) states: "Urinary stoppage is due to bladder and kidney heat...heat enters the bladder; great exuberance of hot qi leads to binding, roughness, and urinary stoppage." In *Xie Ying Lu Yi An* (*Xie Ying-Lu's Case Histories*),[10] we find the following reference: "[Whether or not] urination is free-flowing or stopped-up is completely dependent on [whether or not] qi is transforming."

From reading these premodern references, the themes of heat and stoppage emerge as central issues in Chinese-defined diseases which have symptoms similar to acute bacterial prostatitis.

Although Chinese medicine does not have a disease known as prostatic abscess, Ma and An (2001) cite references to two diseases in the premodern literature which are reasonable correlates—suspended welling-abscess (*xuan yong*) and crotch-boring eruption (*chuan dang fa*). Although discussions of suspended welling-abscess first appeared in the Ming dynasty, it is noteworthy that this disease also appears in the Qing dynasty imperial compilation *Yi Zong Jin Jian* (*The Golden Mirror of Orthodox Medicine*).[11] The pathomechanisms for these diseases offered in these texts emphasize the role of damp-heat, depression, heat toxin, and rotting of healthy tissue. It is also interesting to note that these diseases are logically organized under the heading of external medicine (*wai ke*) in the premodern literature.

Disease causes and pathomechanisms

In Chinese medicine, the primary disease mechanism in acute bacterial prostatitis

---

[10] Publication date unknown.

[11] *Yi Zong Jin Jian* is an imperial medical compilation ordered by the Qing emperor and published in 1742. It represents one of a series of efforts undertaken by the Chinese government at different times during the history of Chinese medicine aimed at codifying and standardizing medical curriculum and practice.

is brewing and binding of damp-heat.[12] However, it is not uncommon to see patients who have an acute bacterial prostatitis superimposed upon a background of chronic prostatitis. In such cases, while the repletion-tip (damp-heat, heat toxin, and qi stagnation and blood stasis) is the clinical priority, one should consider the root-vacuity (usually spleen-kidney qi vacuity) when determining choice and dosages of medicinals, and duration of therapy. In acute bacterial prostatitis, heat toxin, blood heat, and blood stasis and qi stagnation often arise as complications of the brewing and binding of damp-heat.

In summary, in acute prostatitis the main disease causes are damp-heat, heat toxin, blood heat, and qi stagnation and blood stasis. In chronic prostatitis, while repletion factors are often present, spleen and kidney vacuity are invariably present in varying degrees in the same patient. A common set of patterns in these patients is damp-heat harassing the essence chamber, liver depression and qi stagnation, blood stasis, and spleen and kidney vacuity. These disease causes and pathomechanisms are explained further below.

• Brewing and binding of damp-heat

This pattern is caused by eating rich, greasy, spicy, and roasted foods as well as by drinking large amounts of alcohol. Such dietary indiscretions damage the spleen and stomach and cause loss of splenic movement and transformation; this leads to the internal engenderment of water-dampness. Enduring depressed dampness transforms heat which then combines with dampness and forms the complex of damp-heat. Additionally, damp-heat may also come about as a result of fire transforming from depression of the seven affects. For example, hyperactive heart or liver fire from emotional upset may conduct downwards to the anterior yin through the small intestine or liver channel. There, it scorches and decocts local physiological fluids into evil damp-heat. External contraction of damp-heat fire toxin is usually associated with poor hygiene and/or sexual transmission. In all of these cases—regardless of its origin—damp-heat binds and brews in the essence chamber (*i.e.*, the prostate) and in the bladder, obstructs triple burner and bladder qi transformation, and inhibits the waterways.

• Heat toxin and blood heat

The classic symptoms and signs of heat toxin (or fire toxin if more severe) in Chinese medicine are redness, sensations of heat, swelling, pain, and pus. In acute bacterial prostatitis, depressed heat and fire-toxin evil in the essence chamber scorches and vanquishes blood and may rot healthy tissue. This pathomechanism creates blood stasis as well as pus and bleeding, just as it does in the formation of any welling-abscess, no matter where it is located.

As discussed previously, prostatic abscess—a clear example of fire toxin—is a potential complication of acute bacterial prostatitis. Although cases without prostatic abscess comprise less dramatic examples of heat toxin, the swelling

---

[12] The main disease mechanisms in chronic prostatitis involve root vacuity (kidney vacuity; very often spleen-kidney vacuity) and tip repletion (damp-heat, blood stasis, and qi stagnation; very often all three).

and heat sensations that are almost universally present in acute bacterial prostatitis still suggest heat toxin (albeit milder than in welling-abscess) as well as blood stasis and blood heat. We should recognize these factors and treat accordingly. It is important to note that fire toxin may either attack from the exterior and then directly strike the essence chamber or it may transform from internally-engendered depressed damp-heat.

• Qi and blood stasis and stagnation

Qi and blood stasis and stagnation in the anterior yin can either arise directly or indirectly. Direct causes include external trauma to the lower abdomen or perineal region, and sitting, driving, or riding a bicycle for long periods of time. Direct trauma—such as that which might occur during sporting activities like football or baseball—damages the channels and network vessels and obstructs the free flow of qi and blood in and around the prostate. And pressure placed on the perineum and buttocks by prolonged sitting, driving, or riding also impairs local free flow of qi and blood. Indirect causes of stasis and stagnation include other evils and their related pathomechanisms such as dampness, heat, and phlegm.

When there is dampness and heat brewing and binding in the anterior yin, dampness—a yin evil—obstructs qi transformation, and heat—a yang evil—scorches blood and fluids. This combination of depressed dampness and qi and blood stagnation also inflames ministerial fire and leads to further heat.[13] Additionally, environmental contraction of cold damp evil may also result in this pattern. Depressed cold and damp evils give rise to damp-natured greasy stagnation which obstructs the flow of qi and blood within the reverting yin liver channel and in its associated network vessels.

As we recall the guidance of the Jin-Yuan physician Zhu Dan-Xi,[14] we are reminded that any of the six depressions can mutually transform into one another. Hence, we should have no trouble seeing the mutually-transforming relationship between damp-heat and qi stagnation and blood stasis, which are

---

[13] As an aside, this can legitimately be called a repletion pathomechanism of the kidney, as long as we shed the assumption that there is no such thing as repletion of the kidney. The influential Song dynasty physician Qian Yi, in his pediatric text called *Xiao Er Yao Zheng Zhi Jue* (*Key to Diagnosis and Treatment of Children's Diseases*), stated: "The kidney governs vacuity; [it has] no repletion." This statement became the locus classicus for later doctors' assertions that there can be no repletion pathomechanisms of the kidney. However, a closer look at the wider breadth of texts preceding the Song reveals discussions of damp-heat brewing in the kidney, cold-dampness affecting the kidney, blood stasis obstructing the kidney, and wind evil invading the kidney—all repletion pathomechanisms (Wang, 2001).

[14] Zhu Dan-Xi was the last of the Four Great Masters of the Jin-Yuan dynasties (*Jin Yuan Si Da Jia*). While he is most noted for his theories on the prevalence of yin vacuity as reflected in his statement "yang is often in superabundance and yin is often insufficient," his contributions far exceed this narrow understanding of his work. For a presentation of his approach to spleen-stomach disease, see Ni and Damone (1992).

the two primary factors in acute bacterial prostatitis and the two ever-present secondary factors in chronic prostatitis. It is also important to note that according to Zhu Dan-Xi, among the six depressions, qi depression is primary.

• Spleen and kidney vacuity and detriment

In conditions such as chronic prostatitis, unresolved damp-heat consumes and damages right qi. Moreover, aging, enduring disease and bodily weakness, overtaxation, sexual intemperance (including excessive masturbation), and sexual taxation while under the influence of alcohol or drugs can all lead to depletion and vacuity of the spleen and kidney. The presence of spleen and kidney vacuity helps to explain why in chronic prostatitis, symptoms such as abdominal distention and pain, fatigue, soreness and weakness of the lumbus and knees, yang wilt, seminal emission, and premature ejaculation often occur. Furthermore, due to spleen and kidney vacuity—and by extension right qi vacuity—evils such as damp-heat and toxin are more likely to invade and lead to either acute prostatitis or to an acute exacerbation within the course of chronic prostatitis.

Spleen qi vacuity leads to movement and transformation failure and depression of the resulting dampness leads to phlegm and damp-heat. Once damp-heat forms in the center burner it may pour downward into the lower burner and obstruct bladder and kidney qi transformation. As a yin evil, phlegm obstructs free flow and thus leads to qi stagnation and blood stasis, and may also transform heat. Further, center qi fall—a complication of spleen qi vacuity—leads to chaotic qi dynamic[15] in that the clear is not borne upward and the turbid is not borne downward and therefore to inefficient expulsion of urine by underpowered lung, bladder, triple burner, and kidney qi transformation. This explains the various urinary complaints of the patient with chronic prostatitis. Depletion and vacuity of kidney qi and insecurity of the lower origin result in an inability to process humor (*ye*), which drains downward and mixes with urine and makes it murky and turbid. This is characteristic of the pattern of unctuous strangury (*gao lin*) and remains a good model for the evaluation of chronic prostatitis with penile discharge. When depletion and vacuity of kidney yin results in vacuity fire which scorches the network vessels in the essence chamber (*i.e.*, the prostate), the semen may contain blood. This provides an explanation for the hematospermia sometimes reported by men with acute or chronic prostatitis.

Pattern discrimination

Acute bacterial prostatitis

I. Damp-heat pouring downward

Main symptoms: Acute onset of frequent, urgent, and painful urination, possible hematuria, a scorching sensation in the urethra, yellowish-red or cloudy urine, drooping distention and pain of the perineum, scrotal dampness, possible heat effusion and aversion to cold, soreness of the body and cumbersome

---

[15] Any discussion of chaotic qi dynamic pertains to failures of upbearing, downbearing, exit, or entry.

limbs, enlarged painful prostate on palpation, red tongue with slimy yellow fur, and wiry slippery rapid pulse.

Treatment principles: Clear heat and disinhibit dampness, free strangury and resolve toxicity

Guiding formula: Modified *Ba Zheng San* (Eight Corrections Powder)

Ingredients:
Mu Tong (Akebiae Trifoliatae Caulis), 10g
Qu Mai (Dianthi Herba), 12g
Bian Xu (Polygoni Avicularis Herba), 12g
Che Qian Zi (Plantaginis Semen), 15g
Hua Shi (Talcum), 12g
Gan Cao (Glycyrrhizae Radix), 6g
Da Huang (Rhei Radix et Rhizoma), 6g
Deng Xin Cao (Junci Medulla), 12g
Jin Yin Hua (Lonicerae Flos), 30g
Lian Qiao (Forsythiae Fructus), 15g
Bai Jiang Cao (Patriniae Herba), 15g
Bai Hua She She Cao (Oldenlandiae Diffusae Herba), 15g
Hu Zhang (Polygoni Cuspidati Rhizoma), 12g
Shan Zhi Zi (Gardeniae Fructus), 10g
Long Dan Cao (Gentianae Radix), 10g

Modifications: For hematuria, add *Bai Mao Gen* (Imperatae Rhizoma), 15g, *Xiao Ji* (Cirsii Herba), 15g, *Sheng Qian Cao Gen* (Rubiae Radix Crudum), 12g, and *Sheng Pu Huang* (Typhae Pollen Crudum), 12g. For severe pain, add *Yan Hu Suo* (Corydalis Rhizoma), 12g, *Chuan Lian Zi* (Toosendan Fructus), 12g, and *Zhi Ru Xiang* (Olibanum Praeparatum), 9g.

2. Heat toxin congesting

Signs: Signs of the damp-heat pouring downward pattern plus unremitting fever, redness, swelling, and heat sensations in the perineum, dribbling and rough micturition or even urinary block (*i.e.*, urinary retention), thirst for cool fluids, constipation, a markedly swollen and hot prostate upon palpation, red tongue with yellow fur, and slippery rapid pulse.

Treatment principles: Clear heat and drain fire, resolve toxicity and disinhibit dampness

Guiding formula: Modified *Long Dan Xie Gan Tang* (Gentian Liver-Draining Decoction)

Ingredients:
Long Dan Cao (Gentianae Radix), 15g
Huang Qin (Scutellariae Radix), 10g
Chai Hu (Bupleuri Radix), 10g

Mu Tong (Akebiae Trifoliatae Caulis), 10g
Ze Xie (Alismatis Rhizoma), 15g
Che Qian Zi (Plantaginis Semen), 15g
Jin Yin Hua (Lonicerae Flos), 12g
Lian Qiao (Forsythiae Fructus), 12g
Pu Gong Ying (Taraxaci Herba), 12g
Bai Hua She She Cao (Oldenlandiae Diffusae Herba), 30g
Bai Jiang Cao (Patriniae Herba), 15g
Tian Hua Fen (Trichosanthis Radix), 12g
Da Huang (Rhei Radix et Rhizoma), 6g

Modifications: For more effulgent heat, add *Shi Gao* (Gypsum Fibrosum), 30g
and *Zhi Mu* (Anemarrhenae Rhizoma), 12g. For cases in which there is pus
forming, add *Bai Zhi* (Angelicae Dahuricae Radix), 12g, *Zao Jiao Ci* (Gleditsiae
Spina), 12g, and *Ru Xiang* (Olibanum), 12g. For cases in which evil heat falls
inward to the construction and blood aspects, use a modification of *Qing Ying
Tang* (Construction-Clearing Decoction) containing the following medicinals:
Shui Niu Jiao (Bubali Cornu), 30g
Sheng Di Huang (Rehmanniae Radix Exsiccata seu Recens), 12g
Xuan Shen (Scrophulariae Radix), 12g
Mai Men Dong (Ophiopogonis Radix), 15g
Jin Yin Hua (Lonicerae Flos), 30g
Dan Shen (Salvia Miltiorrhizae Radix), 20g
Lian Qiao (Forsythiae Fructus), 12g
Huang Lian (Coptidis Rhizoma), 6g
Zhu Ye Xin (Lophatheri Folium Immaturum), 10g
Bai Jiang Cao (Patriniae Herba), 30g
Sheng Gan Cao (Glycyrrhizae Radix Cruda), 6g
Shi Gao (Gypsum Fibrosum), 30g
Zhi Mu (Anemarrhenae Rhizoma), 12g
Tian Hua Fen (Trichosanthis Radix), 12g

Acumoxa therapy for acute bacterial prostatitis

Main points: *Hui Yin* (CV-1), *Zhong Liao* (BL-33), *Yin Ling Quan* (SP-9), *Li
Gou* (LV-5), *Da Dun* (LV-1), *Zhong Ji* (CV-3), *Qi Hai* (CV-6), *Yao Yang Guan*
(GV-3), *Guan Yuan* (CV-4), *Shen Shu* (BL-23), *Ming Men* (GV-4), *Zhi Shi* (BL-
52), *San Yin Jiao* (SP-6), *Zu San Li* (ST-36)

Modifications: For high fever, add *Da Zhui* (GV-14) and *Qu Chi* (LI-11). For
hematuria, add *Xue Hai* (SP-10). For more pronounced urinary frequency and
pain, add *Shui Dao* (ST-28).

Experiential formulas for acute bacterial prostatitis

Clearing heat and drying dampness and clearing heat and resolving toxicity

Ma and An (2001) recommend the following formula (they provide no
specific dosages for the medicinals):

Bai Jiang Cao (Patriniae Herba)
Pu Gong Ying (Taraxaci Herba)
Bai Hua She She Cao (Oldenlandiae Diffusae Herba)
Chuan Xin Lian (Andrographis Herba)
Ya Zhi Cao (Commelinae Herba)
Chi Shao Yao (Paeoniae Radix Rubra)
Da Xue Teng (Sargentodoxae Caulis)
Hu Zhang (Polygoni Cuspidati Rhizoma)
Sheng Da Huang (Rhei Radix et Rhizoma Cruda)
Che Qian Zi (Plantaginis Semen)
Bi Xie (Dioscoreae Hypoglaucae seu Semptemlobae Rhizoma)
Huang Lian (Coptidis Rhizoma)
Huang Bai (Phellodendri Cortex)

Chronic prostatitis

1. Qi stagnation and blood stasis

Signs: Enduring course with the key features of soreness and pain of the lesser abdomen, testes, and lumbus, an obviously painful, unevenly surfaced, but normally-sized and nodular prostate as revealed by digital rectal exam (DRE), low volume or absence of prostatic expressate (but when present often cultures negative), dark tongue body with possible stasis macules, white tongue fur, stringlike slippery or wiry tight pulse.

Treatment principles: Quicken the blood, transform stasis, move qi, stop pain

Guiding formula: Modified *Qian Lie Xian Yan Tang* (Prostatitis Decoction)[16]

Ingredients:
Dan Shen (Saliva Miltiorrhizae Radix), 30g
Chi Shao (Paeoniae Radix Rubra), 12g
Hong Hua (Carthami Flos), 12g
Tao Ren (Persicae Semen), 12g
Ze Lan (Lycopi Herba), 12g
Wang Bu Liu Xing (Vaccariae Semen), 15g
Chuan Shan Jia (Manitis Squama), 15g
Ru Xiang (Olibanum), 12g
Mo Yao (Myrrha), 12g
Yan Hu Suo (Corydalis Rhizoma), 12g
Chuan Lian Zi (Toosendan Fructus), 12g
Bai Zhi (Angelicae Dahuricae Radix), 10g
Qing Pi (Citri Reticulatae Pericarpium Viride), 12g
Pu Gong Ying (Taraxaci Herba), 30g
Bai Jiang Cao (Patriniae Herba), 30g

---

[16] Guo et al. (1999)

Yi Mu Cao (Leonuri Herba), 12g
Hu Zhang (Polygoni Cuspidati Rhizoma), 12g
Jin Qian Cao (Lysimachiae Herba), 30g
Bai Hua She She Cao (Oldenlandiae Diffusae Herba), 30g
Sheng Gan Cao (Glycyrrhizae Radix Cruda), 6g

Modifications: For patients with piercing pain in the perineum, add *Pu Huang* (Typhae Pollen), 12g, *Wu Ling Zhi* (Trogopteri Faeces), 12g, and *Chen Xiang* (Aquilariae Lignum Resinatum), 10g. For a prostate that feels hard and especially nodulated on palpation, add *San Leng* (Sparganii Rhizoma), 12g, *E Zhu* (Curcumae Rhizoma), 12g, and *Zao Jiao Ci* (Gleditsiae Spina), 12g. For rough and painful micturition, add *Hua Shi* (Talcum), 12g, *Bian Xu* (Polygoni Avicularis Herba), 12g, *Qu Mai* (Dianthi Herba), 12g, and *Che Qian Zi* (Plantaginis Semen), 15g.

2. Turbid dampness pouring downward

Signs: Cloudy turbid urine that looks like water in which rice has been washed, discharge of whitish fluid from the urethra either during bowel movement or just prior to urination, relative absence of pain or other discomfort during urination, pale red tongue with slimy fur, soggy pulse.

Treatment principles: Dry dampness and drain turbidity

Guiding formula: Modified *Er Chen Tang* (Two Matured Ingredients Decoction)

Ingredients:
Fa Ban Xia (Pinelliae Rhizoma Praeparatum), 12g
Chen Pi (Citri Reticulatae Pericarpium), 10g
Fu Ling (Poria), 15g
Zhi Gan Cao (Glycyrrhizae Radix cum Liquido Fricta), 6g
Bi Xie (Dioscoreae Hypoglaucae seu Semptemlobae Rhizoma), 20g
Bai Hua She She Cao (Oldenlandiae Diffusae Herba), 30g
Dan Shen (Salviae Miltiorrhizae Radix), 15g
Che Qian Zi (Plantaginis Semen), 15g

Modifications: For those with spleen-stomach damp-heat and damp-heat pouring downward who have turbid urine and a scorching heat sensation in the urethra when urinating, dry mouth and bitter oral taste, slimy yellow tongue fur, and soggy rapid pulse, add *Huang Bai* (Phellodendri Cortex), 12g, *Deng Xin Cao* (Junci Medulla), 10g. Or, use *Bi Xie Fen Qing Yin* (Fish Poison Yam Clear-Turbid Separation Beverage) as the guiding formula instead. In enduring cases with additional signs of spleen vacuity and center qi fall such as fatigue, pale white facial complexion and pale tongue, sloppy stool, and vacuous pulse, combine with *Bu Zhong Yi Qi Tang* (Center-Supplementing Qi-Boosting Decoction).

Bi Xie Fen Qing Yin (Fish Poison Yam Clear-Turbid Separation Beverage)[17]

Bi Xie (Dioscoreae hypoglaucae Rhizoma), 15g
Huang Bai (Phellodendri Cortex), 10g
Shi Chang Pu (Acori tartarinowii Rhizoma), 10g
Fu Ling (Poria), 12g
Bai Zhu (Atractylodis macrocephalae Rhizoma), 12g
Lian Zi Xin (Nelumbinis Plumula), 6g
Dan Shen (Salvia miltiorrhizae Radix), 10g
Che Qian Zi (Plataginis Semen), 15g

Bu Zhong Yi Qi Tang (Center-Supplementing Qi-Boosting Decoction)

Chai Hu (Bupleuri Radix), 6g
Sheng Ma (Cimicifugae Rhizoma), 6g
Ren Shen (Ginseng Radix), 10g
Huang Qi (Astragali Radix), 15g
Bai Zhu (Atractylodis Macrocephalae Rhizoma), 12g
Dang Gui (Angelicae Sinensis Radix), 10g
Chen Pi (Citri Reticulatae Pericarpium), 6g
Zhi Gan Cao (Glycyrrhizae Radix cum Liquido Fricta), 3g

3. Kidney yin vacuity

Signs: Usually occurs in middle-aged men. During bowel movement and just prior to urinating there may be whitish or clear penile discharge. Or, at the initiation of sexual activity, there may be spontaneous discharge of fluid. Other signs include soreness and weakness of the lumbus and knees, five center vexation and heat, insomnia, seminal emission and premature ejaculation, occasional bloody ejaculate, terminal dribbling, and penile pain, normal-sized and only slightly painful prostate on digital examination. Relatively scanty prostatic expressate that sometimes cultures positive for bacteria, red tongue body with white fur, fine slightly rapid pulse.

Treatment principles: Enrich kidney and nourish yin, clear and drain ministerial fire

Guiding formulas: Modified *Zhi Bai Di Huang Wan* (Anemarrhena, Phellodendron, and Rehmannia Pill) and *Da Bu Yin Wan* (Major Yin Supplementation Pill)

Ingredients:
Zhi Mu (Anemarrhenae Rhizoma), 12g
Huang Bai (Phellodendri Cortex), 12g
Shu Di Huang (Rehmanniae Radix Praeparata), 20g
Shan Yao (Dioscoreae Rhizoma), 15g
Shan Zhu Yu (Corni Fructus), 15g

---

[17] Note that this version of the formula derives from *Yi Xue Xin Wu* (*Medical Insights*), written by Cheng Guo-Peng in 1732, during the Qing dynasty.

Fu Ling (Poria), 10g
Ze Xie (Alismatis Rhizoma), 10g
Mu Dan Pi (Moutan Cortex), 10g
Gui Ban (Testudinis Carapax et Plastrum), 20g

Modifications: For patients with insomnia and copious dreaming, red tongue and possible mouth sores due to hyperactive sovereign fire from noninteraction of the heart and kidney, remove *Shu Di Huang* (Rehmanniae Radix Praeparata), and add *Sheng Di Huang* (Rehmanniae Radix Exsiccata seu Recens), 15g, *Dan Zhu Ye* (Lophatheri Herba), 9g, *Gan Cao* (Glycyrrhizae Radix), 6g, and *Niu Xi* (Achyranthis Bidentatae Radix), 10g, to clear the heart and downbear fire, and to conduct the fire downwards. For those with seminal efflux or premature ejaculation, add *Jin Ying Zi* (Rosae Laevigatae Fructus), 15g, *Long Gu* (Mastodi Ossis Fossilia), 30g, and *Mu Li* (Ostreae Concha), 30g, to boost the kidney and secure essence. For those with a slimy yellow tongue fur, remove *Shan Zhu Yu* (Corni Fructus) and add *Cang Zhu* (Atractylodis Rhizoma), 9g, *Yi Yi Ren* (Coicis Semen), 15g, *Niu Xi* (Achyranthis Bidentatae Radix), 10g, *Lu Gen* (Phragmitis Rhizoma), 15g, and *Gan Cao* (Glycyrrhizae Radix), 6g, to eliminate dampness and clear heat.

4. Kidney yang vacuity

Signs: Whitish urethral dribbling at the end of urination, soreness and lack of strength in the lumbus and knees, listlessness and low spirits, hypertonicity of the lower abdomen, cold extremities, frequent urination, dribbling and incomplete urination, and lack of firmness of erection, a relatively small and non-painful prostate upon digital examination, relatively scanty prostatic expressate that often cultures negative and that lacks leukocytes, pale tongue that is enlarged and has tooth marks, thin white fur, fine weak pulse.

Treatment principles: Warm and supplement kidney yang, secure essence and stop turbidity

Guiding formulas: Modified *You Gui Wan* (Right-Restoring [Life Gate] Pill) with *Jin Suo Gu Jing Wan* (Golden Lock Essence-Securing Pill)

Ingredients:
Fu Zi (Aconiti Radix Lateralis Praeparata), 6g
Rou Gui (Cinnamomi Cortex), 6g
Shu Di Huang (Rehmanniae Radix Praeparata), 20g
Shan Yao (Dioscoreae Rhizoma), 15g
Shan Zhu Yu (Corni Fructus), 15g
Gou Qi Zi (Lycii Fructus), 12g
Tu Si Zi (Cuscutae Semen), 15g
Du Zhong (Eucommiae Cortex), 15g
Dang Gui (Angelicae Sinensis Radix), 12g
Sha Yuan Zi (Astragali Complanati Semen), 15g
Qian Shi (Euryales Semen), 15g
Lian Xu (Nelumbinis Stamen), 12g

Duan Long Gu (Mastodi Ossis Fossilia Calcinata), 30g
Duan Mu Li (Ostreae Concha Calcinata), 30g

Modifications: For patients with unsmooth urination, add *Ze Xie* (Alismatis Rhizoma), 10g, *Fu Ling* (Poria), 10g, *Niu Xi* (Achyranthis Bidentatae Radix), 10g, and *Che Qian Zi* (Plantaginis Semen), 12g, to disinhibit urine. For premature ejaculation, add *Fu Pen Zi* (Rubi Fructus), 15g, to further secure essence.

Acumoxa therapy for chronic prostatitis

Main points: *Tai Chong* (LV-3), *Zhi Bian* (BL-54), *Guan Yuan* (CV-4), *Zhong Ji* (CV-3), *Tai Xi* (KI-3), *Hui Yin* (CV-1), *Shen Shu* (BL-23), *San Yin Jiao* (SP-6), *Yong Quan* (KI-1), *Yin Gu* (KI-10), *Ming Men* (GV-4), *Guan Yuan Shu* (BL-26)

Experiential formulas for chronic prostatitis

Clearing heat and drying dampness, enriching kidney yin, and moving qi and quickening blood

For chronic prostatitis with a combination of damp-heat, kidney yin vacuity, and qi and blood stasis and stagnation, use *Qian Lie Xian Yan Tang* (Prostatitis Decoction):[18]

Huang Bai (Phellodendri Cortex)
Shu Di Huang (Rehmanniae Radix Praeparata)
He Huan Pi (Albizziae Cortex)
Tu Fu Ling (Smilacis Glabrae Rhizoma)
Bai Hua She She Cao (Oldenlandiae Diffusae Herba)
Di Long (Pheretima)
Wu Gong (Scolopendra)
Bie Jia (Trionycis Carapax)
Chuan Shan Jia (Manitis Squama)
Huang Qi (Astragali Radix)
Wang Bu Liu Xing (Vaccariae Semen)
Tu Si Zi (Cuscutae Semen)
Nu Zhen Zi (Ligustri Lucidi Fructus)
Bian Xu (Polygoni Avicularis Herba)
Gan Cao (Glycyrrhizae Radix)

Moving qi and quickening blood and transforming stasis

For the qi and blood stasis and stagnation pattern of chronic prostatitis, Tan and Tao (1999) use *Fu Fang Di Hu Tang* (Compounded Earth and Tiger Decoction):

Huang Qi (Astragali Radix)
Yan Hu Suo (Corydalis Rhizoma)
Di Long (Pheretima)
Hu Zhang (Polygoni Cuspidati Rhizoma)
Bai Hua She She Cao (Oldenlandiae Diffusae Herba)

[18] Tan and Tao (1999)

Chuan Shan Jia (Manitis Squama)
Lai Fu Zi (Raphani Semen)
Chi Shao (Paeoniae Radix Rubra)
Ru Xiang (Olibanum)
Mo Yao (Myrrha)
Bian Xu (Polygoni Avicularis Herba)
Gan Cao (Glycyrrhizae Radix)

External treatments for acute and chronic prostatitis

Retention enemas

1. Mix *Jin Huang San* (Golden Yellow Powder),[19] 30g, with a suitable amount of powdered *Shan Yao* (Dioscoreae Rhizoma) to make a thin paste when mixed with 200 ml of water. Heat until warm (40°C) and use as a retention enema solution to be retained in the rectum for as long as 2–4 hours. Use once per day, 14 days comprising one course of therapy. Used for damp-heat and heat toxin patterns.

2. Mix the medicinals listed below with 600 ml of water and decoct down to 100 ml. Use the resulting solution at 40°C once every other day and retain for 2–4 hours, ten days comprising one course of therapy. Used for damp-heat patterns complicated by qi stagnation and blood stasis.
   Da Huang (Rhei Radix et Rhizoma), 15g
   Huang Bai (Phellodendri Cortex), 15g
   San Leng (Sparganii Rhizoma), 10g
   Yu Jin (Curcumae Rhizoma), 10g
   Mao Dong Qing (Ilicis Pubescentis Radix), 30g
   Huang Qi (Astragali Radix), 20g
   Mu Xiang (Aucklandiae Radix), 10g

Sitz bath formulas (Chen and Jiang, 2000)

1. Bathe in plain hot water for 30 minutes 2–3 times per day. This is used for all types of prostatitis, however, it should be avoided by men who have impaired fertility because when the testes are heated spermatogenesis and sperm vitality are impaired.

2. For damp-heat and heat toxin patterns, decoct the medicinals listed below in enough water to yield 1500–2000ml of medicinal solution. Use as a hot sitz bath for 30 minutes once per day.
   Ye Ju Hua (Chrysanthemi Indici Flos), 30g
   Ku Shen (Sophorae Flavescentis Radix), 30g

[19] To make 200g of *Jin Huang San* (Golden Yellow Powder), grind together 25g each of *Da Huang* (Rhei Radix et Rhizoma), *Huang Bai* (Phellodendri Cortex), *Jiang Huang* (Curcumae Longae Rhizoma), and *Bai Zhi* (Angelicae Dahuricae Radix), 12.5g each of *Tian Nan Xing* (Arisaematis Rhizoma), *Chen Pi* (Citri Reticulatae Pericarpium), *Hou Po* (Magnoliae Officinalis Cortex), and *Gan Cao* (Glycyrrhizae Radix), and 50g of *Tian Hua Fen* (Trichosanthis Radix).

Ma Chi Xian (Portulacae Herba), 30g
Bai Jiang Cao (Patriniae Herba), 30g
Yan Hu Suo (Corydalis Rhizoma), 15g
Dang Gui (Angelicae Sinensis Radix), 12g
Bing Lang (Arecae Semen), 10g

3. For damp-heat and heat toxin patterns, decoct the medicinals listed below in enough water to yield 1500–2000 ml of medicinal solution. Use as a hot sitz bath solution for 30 minutes once per day.
Pu Gong Ying (Taraxaci Herba), 30g
Bai Zhi (Angelicae Dahuricae Radix), 30g
Da Huang (Rhei Radix et Rhizoma), 30g
Gan Cao (Glycyrrhizae Radix), 10g
Bi Xie (Dioscoreae Hypoglaucae seu Semptemlobae Rhizoma), 30g

Suppository formula

For heat toxin pattern, use a suppository made from *Ye Ju Hua* (Chrysanthemi Indici Flos) inserted into the rectum to a depth of 2–3 cm, once per day. One month comprises one course of treatment (Chen and Jiang, 2000 and Tan and Tao, D. 1999).

Fumigation and wash formulas

This method consists of placing a basin or pot of steaming decoction (care should be taken to ensure that the temperature of the decoction is not too hot to avoid steam burns) beneath the perineum and using a cloth to repeatedly bathe the perineum and scrotal area with the decoction once per day for 30 minutes.

Fumigation and wash formula #1: For damp-heat, blood stasis, and heat toxin patterns
Ku Shen (Sophorae Flavescentis Radix), 20g
Dang Gui (Angelicae Sinensis Radix), 20g
She Chuang Zi (Cnidii Fructus), 20g
Jin Yin Hua (Lonicerae Flos), 20g
Pu Gong Ying (Taraxaci Herba), 20g
Huang Bai (Phellodendri Cortex), 20g
Hong Hua (Carthami Flos), 10g
Gan Cao (Glycyrrhizae Radix), 10g

Fumigation and wash formula #2: For damp-heat and heat toxin patterns
Long Dan Cao (Gentianae Radix), 20g
Shan Zhi Zi (Gardeniae Fructus), 20g
Huang Qin (Scutellariae Radix), 20g
Huang Bai (Phellodendri Cortex), 20g
Bi Xie (Dioscoreae Hypoglaucae seu Semptemlobae Rhizoma), 20g
Sheng Di Huang (Rehmanniae Radix Exsiccata seu Recens), 20g
Tu Fu Ling (Smilacis Glabrae Rhizoma), 20g
Che Qian Cao (Plantaginis Herba), 20g

Preventive measures and lifestyle modifications _____

1. Rule out primary infections in other regions of the body

Sometimes patients with bacterial prostatitis have a primary infection in another region of their body such as in their tonsils, gums, sinuses, or intestines. Appropriate screening and treatment measures should be explored in recalcitrant cases.

2. Sexual moderation

During an episode of acute bacterial prostatitis, it is better to avoid sexual activity until the symptoms resolve. However, for patients with chronic prostatitis, maintaining normal levels of sexual activity can help to drain the prostate and thus provides some symptomatic relief. In cases where bacterial infection is known or suspected, it is prudent to use a condom to avoid passing the infection to one's partner, but patients with nonbacterial prostatitis do not need to follow this precaution if they are neither trying to prevent pregnancy nor protecting themselves from sexually-transmitted diseases (*i.e.*, if they are in a long-term committed and monogamous relationship with a partner known not to have any sexually-transmitted diseases). Some Chinese authors, including Chen and Jiang (2000) suggest that masturbation could have a deleterious effect on patients with prostatitis, but it is frankly difficult to determine if this negative attitude towards masturbation is culturally or medically driven. Some men, however, do anecdotally report that they notice a distinct difference between the quality of the sexual experience they share with a caring partner in comparison to that experienced alone, in that they find sex with a caring partner more "nurturing" and therefore less "draining."

For men with or without partners, it is prudent to maintain a moderately-paced sexual life, neither emphasizing complete abstinence nor overly frequent activity. Generally speaking, for patients with chronic prostatitis, having sex with ejaculation once or twice per week constitutes a moderate sexual life. Of course, the frequency with which any given man should have sex depends on his age and constitution, and this rate should naturally vary with the season of the year, being slightly less frequent in winter and slightly more frequent in spring and summer. Further, for the health of the prostate it is generally unwise for men to engage in seminal retention practices as these may prevent normal and healthy draining of the prostate and may encourage the development of prostatitis or exacerbate the symptoms of existing prostatitis.

3. Balance activity and rest

To avoid the weakening of right qi and to maintain its ability to resist evils, it is important to avoid overwork, staying up too late at night and becoming sleep-deprived, catching cold, and skipping meals. These are common sense recommendations, but many Western men have not been socialized into taking care of themselves and thus expect their body to perform optimally at all times even without following such basic life-nourishing (*yang sheng*) principles. Success of initial therapy and the maintenance of positive results is at stake.

4. Maintain comfortable and healthy conditions for the pelvic and perineal region

Sitting for long periods of time, riding bicycles excessively, driving for many hours, wearing tight clothing or undergarments, and being immersed in cold water for long periods of time (as during swimming and surfing) all can either directly or indirectly cause stagnation of qi and stasis of blood by placing undue pressure on the local region or by slowing the local flow of qi and blood. It follows logically that men with prostatitis (or those wishing to prevent its occurrence) who sit for long periods should get up frequently to stretch and move about, and should consider the use of pressure-relieving seat "donuts" when practical. Men who ride bicycles should use bike seats equipped with a "prostate relief zone." Avoiding the use of undergarments completely or choosing boxer shorts instead of briefs is also prudent, especially for men who also have impaired fertility. Further, men who surf should take care to keep their bodies and feet warm with thermal protective clothing while surfing.

5. Dietary modifications

As many cases of prostatitis have a repletion component in the form of damp-heat and stasis and stagnation, dietary modification is absolutely necessary in order to achieve and maintain clinical results. Therefore, all foods and beverages which increase dampness or heat should be either avoided completely or severely limited. The usual culprits for damp-heat include alcohol, greasy-fried foods, refined sugars, and dairy products. And patients with damp-heat should also be advised to avoid excessive consumption of spicy-hot or overly-warm and supplementing foods and medicinals such as dishes made with chile peppers, hot salsa, venison, and lamb, and should not take supplementing medicinals such as *Hong Ren Shen* (Ginseng Radix Rubra). Rather, one should adopt a clear-bland (*qing dan*) and balanced diet devoid of the foods implicated above and rich in fresh cooked vegetables, whole grains, legumes, lean meats, poultry, and fish, unsaturated fats and oils, moderate amounts of fresh fruit, etc. For those with chronic prostatitis—which is usually complicated by spleen and kidney vacuity—who lack significant amounts of damp-heat, spleen and kidney nourishing foods such as venison, beef, chicken, and seafood should be included in the diet.

6. Mental outlook

Chronic prostatitis is an enduring condition which requires long-term treatment, is difficult to cure, and may reduce a man's sexual and reproductive capacity; thus, anxiety, depression, and other mood disorders are commonly seen. In terms of Chinese medicine these emotional changes may reflect complex pathomechanisms, but binding depression of liver qi (often with depressed heat harassing the ethereal soul [*hun*]) and heart qi depression with depressed fire agitating the spirit [*shen*]) is usually present; hence, treatment should also be aimed at these patterns. Moreover, the doctor should encourage the patient to persist in pursuing treatment and in maintaining the recommended lifestyle modifications even when clinical results are slow or when relapse occurs. Of key importance is clearly educating the patient about the connection between his life habits and his condition and motivating him to change, which are often not easy tasks. Psychotherapy should also be considered.

Representative Chinese Research

Clearing heat and resolving toxicity, and disinhibiting water and dampness

Zhou *et al.* (1998) reported on the effectiveness of using *Ba Zheng San* (Eight Corrections Powder) in 26 cases of chronic prostatitis. This formula represented an application of the methods of clearing heat and resolving toxicity, and disinhibiting water and dampness. The medicinals used were:

Che Qian Zi (Plantaginis Semen)
Mu Tong (Akebiae Trifoliatae Caulis)
Qu Mai (Dianthi Herba)
Bian Xu (Polygoni Avicularis Herba)
Hua Shi (Talcum)
Shan Zhi Zi (Gardeniae Fructus)
Da Huang (Rhei Radix et Rhizoma)
Gan Cao (Glycyrrhizae Radix)

Results: The control group consisted of 26 patients with chronic prostatitis who took a Western pharmaceutical agent. After treatment, the investigators compared the results of a digital prostate examination in both groups, and found that the treatment group exhibited an 88.5% (23/26) amelioration rate as compared to a 53.8% (14/26) amelioration rate in the control group. In terms of reduction of symptoms, the treatment group experienced a 76.9% (20/26) reduction in symptoms as compared to the control group, which experienced a 53.8% (14/26) reduction in symptoms. Further, the researchers also compared the rate at which the number of leukocytes in the prostatic fluid reduced to below 10/HP and found that the treatment group exhibited such a change at a rate of 53.8% (14/26), while the control group changed at a rate of 30.8% (8/26).

Warming yang and disinhibiting water, and eliminating blood stasis

Zhang (1999) used a self-composed formula to treat 125 cases of chronic prostatitis. The therapeutic methods used in the formula consisted of warming yang and disinhibiting water, and eliminating blood stasis. The ingredients of the formula are:

Yi Zhi Ren (Alpiniae Oxyphyllae Fructus)
Rou Cong Rong (Cistanches Herba)
Bi Xie (Dioscoreae Hypoglaucae seu Semptemlobae Rhizoma)
Shi Chang Pu (Acori Tatarinowii Rhizoma)
Tao Ren (Persicae Semen)
Tu Fu Ling (Smilacis Glabrae Rhizoma)
Chai Hu (Bupleuri Radix)
Bai Shao (Paeoniae Radix Alba)
Chuan Shan Jia (Manitis Squama)
Wang Bu Liu Xing (Vaccariae Semen)

Results: The treatment group consisted of 87 patients who used the formula for one month; they reported an overall amelioration rate of 62.21%.

Coursing the liver and rectifying qi, quickening blood and harmonizing the network vessels, and resolving tetany

For effective treatment of chronic prostatitis, Qin (1999) advocates the use of a standard formula which should be modified according to the pattern. In his formula, he includes the methods of coursing the liver and rectifying qi, quickening blood and harmonizing the network vessels, and resolving tetany. The formula consists of the following medicinals:

Chai Hu (Bupleuri Radix)
Chi Shao (Paeoniae Radix Rubra)
Bai Shao (Paeoniae Radix Alba)
Xiang Fu (Cyperi Rhizoma)
Yu Jin (Curcumae Radix)
Chuan Lian Zi (Toosendan Fructus)
Yan Hu Suo (Corydalis Rhizoma)
Chuan Shan Jia (Manitis Squama)
Lu Lu Tong (Liquidambaris Fructus)
Shui Zhi (Hirudo)
Tao Ren (Persicae Semen)
Hong Hua (Carthami Flos)
Xi Xin (Asari Herba)
Chuan Xiong (Chuanxiong Rhizoma)
Si Gua Luo (Luffae Fructus Retinervus)
Da Huang (Rhei Radix et Rhizoma)

Chinese medicinal enema

Luo and Zhang (1998) reported a 100% effectiveness rate in 96 cases of chronic bacterial prostatitis with the use of a retention enema formula called *Pen Yan Ling* (Pelvic Inflammation Magic Medicine). The ingredients were:

Chi Shao (Paeoniae Radix Rubra)
Yan Hu Suo (Corydalis Rhizoma)
San Leng (Sparganii Rhizoma)
Dang Gui (Angelicae Sinensis Radix)
Wu Yao (Linderae Radix)
Bai Jiang Cao (Patriniae Herba)
Huang Qin (Scutellariae Radix)
Mu Dan Pi (Moutan Cortex)
Gan Cao (Glycyrrhizae Radix)
Xiang Fu (Cyperi Rhizoma)
Da Xue Teng (Sargentodoxae Caulis)

Acumoxa therapy

Using the conception vessel and the bladder channel

Wang *et al.* (2003) reported on the treatment of chronic prostatitis with acumoxa therapy. They compared the effects on patients who received acumoxa therapy with those who received medicinal treatment in 30 patients with chronic prostatitis. The acumoxa points used in the treatment group were organized into two combinations and consisted of: 1) *Zhong Ji* (CV-3), *Guan Yuan* (CV-4), and *Qi Hai* (CV-6) and; 2) *Ci Liao* (BL-32), *Zhong Liao* (BL-33), and *Xia Liao* (BL-34).

Results: The authors reported a 96% amelioration rate in the treatment group as opposed to an 80% effectiveness rate in the control group.

Using the conception vessel, the bladder channel, and the spleen channel

Liu et al (2002) reported a 92.8% overall amelioration rate for acumoxa therapy in the treatment of 28 cases of chronic prostatitis. The points investigated were *Guan Yuan* (CV-4), *Qi Hai* (CV-6), *Shen Shu* (BL-23), *Ci Liao* (BL-32), and *San Yin Jiao* (SP-6).

Representative Case Studies

Liver channel damp-heat and depression obstructing bladder qi transformation

Liu Du-Zhou, in Peng (1998), reported the treatment of one case of presumed acute prostatitis occurring in a 39 year-old male in 1993. The patient had a three-year history of chronic prostatitis and presented with a chief complaint of a sudden protrusion on his left testicle with intense pain that referred upwards into his lesser abdomen. There was also inhibited urination, thirst, and heart vexation; the tongue was enlarged and the tongue fur was white, and the pulse was sinking stringlike. Dr. Liu diagnosed liver channel damp-heat and depression obstructing bladder qi transformation. The treatment principle was to course the liver and disinhibit dampness, and to free yang and disinhibit water. He used a variation of *Hui Lian Wu Ling San* (Fennel and Toosendan Poria Five Powder) with the following ingredients:

Fu Ling (Poria), 30g
Zhu Ling (Polyporus), 16g
Bai Zhu (Atractylodis Macrocephalae Rhizoma), 10g
Ze Xie (Alismatis Rhizoma), 10g
Gui Zhi (Cinnamomi Ramulus), 4g
Chuan Lian Zi (Toosendan Fructus), 10g
Mu Tong (Akebiae Trifoliatae Caulis), 10g
Xiao Hui Xiang (Foeniculi Fructus), 3g
Qing Pi (Citri Reticulatae Pericarpium Viride), 6g
Tian Xian Teng (Aristolochiae Herba), 20g

The patient experienced partial relief of pain after taking one packet of medicine, and after three packets his urination was free-flowing. The condition completely resolved after seven packets.

In his commentary on this case, Dr. Liu informs us that he treated this case by seeing resonance with the premodern disease category of dribbling mounting (*long shan*) and the disease pattern of liver channel qi depression inhibiting bladder qi transformation. The contents of his prescription, and especially the presence of liver-coursing medicinals such as *Qing Pi* (Citri Reticulatae Pericarpium Viride), *Xiao Hui Xiang* (Foeniculi Fructus), and *Chuan Lian Zi* (Toosendan Fructus), reflect his understanding of the role of free-flowing liver qi in the maintenance of bladder qi transformation. Further, *Wu Ling San* (Poria Five Powder), is one of the building blocks of his prescription, and is a well-known formula for transforming bladder qi by warming yang and disinhibiting water. Liu suggests that *Tian Xian Teng* (Aristolochiae Herba) was especially effective in this case because its functions are to quicken blood and free the network vessels and to move qi and disinhibit water.

Kidney vacuity with dampness and disharmony in the channels and network vessels

Zou (1981) reported the treatment of a 42 year-old male in 1960 who was complaining of a seven-year history of soreness and pain in the lumbus, scorching pain of the urethra and milky-white penile discharge, and occasional dark-colored or turbid urine. Additional symptoms included generalized joint soreness and pain, spontaneous sweating, insomnia, a fine stringlike pulse and thin yellow tongue fur. The patient had a Western medical diagnosis of prostatitis, which was confirmed by many laboratory analyses, though no specific details about the findings were given. He had taken antibiotic therapy before and also had previously taken kidney supplementing as well as clearing and disinhibiting medicine; neither therapies had any salubrious effect.

Dr. Zou diagnosed kidney vacuity with dampness and disharmony in the channels and network vessels, and he decided to simultaneously treat the root and the tip of the problem. Over a period of five visits spanning a few months, with careful tracking of the patient's progress and with corresponding adjustments to the herbal prescription, the symptoms completely resolved. Of particular note, and conforming with my own clinical experience that as dampness is expelled from the body the patient expels turbid-colored urine, the patient had an increased flow of turbid and foul-smelling urine after taking the first prescription. A brief synopsis of the progress of treatment and the prescriptions used follows below.

At the first visit, he prescribed three packets of the following medicinals:
   Sang Ji Sheng (Taxilli Herba), 15g
   Niu Xi (Achyranthis Bidentatae Radix), 9g
   Du Huo (Angelicae Pubescentis Radix), 3g
   Cang Zhu (Atractylodis Rhizoma), 3g
   Fa Ban Xia (Pinelliae Rhizoma Praeparatum), 5g
   Fu Ling (Poria), 3g
   Mu Li (Ostreae Concha), 12g
   Tian Hua Fen (Trichosanthis Radix), 6g
   Fu Ling (Poria), 9g
   Yi Yi Ren (Coicis Semen), 9g

He Ye (Nelumbinis Folium), 9g
Xian Lu Gen (Phragmitis Rhizoma Recens), 2 lengths (remove the nodes)
Liu Yi San (Six-to-One Powder), 9g

Second visit: There was reduction of the sagging pain in the lumbus, and there was excretion of turbid and foul-smelling urine. Zou prescribed three packets of the following prescription:
   Sang Ji Sheng (Taxilli Herba), 15g
   Niu Xi (Achyranthis Bidentatae Radix), 12g
   Gou Qi Zi (Lycii Fructus), 6g
   Ba Ji Tian (Morindae Officinalis Radix), 6g
   Du Huo (Angelicae Pubescentis Radix), 3g
   Fa Ban Xia (Pinelliae Rhizoma Praeparatum), 3g
   Xian Lu Gen (Phragmits Rhizoma Recens), 3 lengths (remove nodes)
   Cang Zhu (Atractylodis Rhizoma), 3g
   Huang Qin (Scutellariae Radix), 3g
   Yi Yi Ren (Coicis Semen), 9g
   Fu Ling (Poria), 9g
   Mai Men Dong (Ophiopogonis Radix), 9g
   Liu Yi San (Six-to-One Powder), 9g
   Mu Li (Ostreae Concha), 12g, predecocted
   Xian He Ye (Nelumbinis Folium Recens), 9g
   Tian Hua Fen (Trichosanthis Radix), 6g

Third visit: After the first and second packets of medicine, the pain in the lumbus was still present, the urine became turbid white, and there was no scorching sensation in the urethra. After taking the third packet of medicine, the urine became clear, the lumbus felt lighter and less painful, and the generalized soreness and pain in the joints had improved. There was still spontaneous sweating. The pulse was fine stringlike and the tongue fur was slightly yellow. The turbid dampness was 80–90% gone, but there was still evidence of kidney vacuity. He used the following prescription:
   Sang Ji Sheng (Taxilli Herba), 15g
   Niu Xi (Achyranthis Bidentatae Radix), 12g
   Gou Qi Zi (Lycii Fructus), 9g
   Huang Qin (Scutellariae Radix), 3g
   Tian Hua Fen (Trichosanthis Radix), 6g
   Mai Men Dong (Ophiopogonis Radix), 2g
   Mu Li (Ostreae Concha), 12g, predecocted
   Xian Lu Gen (Phragmits Rhizoma Recens), 1 length (remove the nodes)
   Xian He Ye (Nelumbinis Folium Recens), 5g
   Yi Yi Ren (Coicis Semen), 5g
   Liu Yi San (Six-to-One Powder), 5g

Fourth visit: The pain in the lumbus was greatly reduced, the urine was clear, and there was no turbid discharge. Further, there was no generalized soreness and pain. However, there was still spontaneous sweating and insomnia. The tongue fur was slightly yellow and the pulse was fine. He changed the formula to a modification of *Gan Mai Da Zao Tang* (Licorice, Wheat, and Jujube Decoction) with the following ingredients:

Fu Xiao Mai (Tritici Fructus Levis), 15g

Zhi Gan Cao (Glycyrrhizae Radix cum Liquido Fricta), 3g

Da Zao (Jujubae Fructus), 4 pieces, cut open

Bai Shao (Paeoniae Radix Alba), 9g

Duan Mu Li (Ostreae Concha Calcinata), 12g, predecocted

Long Gu (Mastodi Ossis Fossilia), 15g, predecocted

Long Chi (Mastodi Dentis Fossilia), 15g, predecocted

Gou Qi Zi (Lycii Fructus), 5g

Sheng Di Huang (Rehmanniae Radix Exsiccata seu Recens), 5g

Sha Yuan Zi (Astragali Complanati Semen), 5g

Fu Ling (Poria), 9g

Deng Xin Cao (Junci Medulla), 9g

Fifth visit: The sweating and sleep had improved, the lumbus was much more comfortable, the urine was clear, and the tongue and pulse were normal. The medicinals below were ground into powder, boiled with 1 (*zhang*)[20] of *Deng Xin Cao* (Junci Medulla), along with 180g each of *Long Gu* (Mastodi Ossis Fossilia) and *Long Chi* (Mastodi Dentis Fossilia), and 120g of *Duan Mu Li* (Ostreae Concha Calcinata). The resulting mass was formed into pills the size of a mung bean to be taken with warm water at a dosage of 4.5 grams a day, twice a day. The ingredients were:

Sha Yuan Zi (Astragali Complanati Semen), 120g

Gan Di Huang (Rehmanniae Radix), 60g

Gou Qi Zi (Lycii Fructus), 60g

Ai Ye (Artemisiae Argyi Folium), 120g

Fu Ling (Poria), 30g

Fa Ban Xia (Pinelliae Rhizoma Praeparatum), 30g

Zhi Gan Cao (Glycyrrhizae Radix cum Liquido Fricta), 60g

Fu Xiao Mai (Tritici Fructus Levis), 90g

Xian He Ye (Nelumbinis Folium Recens), 30g

Da Zao (Jujubae Fructus), 20 pieces

The patient took two courses of this therapy at the recommended dosage over a period of eight months. Follow-up four years later revealed no recurrence of the symptoms.

Brewing and binding of damp-heat in the lower burner with qi stagnation and blood stasis

Shen Qu-Qiao, in Dai and Liu (1990), report on a case of acute prostatitis complicating a case of chronic prostatitis in a 27 year-old male. The chief complaint was the sudden onset of painful urination and perineal distention and pain. Dur-

---

[20] One *zhang* is a traditional Chinese measurement roughly equivalent to 3.3 meters.

ing the week prior to the first visit, due to some unspecified deleterious alterations in lifestyle, the patient experienced sudden onset of pain during urination, distention in the lesser abdomen and perineum, slight urethral discharge from the urethra immediately after he bore down to have a bowel movement, soreness and limpness of the lumbus and knees, and fatigued spirit and lack of strength. He had not been satisfied with the results of Western medical treatment and had decided to seek treatment with Chinese medicine. Upon digital examination, his prostate was enlarged, swollen, and relatively firm, and it was painful when intrarectal digital pressure was applied; further, its surface was smooth and indurated. Laboratory evaluation of the prostatic expressate revealed leukocytosis and red blood cells. The pulse was wiry slippery and the tongue fur was thick slimy.

Dr. Shen diagnosed brewing and binding of damp-heat in the lower burner accompanied by qi stagnation and blood stasis. He therefore designed a prescription to clear heat, resolve toxicity, and disinhibit dampness, as well as to quicken blood and transform stasis. Below, is a brief synopsis of the progress of treatment and the medicinals he used to treat this case.

First visit:

    Dang Gui (Angelicae Sinensis Radix), 10g

    Chi Shao Yao (Paeoniae Radix Rubra), 10g

    Wang Bu Liu Xing (Vaccariae Semen), 10g

    Mu Dan Pi (Moutan Cortex), 10g

    Huang Lian (Coptidis Rhizoma), 1.5g

    Huang Bai (Phellodendri Cortex), 6g

    Jin Yin Hua (Lonicerae Flos), 15g

    Gan Cao (Glycyrrhizae Radix), 6g

    Fu Ling (Poria), 10g

    Ze Xie (Alismatis Rhizoma), 10g

    Ma Bian Cao (Verbenae Herba), 15g

Second visit: The patient had taken 18 packets of the prescription above and had experienced a gradual reduction in his symptoms, and in particular his urination had normalized. However, he still had soreness and limpness of the lumbus and knees, fatigued spirit and lack of strength, and the penile discharge following bowel movements. The pulse was fine stringlike rapid, and the tongue fur was slightly slimy. Since there was still uncleared damp-heat along with dual vacuity of the spleen and kidneys, Dr. Shen designed a prescription to regulate and supplement the spleen and kidneys, as well as to clear heat and disinhibit dampness. The patient took the following prescription for one month and there were no further symptoms. Two follow-up laboratory examinations of the prostate expressate were normal.

    Dang Shen (Codonopsis Radix), 15g

    Shan Yao (Dioscoreae Rhizoma), 15g

    Gou Qi Zi (Lycii Fructus), 10g

    Fu Pen Zi (Rubi Fructus), 10g

    Mu Dan Pi (Moutan Cortex), 10g

Zhi Mu (Anemarrhenae Rhizoma), 10g
Yu Zhu (Polygonati Odorati Rhizoma) 10g
Jin Yin Hua (Lonicerae Flos), 15g
Bai Mao Gen (Imperatae Rhizoma), 10g
Fu Ling (Poria), 10g

Warming and supplementing liver and kidney yang

Dr. Pan Xue-Zhu (1995) used the method of warming and supplementing liver and kidney yang to treat a case of chronic prostatitis occurring in a 27 year-old male. Five months prior to the first visit, he experienced the onset of the following symptoms: ungratifying micturition; soreness and limpness of the lumbus and knees and; infertility. He sought Western medical care and thus received antibiotic therapy (though the specific drug was not specified in the case report) as well as prostatic massage for over a month without any marked beneficial effects. After that, he sought treatment with Chinese medicine, and was placed on a one-month course of heat-clearing and toxin-resolving medicinals while he continued with the Western treatment; still no relief was obtained. At that time, his prostate lab values revealed a pH of 7.0, and there were also leukocytes in the prostatic expressate.

At the first visit, Dr. Pan noted that the patient appeared to have constitutional kidney weakness which led to enduring soreness and weakness of the lumbus and knees and lack of strength. He also noted that there was coldness of both legs, reduced appetite, vertigo, insomnia, distention and pain of the testes, cold and retracted penis and scrotum, occasional painful urination with pain referring into the lesser abdomen, an occasional sense of incomplete emptying of his bladder, periodic leakage of white turbid fluid from the penis after urinating, thin sloppy stools, and infertility for three years. The tongue was pale and the tongue fur was slightly slimy, and the pulse was sinking fine. Upon digital palpation, the prostate felt enlarged, slightly tough, and there was pain with pressure. The pH of the prostatic expressate was 7.0, and there was leukocytosis. The diagnosis was liver and kidney yang vacuity with yin-cold in the channels (liver and kidney channels especially). Seeking to warm the liver and dissipate cold and to free the channels, Dr. Pan used a variation of *Nuan Gan Jian* (Liver-Warming Brew). The ingredients were:

Wu Zhu Yu (Evodiae Fructus), 9g
Shu Fu Zi (Aconiti Radix Lateralis Conquita), 9g
Mu Xiang (Aucklandiae Radix), 6g
Chuan Lian Zi (Toosendan Fructus), 6g
Yan Hu Suo (Corydalis Rhizoma), 6g
Bi Xie (Dioscoreae Hypoglaucae seu Semptemlobae Rhizoma), 9g
Shui Zhi (Hirudo), 9g
Li Zhi He (Litchi Semen), 9g
Qing Pi (Citri Reticulatae Pericarpium Viride), 6g

In addition to having the patient take the prescription internally, Pan also instructed the patient to fumigate the anterior yin region with the dregs of the decoction after the medicinal juice was strained off in order to quicken the blood and accelerate the reabsorption of any inflammatory by-products and to warm and free the channels and smooth the outflow of turbid material. By continuing with essentially the same prescription (with the notable addition of *Huang Qi* [Astragali Radix], 20g and the cessation of the external fumigation at the third visit), for a period of roughly four months, this patient's symptoms all disappeared, his prostate physical examination and laboratory values normalized, and he and his wife were able to conceive a child.

It is very interesting to note that in the commentary Dr. Pan asserts that it is unwise to rigidly adhere to the statement "the liver is often in surplus," and to thus ignore the fact that liver yang can be vacuous and cold. He claims that liver yang is an important source of physiological activity for the entire body and is of special importance in the treatment of both chronic prostatitis and male infertility.

Kidney yin vacuity with hyperactive heart fire

Dr. Tu, in Zhong (1997), cited effective treatment of one case of chronic prostatitis in a 45 year-old male with a diagnosis of kidney yin vacuity and hyperactive heart fire. The patient, who had a two-year history of frequent and urgent micturition, presented with the following symptoms: lesser abdominal pain refusing pressure; an occasional sensation of drooping pain in the abdomen; thirst; susceptibility to vexation and agitation and; a history of seminal emission in youth. He also underwent a varicocelectomy in 1960. The pulse was stringlike slippery rapid, the tongue fur was slightly yellow, and the tongue body had pale purple macules. The diagnosis was kidney yin vacuity and hyperactive heart fire and the treatment principle was to enrich and nourish kidney water and to clear the heart and quiet the spirit. After taking the recommended prescription, all the symptoms completely disappeared.

First visit: Two months of the following prescription was prescribed:
    Sheng Di Huang (Rehmanniae Radix Exsiccata seu Recens), 12g
    Mu Dan Pi (Moutan Cortex), 12g
    Fu Ling (Poria), 10g
    Rou Gui (Cinnamomi Cortex), 4g
    Ze Xie (Alismatis Rhizoma), 10g
    Huang Bai (Phellodendri Cortex), 12g
    Zhi Mu (Anemarrhenae Rhizoma), 12g
    Gan Cao Shao (Glycyrrhizae Radix Tenuis), 15g
    Di Long (Pheretima), 12g
    Bai Zi Ren (Platycladi Semen), 12g
    Huang Lian (Coptidis Rhizoma), 4g

Second visit: After taking the following prescription for over one month, all the symptoms disappeared. The ingredients are as follows:
    Sheng Di Huang (Rehmanniae Radix Exsiccata seu Recens), 20g
    Mu Dan Pi (Moutan Cortex), 12g
    Fu Ling (Poria), 10g

Ze Xie (Alismatis Rhizoma), 10g
Shan Zhu Yu (Corni Fructus), 10g
Zhi Mu (Anemarrhenae Rhizoma), 12g
Huang Bai (Phellodendri Cortex), 10g
Sheng Gan Cao (Glycyrrhizae Radix Cruda), 12g
Bai Zi Ren (Platycladi Semen), 10g
Che Qian Cao (Plantaginis Herba), 30g

Benign Prostatic Hyperplasia (BPH)

Western Medicine

Benign Prostatic Hyperplasia (BPH) is characterized by a nonmalignant increase in-growth of the prostate. This growth is thought to be stimulated by dihydrotestosterone—which mediates prostate growth and is present in the male body from the onset of puberty. Dihydrotestosterone is produced in prostate tissue from testosterone through the mediation of the enzyme 5 alpha-reductase. The prostate growth-mediating action of dihydrotestosterone is enhanced by the progressively increasing presence (in the bodies of men over forty-five years of age) of prostate-proliferative estradiol.

According to Fauci *et al.* (1998), 90% of men in their eighties have prostate hyperplasia at autopsy. As the hyperplasia begins earlier in life (often at about forty-five years of age), and usually progresses slowly, it is a significant cause of urinary symptoms in men from the age of forty-five onward. Because the prostate surrounds the urethra, the enlarged prostate causes urethral outlet obstruction and urethral irritation, and hence leads to progressive urinary frequency, urgency, hesitancy, and incontinence, as well as to nocturia, decreased urinary stream strength, split-stream voiding, hematuria, and terminal dribbling (Penson, 2001). Untreated and severe cases may progress to the point of complete urinary obstruction with secondary hydronephrosis and renal failure. According to Beers and Berkow (1999), symptoms can be exacerbated by attempts to delay urination for long periods of time, taking sympathomimetic drugs (including over-the-counter decongestants such as pseudoephedrine), anticholinergic drugs (including antidepressants, antipsychotics, and antispasmodics), exposure to cold, and consumption of alcohol.

Diagnosis

The self-administered symptom score questionnaire provided by the American Urological Association and printed below is of great assistance in quantifying the clinical symptoms of BPH (Barry and O'Leary, 1992). It provides a subjective measurement of the severity of the lower urinary tract symptoms (LUTS) exhibited by a given patient. And it can be used as a means of tracking clinical results in that a change of three points or more is considered clinically significant.

American Urological Association (AUA) symptom index

A scale of 0–6 is used to rate the severity of symptoms in the form of a response to questions 1–6 below. Circle the number that most applies:

Not at all	Less than 1 time in 5	Less than half the time	About half the time	More than half the time	Almost always
0	1	2	3	4	5

1. Over the past month, how often have you had the sensation of not emptying your bladder completely after you finished urinating?

0	1	2	3	4	5

2. Over the past month, how often have you had to urinate again less than two hours after you finished urinating?

0	1	2	3	4	5

3. Over the past month, how often have you found you stopped and started again several times when you urinated?

0	1	2	3	4	5

4. Over the past month, how often have you found it difficult to postpone urination?

0	1	2	3	4	5

5. Over the past month, how often have you had a weak urinary stream?

0	1	2	3	4	5

6. Over the past month, how often did you push or strain to begin urination?

0	1	2	3	4	5

A scale of 0–6 is used to rate the frequency of nocturia in response to question 7 below:

None	1 time	2 times	3 times	4 times	5 or more times
0	1	2	3	4	5

7. Over the past month, how many times did you most typically get up to urinate from the time you went to bed at night until the time you got up in the morning?

0	1	2	3	4	5

The sum of the answers to questions 1–7 comprises the patient's AUA score.
The severity of symptoms may be classified as follows:

0–7: Mild symptoms   8–19: Moderate symptoms   20–35: Severe symptoms

---

• (DRE) Digital rectal examination of the prostate

Although physical examination of the prostate via digital rectal examination is recommended for the evaluation of men with suspected BPH, the size of the prostate is not always directly correlated with the severity of symptoms. Numerous sources report that many men with small prostates have relatively severe symptoms and conversely that some men with an enlarged prostate have few if any symptoms. This suggests that the severity of symptoms has more to do with the location—rather than the degree of hyperplasia—and that centrally-located and therefore nonpalpable hyperplastic prostate tissue exerts a greater narrowing influence on the patency of the urethral lumen than does hyperplasia in other regions of the gland. Diffuse enlargement of the prostate may be present, stony-hard nodules are absent unless cancer or prostatic calculi are present, and the median furrow may be obscured. Further, a boggy and tender prostate suggests prostatitis rather than BPH.

• *Laboratory findings*

In terms of laboratory findings, the serum prostate-specific antigen (PSA) level may be elevated in 30–50% of men with BPH, and does seem to correlate positively with the degree of symptoms and the size of the prostate.[1] Moreover, a PSA level is helpful to rule out prostate cancer—which may present with similar symptoms as BPH (Beers and Berkow, 1999). Other tests are also often used in the evaluation of patients with BPH including: 1) urinalysis and culture when secondary prostate or bladder infection is suspected; 2) transrectal ultrasound of the prostate to more definitively determine the size of the prostate, and to detect cancer or stones; 3) serum creatinine levels to rule out and/or quantify compromised renal function and; 4) urine flowmetry to measure the degree of post-voiding urinary retention.

• *Differential diagnosis*

The differential diagnosis of BPH includes other causes of urethral obstruction such as urethral stricture—which may be associated with gonococcal infection or a previous history of urethral catheterization or other such procedures, prostatic cancer, diabetes, and congestive heart failure (Penson, 2001). Hoole *et al.* (1999) provide the useful clinical hint that patients with diabetes or congestive heart failure generally void large amounts of urine whereas patients with BPH generally experience frequent and difficult voiding of small volumes of urine.

Treatment
• *General*

Men with BPH should be advised that their symptoms may worsen with the ingestion of medications such as over-the-counter decongestants,[2] antidepressants, antipsychotics, and antispasmotic drugs.

• *Watchful waiting*

For men with an AUA score of 7 or less, a PSA ≤4 ng/ml, who have relatively mild LUTS, physicians generally adopt a watchful waiting stance. This means that the patient is advised to track the severity of his symptoms and that the

---

[1] A normal PSA value is under 4 ng/ml.

[2] This raises an interesting question about the use of *Ma Huang* (Ephedrae Herba)—which contains ephedrine—in this condition. In Chinese medicine, *Ma Huang* is sometimes used as a medicinal in formulas to treat BPH. Such use reflects the treatment principle of freeing the upper source of water (the lung) to free the lower source of water (the kidney).

physician will perform digital rectal examination and serum PSA analysis annually (or perhaps more often in certain cases). Should the symptoms worsen, then the other medical therapies listed below are considered.

• Medications

Western medical therapy of BPH consists of mainly three broad strategies, which are adopted in accordance with the severity of lower urinary tract symptoms (LUTS) and the physical and laboratory findings: 1) watchful waiting; 2) alpha-adrenergic blockers or; 3) 5-alpha-reductase inhibitors (Penson, 2001). It should also be noted that a recent study by McConnell *et al.* (2003) suggested that alpha blockers in combination with 5-alpha-reductase inhibitors may be superior to either regimen alone.

• Alpha-adrenergic blockers

When a man has especially bothersome lower urinary tract symptoms, physicians consider the adoption of an alpha-adrenergic blocker such as prazosin, doxazosin, terazosin, or tamsulosin. The mode of action of these medications is to relax the smooth muscle of the bladder neck—which is rich in alpha-1 adrenergic receptors—to increase peak urinary flow rate. According to Fauci *et al.* (1998), there is no reason to believe that such medications will halt the progress of the disease, though they may provide symptomatic relief. In some cases, these medications are associated with significant orthostatic hypotension as well as dizziness.

• 5-alpha-reductase inhibitors

Men who have markedly enlarged prostates and who have not experienced significant relief of LUTS from alpha-adrenergic blocker therapy are generally commenced on a trial of therapy with Finasteride—a 5-alpha-reductase inhibitor. 5-alpha-reductase inhibitors block the conversion of testosterone into dihydrotestosterone which is thought to be responsible for proliferation of prostatic tissue. Although some sources report that the incidence of side effects for Finasteride is low, Penson (2001) reports erectile dysfunction and decreased libido. Penson also states that alpha adrenergic-blockers are generally preferred to Finasteride, yet it still remains the drug of choice for second-line therapy when alpha blockers fail. Hoole *et al.* (1999) question its efficacy, however, and state that it has little benefit in comparison with placebo.

• Surgery

Transurethral resection of the prostate (TURP) is the preferred surgical procedure and does offer considerable chances for LUTS relief, but it is also associated with the highest rate of worrisome complications such as erectile dysfunction, stress incontinence, and retrograde ejaculation. Generally speaking, TURP is considered in a few circumstances including when: 1) medical therapy fails; 2) bladder outlet obstruction has progressed to the point of obstructive uropathy with elevated serum creatinine levels or repeated urinary tract infections and; 3) bladder stones have developed. Penson (2001) reports that other less-invasive therapies are currently being studied for the treatment of BPH, including transurethral microwave thermotherapy, laser prostatectomy, transurethral needle ablation of the prostate, and transurethral incision.

Western Complementary Medicine

There are many products offered on the complementary medicine market which claim to treat BPH, including Saw Palmetto (Serenoa ripens) extract, African Plum (Pygeum Africanum Fructus), Zinc, Rye Grass Pollen (Secale Cereale), and Pumpkin seeds (Curcubita Semen). Among these, Saw Palmetto, African Plum, and Rye Grass Pollen have been the most widely studied.

• *Saw Palmetto*

In a systematic review of the literature on Saw Palmetto, Wilt *et al.* (2002) concluded that it "provides mild to moderate improvement in urinary symptoms and flow measures," and that it "produced similar improvement in urinary symptoms and flow compared to Finasteride and is associated with fewer adverse treatment events." However, a recent study reported in the *New England Journal of Medicine* suggested that Saw Palmetto was not more effective than placebo in reducing the symptoms of moderate to severe BPH (Bent *et al.*, 2006).

• *African Plum*

Extracts of African Plum (Pygeum Africanum Fructus) have gained attention as a possible treatment for BPH. Although citing the need for better-refined studies that employ a standardized extract of the plant material, Wilt and Ishani *et al.* (1998) found that African Plum may be useful in the reduction of BPH symptoms such as nocturia and residual urine volume with few if any side effects.

• *Rye Grass Pollen*

A review of the available literature on Rye Grass Pollen (Secale Cereale) concluded that it was effective in reducing nocturia associated with BPH, but failed to show significant effects on improving urinary flow rates, residual volume, or prostate size (Wilt and McDonald *et al.*, 1998).

Chinese Medicine

Disease discrimination

In Chinese medicine, the symptoms and signs of BPH largely fall under the premodern disease categories of dribbling urinary block (*long bi*) and—to a lesser extent—either essence dribbling [block] (*jing long*) or essence turbidity (*jing zhuo*). As the latter two diseases are characterized by a milky-white penile discharge—a sign more often associated with prostatitis rather than prostatic hyperplasia—dribbling urinary block is by far the most relevant Chinese disease category to use when reframing BPH in a Chinese medical framework.

The premodern disease category dribbling urinary block (*long bi*) was first mentioned in the *Huang Di Nei Jing (Yellow Emperor's Inner Canon)* and it contains many passages which give insight into the analysis of this condition. For example, chapter 25 of *Su Wen (Plain Questions)*[3] states: "Inhibition of the bladder leads to [urinary] dribbling," and chapter 65 of *Su Wen* states: "[When] the bladder is diseased, [there will be] urinary block." Dribbling urinary block presents with scanty urine and slight urinary dripping in mild cases. In more serious cases, however, there is complete blockage of urinary outflow.

Although both conditions share the common symptoms of encumbered and difficult urination, urinary dribbling and urinary block were originally considered separate and distinct diseases, yet over time, doctors began to see the close relationship between the two conditions and to discuss them together under the same heading; in essence, dribbling (*long*) and block (*bi*) differ primarily in terms of degree of failure of the bladder and triple burner qi transformation. Taken as a separate disease, dribbling is a relatively mild condition that does not require immediate attention and is characterized by inhibited urination, scanty urination, and slight urinary dripping. However, urinary block is a more serious condition. Its clinical features include slight urinary dripping and urinary retention. The clinical resemblance between the symptoms of dribbling urinary block and those experienced by patients with BPH is clear; thus, this condition serves as a conceptual and clinically-useful model for the treatment of such patients.

On a historical note, in his well-known text *Qian Jin Yao Fang (A Thousand Gold Pieces Formulary)*,[4] the preeminent Tang dynasty physician Sun Si-Miao described the use of catheterization for the treatment of urinary block in the following passage: "...use a scallion leaf with the head removed and deeply insert it into the head of the penis [to a depth of] about three *cun*. Blow into it slightly until the bladder becomes distended, there will be a great flow of fluids, and the condition will be cured."

Disease causes and pathomechanisms

The fundamental disease cause of BPH is kidney vacuity and the main pathomechanism is blood stasis caused by kidney qi vacuity (Tan and Tao, 1999). When the kidney becomes weak, there is a lack of harmony of yin and yang, and qi and blood are likely to become depressed and static. Owing to kidney vacuity, bladder and kidney qi transformation lack power and blood stasis binds and forms concretions; this leads to obstruction of the waterways and thus to a failure of triple burner qi transformation.

---

[3] *Su Wen* is the first section of the *Huang Di Nei Jing (Yellow Emperor's Inner Canon)*, which was published in the 1st century CE, during the Eastern Han dynasty.

[4] Sun Si-Miao (581–682 CE) was one of the most famous physicians of the Tang dynasty. Among his contributions are the influential texts *Qian Jin Yao Fang (A Thousand Gold Pieces Formulary)* and *Qian Jin Yi Fang (Wings of the Thousand Gold Pieces Formulary)*.

• Kidney yang vacuity

Kidney yang vacuity may come about as a result of aging and from sexual taxation. When kidney yang is vacuous and cold, and thus kidney qi is relatively debilitated, the bladder loses its warmth and power. As a result, bladder qi transformation is unable to maintain its normal function of smoothly and completely excreting urine. *Zheng Yin Mai Zhi* (*Pathoconditions: Causes, Pulses, and Treatments*)[5] states: "[When there is] kidney true yang vacuity, the [water] gate fails to open; this gathered water engenders disease, and causes inhibited urination."

• Kidney yin vacuity

The causes of kidney yin vacuity include constitutional kidney yin vacuity (either inherited as natural endowment insufficiency or acquired through careless living), enduring heat disease which consumes yin, and sexual taxation. When there is kidney yin vacuity, ministerial fire becomes hyperactive and flames unchecked and consumes yin-fluids further. When there is no yin, yang is unable to transform, and fluids do not flow downward to the bladder. This leads to short rough voiding of reddish urine. *Zheng Yin Mai Zhi* states: "The kidney governs the [water] gate. [When] kidney yin is insufficient, [there is] exhaustion of water in the lower [burner]; this causes inhibited urination."

• Qi stagnation and blood stasis

Beyond the pathomechanism of kidney vacuity leading to blood stasis, binding depression of liver qi is the main cause of qi stagnation and blood stasis in BPH. As a result of affect-mind damage, liver's free coursing of qi, blood, and fluids becomes depressed. Also, fulminant outbursts of anger can acutely damage the liver and lead to counterflow of qi and stasis of blood. Because the liver channel skirts the genitals and because liver's free coursing is essential to bladder qi transformation, binding depression of liver qi commonly leads to inhibited urination. Liver depression leads to blood stasis, and blood stasis leads to concretions and binds which obstruct the waterways and cause painful urination and/or urinary incontinence. In severe cases, qi stagnation and blood stasis form such a significant obstruction to bladder and triple burner qi transformation that urinary blockage which allows only slight dribbling of urine occurs.

• Lung heat and qi congestion

When either enduring depressed wind-cold transforms heat, or when wind-heat or dryness-heat become depressed in the lung, the condition of lung heat qi congestion can occur. As a result, the lung loses its governance and control as well as its function of depurative downbearing. Thus, the lung is unable to regulate the waterways and to transport fluids downward to the bladder; this results in inhibited urination. Further, if exuberant heat continues to conduct downward from the lung into the bladder over a long period of time, blocked and depressed heat in both the upper and lower burners results in difficult and

---

[5] *Zheng Yin Mai Zhi* was written by Qin Jing-Ming and published in 1641, during the Ming dynasty.

painful urination with a scorching sensation in the urethra. *Zheng Yin Mai Zhi* states: "The lung governs the regulation of the waterways, and the stomach and intestines govern the conveyance and transformation of water and grain. When the upper burner loses its authority for clearing and transforming, it is unable to conduct [water] downward to the bladder; this leads to inhibited urination."

• Damp-heat pouring downward

Dietary irregularities such as overconsumption of greasy, rich, and sweet foods and fluids damage the spleen and result in splenic movement and transformation failure. They also impair the stomach functions of intake and decomposition. The resulting collection of water-damp and food stagnation in the center burner—when enduring or severe—will transform heat, which combines with dampness to form damp-heat. Once damp-heat forms in the center burner, dampness (a yin evil) has a tendency to pour downward into the lower burner, which is referred to as a "sluice"[6] in many premodern sources. The 31st Difficulty of the *Nan Jing* (*Classic of Difficult Issues*)[7] states: "The lower burner... governs the separation of clear and turbid. It governs exit and not intake and serves as a conveyer [of waste]." If this means of conveyance of waste is obstructed, and specifically bladder qi transformation fails, urine and fluids cannot be distributed. Bladder qi transformation failure obstructing urinary function leads to symptoms such as unsmooth urinary flow, frequent urination with scorching hot urine, and dribbling urination. Because bladder qi transformation has a role in the spread of physiological fluids as well as urine, damp-heat obstructing bladder qi transformation also results in dry mouth with lack of desire to drink.

• Spleen qi vacuity and center qi fall

When aging and/or enduring dietary irregularities weaken the spleen, its qi falls downward and it loses its ability to upbear the clear essence of water and grain. This upsets the qi dynamic of the center burner, and as a result, not only will the clear not be borne upward, but the turbid yin will not be borne downward. Although there are a few different ways in which this pathomechanism is applied in Chinese medicine, in terms of urinary diseases, "turbid" (*zhuo*) refers to urine.

Hence, center qi fall—which we should see as a furthering or as a complication of spleen qi vacuity—leads to difficult, inhibited, and dribbling urination because it implies an inability to upbear the clear and downbear the turbid. Further, included in the small intestine's function of "separating the clear and turbid," is the fact that it absorbs "the clear" (fluid in this context) and sends it to the bladder for further separation of its clear and turbid aspects, including the excretion of urine. According to Wang (2001), this function of the

---

[6] According to *The New Oxford American Dictionary* (2001), a sluice is a "sliding gate or other device for controlling the flow of water, espec[ially] one in a lock gate" (p. 1608).

[7] The *Nan Jing* was published in the 1st century, during the Eastern Han dynasty.

small intestine is largely an expression of splenic movement and transformation and is therefore powered by spleen qi. When there is center qi fall, the small intestine fails to smoothly and efficiently send fluid to the bladder, and this results in bladder qi transformation failure and urinary inhibition, dribbling, and retention, as described in the traditional disease category of dribbling urinary block. Of course, the roles of the spleen and the small intestine here also include—by logical extension—that of the triple burner. Within the section about urinary inhibition caused by qi vacuity, the Ming dynasty text *Zheng Yin Mai Zhi* states: "[Factors such as] constitutional vacuity of original qi (*yuan qi*),[8] excessive sweating and precipitation,[9] weakness of qi resulting from enduring disease, taxation damaging the physical body, careless living, and chaotic triple burner qi all [may lead to the] pathocondition of inhibited urination."

Pattern discrimination

1. Kidney yang vacuity and debility

Signs: Inhibited urination or frequent urination (especially at night), clear white urine that is expelled without force, either difficult urination or uncontrolled spontaneous flow of urine, somber white facial complexion, exhaustion of essence-spirit, timidity and weakness of the spirit, fear of the cold, soreness, weakness, and coldness of the lumbus and knees, cold retracted scrotum and penis, enlarged pale tender tongue with white fur, sinking fine or slow weak pulse.

Treatment principles: Warm and supplement kidney yang, transform qi and move water

Guiding formula: Modified *Ji Sheng Shen Qi Wan* (Life Saver Kidney Qi Pill)

Ingredients:
    Rou Gui (Cinnamomi Cortex), 6g
    Fu Zi (Aconiti Radix Lateralis Praeparata), 6g, predecocted
    Shu Di Huang (Rehmanniae Radix Praeparata), 15g
    Shan Zhu Yu (Corni Fructus), 12g
    Shan Yao (Dioscoreae Rhizoma), 12g
    Fu Ling (Poria), 10g
    Ze Xie (Alismatis Rhizoma), 10g
    Mu Dan Pi (Moutan Cortex), 10g
    Chuan Niu Xi (Cyathulae Radix), 15g
    Che Qian Zi (Plantaginis Semen), 15g
    Sheng Huang Qi (Astragali seu Hedysari Radix Cruda), 30g
    Yi Zhi Ren (Alpiniae Oxyphyllae Fructus), 15g
    Chen Xiang (Aquilariae Lignum Resinatum), 10g

---

[8] Original qi (*yuan qi*) here signifies either kidney qi, spleen qi, or an amalgamation of both.

[9] This implies iatrogenesis through overuse of exterior-resolving and/or precipitating medicinals.

Wang Bu Liu Xing (Vaccariae Semen), 15g
Tao Ren (Persicae Semen), 12g
Hong Hua (Carthami Flos), 12g

Modifications: For patients with spleen qi vacuity and lack of transformation who have poor appetite and exhaustion of essence-spirit, add *Dang Shen* (Codonopsis Radix), 12g, and *Bai Zhu* (Atractylodis Macrocephalae Rhizoma), 9g, to fortify the spleen and boost qi. For those with marked frequent urination, add *Fu Pen Zi* (Rubi Fructus), 15g, and *Sang Piao Xiao* (Mantidis Ootheca), 15g, to secure the kidney and reduce urine.

2. Kidney yin detriment and damage

Signs: Frequent but ungratifying urination, scanty yellowish-red urine, desire to urinate with inability to expel urine, scorching hot sensation in the urethra, frequent urination at night, dry mouth and throat, insomnia and heart vexation, postmeridian reddening of the cheeks, soreness and weakness of the lumbus and knees, dizzy head and tinnitus, dry red tongue with scanty fur, fine rapid pulse.

Treatment principles: Enrich yin and supplement the kidney, transform qi and disinhibit water

Guiding formulas: Modified *Zi Yin Tong Guan Wan* (Yin-Enriching Gate-Opening Pill) with *Zhi Bai Di Huang Wan* (Anemarrhena, Phellodendron, and Rehmannia Pill)

Ingredients:
Huang Bai (Phellodendri Cortex), 10g
Zhi Mu (Anemarrhenae Rhizoma), 15g
Sheng Di Huang (Rehmanniae Radix Exsiccata seu Recens), 15g
Shan Yao (Dioscoreae Rhizoma), 12g
Fu Ling (Poria), 15g
Mu Dan Pi (Moutan Cortex), 12g
Ze Xie (Alismatis Rhizoma), 15g
Bie Jia (Trionycis Carapax), 15g, predecocted
Gui Ban (Testudinis Carapax et Plastrum), 15g, predecocted
Rou Gui (Cinnamomi Cortex), 3g

Modifications: For effulgent fire from yin vacuity and exuberant fire in the lower burner with steaming bone tidal heat effusion, add *Di Gu Pi* (Lycii Cortex), 15g, to clear vacuity heat and cool blood. For patients with marked dry mouth, add *Tian Hua Fen* (Trichosanthis Radix), 30g, to clear heat and engender fluids. For bound stool, add *Da Huang* (Rhei Radix et Rhizoma), 10g, add at the end, to free the bowels.

3. Stasis and stagnation obstructing the urinary pathway

Signs: Difficult excretion of either slight drips of urine or a thin stream of urine (in severe cases, urination can be completely blocked), unsmooth urination, urinary urgency, fullness, distention, and pain of the perineum and lesser abdomen, dark purple tongue with possible stasis macules or stasis points, and a deep stringlike or fine rough pulse.

Treatment principles: Move stasis and dissipate binds, free and disinhibit urination

Guiding formula: Modified *Dai Di Dang Wan* (Substitute Dead-On Pill)

Ingredients:
    Da Huang (Rhei Radix et Rhizoma), 6g
    Sheng Di Huang (Rehmanniae Radix Exsiccata seu Recens), 15g
    Dang Gui Wei (Angelicae Sinensis Radicis Extremitas), 6g
    Tao Ren (Persicae Semen), 10g
    Mang Xiao (Natrii Sulfas), 15g
    Rou Gui (Cinnamomi Cortex), 3g
    Niu Xi (Achyranthis Bidentatae Radix), 12g
    Hu Po (Succinum), 3g, powdered and taken mixed with the strained
        decoction
    Zhe Bei Mu (Fritillariae Thunbergii Bulbus), 15g

Modifications: For patients with hematuria, add *San Qi* (Notoginseng Radix), 3g, *Sheng Pu Huang* (Typhae Pollen Crudum), 12g, *Qian Cao Gen* (Rubiae Radix), 12g, and *Bai Mao Gen* (Imperatae Rhizoma), 30g, to clear heat and cool the blood and to stop bleeding. For patients with enduring disease who have a lusterless facial complexion from dual vacuity of qi and blood, add *Huang Qi* (Astragali Radix), 15g, *Dan Shen* (Salviae Miltiorrhizae Radix), 20g, and *Dang Gui* (Angelicae Sinensis Radix), 10g, to supplement and nourish qi and blood. For urinary stones, add *Jin Qian Cao* (Lysimachiae Herba), 15g, *Dong Kui Zi* (Malvae Semen), 10g, and *Hai Jin Sha* (Lygodii Spora), 15g, to free strangury and expel stones.[10]

4. Lung heat and qi congestion

Signs: Slight dripping and blocked urination, thin-streamed urination, dull pain, distention, and fullness of the lesser abdomen, panting and/or cough, oppression of the chest, dry mouth and throat, vexation and thirst desiring fluid, red tongue with slightly yellow fur, slippery rapid pulse.

---

[10] Guo et al. (1999) suggest that in cases of urinary blockage, one should also swallow a small amount of *She Xiang* (Moschus) with the decoction, but I cannot support the use of this medicinal because it is derived from an endangered species. Synthetic musk is available, but I am not certain of its safety. The principle of aromatic opening for blockage holds potential therapeutic value in this case. Hence, perhaps using another aromatic orifice-opening medicinal such as *Shi Chang Pu* (Acori Tatarinowii Rhizoma) could theoretically produce a similar result, though I have not had that specific experience.

Treatment principles: Clear heat from the lung, disinhibit the waterways[11]

Guiding formula: Modified *Qing Fei Yin* (Lung-Clearing Beverage)

Ingredients:
Huang Qin (Scutellariae Radix), 12g
Sang Bai Pi (Mori Cortex), 12g
Mai Men Dong (Ophiopogonis Radix), 15g
Che Qian Zi (Plantaginis Semen), 15g
Shan Zhi Zi (Gardeniae Fructus), 10g
Mu Tong (Akebiae Trifoliatae Caulis), 10g
Fu Ling (Poria), 15g
Ting Li Zi (Lepidii/Descurainiae Semen), 12g
Jie Geng (Platycodonis Radix), 10g
Wang Bu Liu Xing (Vaccariae Semen), 12g
Yi Mu Cao (Leonuri Herba), 12g
Sheng Gan Cao (Glycyrrhizae Radix Cruda), 6g

Modifications: For patients with bound stool, add *Da Huang* (Rhei Radix et Rhizoma), 6g, add at the end, and *Tao Ren* (Persicae Semen), 10g, to free the bowels. For symptoms indicating the presence of an evil at the exterior, such as heat effusion and aversion to cold, nasal congestion, headache, and superficial pulse, add *Ma Huang* (Ephedrae Herba), 6g, and *Gui Zhi* (Cinnamomi Ramulus), 6g, to resolve the exterior and diffuse the lung and to open the waterways.

5. Damp-heat pouring downward

Signs: Urinary dribbling and unsmooth urinary flow, or possibly frequent urination with scorching hot urine, rough painful urination, yellowish-red urine, distention, pain, and fullness of the lesser abdomen, bitter and sticky taste in the mouth or dry mouth without desire to drink, unsmooth bowel movement or bound stool, heat effusion, red tongue with slimy yellow fur, either slippery rapid or stringlike rapid pulse.

Treatment principles: Clear heat and disinhibit dampness, free strangury

Guiding formula: Modified *Ba Zheng San* (Eight Corrections Powder)

Ingredients:
Mu Tong (Akebiae Trifoliatae Caulis), 12g
Che Qian Zi (Plantaginis Semen), 10g
Qu Mai (Dianthi Herba), 12g
Bian Xu (Polygoni Avicularis Herba), 12g

---

[11] The term "waterways" (*shui dao*) is used here intentionally to indicate both the triple burner (*san jiao*) itself and the lung in its role of regulating the triple burner.

Da Huang (Rhei Radix et Rhizoma), 6g
Shan Zhi Zi (Gardeniae Fructus), 12g
Hua Shi (Talcum), 20g
Sheng Di Huang (Rehmanniae Radix Exsiccata seu Recens), 15g
Dan Zhu Ye (Lophatheri Herba), 10g
Gan Cao Shao (Glycyrrhizae Radix Tenuis), 6g

Modifications: For patients with marked lesser abdominal distention and pain, and bound stool, add *Bing Lang* (Arecae Semen), 12g, and *Zhi Shi* (Aurantii Fructus immaturis), 12g, to break qi and conduct stagnation downward. For urgent painful urination, add *Mu Xiang* (Aucklandiae Radix), 9g, *Hu Po* (Succinum), 3g, taken mixed with the strained decoction, and *Wu Yao* (Linderae Radix), 10g, to move qi, quicken blood, and free strangury. For marked yellow slimy fur, add *Cang Zhu* (Atractylodis Rhizoma), 9g, and *Huang Bai* (Phellodendri Cortex), 12g, to clear and transform damp-heat.

For patients who also have hyperactive heart fire causing heart vexation, and mouth and tongue sores, combine *Ba Zheng San* (Eight Corrections Powder) with *Dao Chi San* (Red-Abducting Powder). For those with symptoms of liver channel damp-heat such as rib-side pain and bitter taste in the mouth, and redness, swelling, and pain in the eyes, combine *Ba Zheng San* (Eight Corrections Powder) with *Long Dan Xie Gan Tang* (Gentian Liver-Draining Decoction). If damp-heat congests the triple burner and inhibits qi transformation, with symptoms such as scanty urine or anuria, dark stagnant complexion, oppression of the chest and heart vexation, nausea and vomiting, the taste of urine in the mouth, and even possibly clouded spirit and delirious speech, use *Huang Lian Wen Dan Tang* (Coptis Gallbladder-Warming Decoction) with *Che Qian Zi* (Plantaginis Semen), 15g, *Bai Mao Gen* (Imperatae Rhizoma), 30g, and *Mu Tong* (Akebiae Trifoliatae Caulis), 10g, to downbear the turbid and harmonize the stomach, and to clear and transform damp-heat (Guo *et al.*, 1999).

6. Liver depression and qi stagnation

Signs: Urinary stoppage or ungratifying urination, distention and pain of the chest and rib-side, sagging distention in the lesser abdomen that is relieved by belching and sighing, dull pain in the genital region (including in the scrotum), emotional repression and depression, vexation, agitation, and irascibility, red tongue with thin yellow fur, and a stringlike pulse.

Treatment principles: Course the liver and rectify qi, free and disinhibit urination

Guiding formula: Modified *Chen Xiang San* (Aquilaria Powder)

Ingredients:
Chen Xiang (Aquilariae Lignum Resinatum), 6g
Shi Wei (Pyrrosiae Folium), 10g
Hua Shi (Talcum), 20g
Qing Pi (Citri Reticulatae Pericarpium Viride), 10g
Bai Shao Yao (Paeoniae Radix Alba), 15g

Tian Kui Zi (Semiaquilegiae Radix), 10g
Wang Bu Liu Xing (Vaccariae Semen), 12g
Dang Gui (Angelicae Sinensis Radix), 6g
Chai Hu (Bupleuri Radix), 6g

Modifications: For patients with depressed liver fire with bitter taste in the mouth, throat pain, and marked painful urination, add *Mu Dan Pi* (Moutan Cortex), 12g, *Shan Zhi Zi* (Gardeniae Fructus), 12g, and *Long Dan Cao* (Gentianae Radix), 12g, to clear and drain liver fire. For marked liver depression, add *Yu Jin* (Curcumae Radix), 12g, *Xiang Fu* (Cyperi Rhizoma), 9g, and *Chuan Lian Zi* (Toosendan Fructus), 12g, to course the liver and rectify qi, and to resolve depression and dissipate binds.

7. Center qi fall

Signs: Sagging distention in the lesser abdomen, desire to urinate with either an inability to expel urine or an inability to expel more than a scanty amount of urine, unsmooth urination, lassitude of essence-spirit, poor appetite, shortness of breath and laziness to speak, faint low voice, sagging sensation in the anus, pale tongue with thin white fur, fine weak pulse.

Treatment principles: Upbear the clear and downbear the turbid, transform qi and disinhibit urine

Guiding formulas: *Bu Zhong Yi Qi Tang* (Center-Supplementing Qi-Boosting Decoction) with *Chun Ze Tang* (Spring Pond Decoction)

Ingredients:

Dang Shen (Codonopsis Radix), 15g
Bai Zhu (Atractylodis Macrocephalae Rhizoma), 12g
Fu Ling (Poria), 15g
Huang Qi (Astragali Radix), 15g
Sheng Ma (Cimicifugae Rhizoma), 6g
Chai Hu (Bupleuri Radix), 6g
Zhu Ling (Polyporus), 15g
Ze Xie (Alismatis Rhizoma), 12g
Gui Zhi (Cinnamomi Ramulus), 10g

Modifications: For symptoms such as abdominal distention, belching, nausea, diarrhea, and white slimy tongue fur, add *Ban Xia* (Pinelliae Rhizoma), 12g, *Mu Xiang* (Aucklandiae Radix), 10g, add at end, and *Sha Ren* (Amomi Fructus), 12g, add at end, to aromatically transform dampness and move qi.

General treatment principles

In addition to the specific treatment protocols discussed above for BPH, there are some other general principles of treatment in Chinese medicine that also apply to this condition.

I. Quickening blood and transforming stasis, transforming phlegm and softening hardness, and dissipating binds

From Western medicine, we do now know that the symptoms experienced by these patients are due to a hyperplasia of the urethral prostate which blocks urinary flow. When digital rectal examination or other diagnostic procedures reveal a palpably firm or enlarged prostate, then we know that phlegm-stasis, congelation, and binding are present. Based on this knowledge we can add specific medicinals aimed at treating this. These include:

> *Tao Ren* (Persicae Semen)
> *Hong Hua* (Carthami Flos)
> *Zhi Ru Xiang* (Olibanum Praeparatum)
> *San Leng* (Sparganii Rhizoma)
> *E Zhu* (Curcumae Rhizoma)
> *Xia Ku Cao* (Prunellae Spica)
> *Xuan Shen* (Scrophulariae Radix)
> *Sheng Mu Li* (Ostreae Concha Cruda)
> *Bei Mu* (Fritillariae Bulbus)
> *Hai Zao* (Sargassum)
> *Kun Bu* (Laminariae/Eckloniae Thallus)

2. "Treat the upper [burner] for diseases of the lower [burner]"

The principle of "treating the upper [burner] for diseases of the lower [burner]" applies to this condition. The following medicinals are commonly used:

> *Jie Geng* (Platycodonis Radix)
> *Xing Ren* (Armeniacae Semen)
> *Jing Jie* (Schizonepetae Herba)
> *Gui Zhi* (Cinnamomi Ramulus)
> *Ma Huang* (Ephedrae Herba)

3. "When one desires downbearing, first upbear"

This method of treatment involves the use of medicinals that upbear center burner qi to promote smooth downbearing of water. Chief among these are:

> *Sheng Ma* (Cimicifugae Rhizoma)
> *Chai Hu* (Bupleuri Radix)
> *He Ye* (Nelumbinis Folium)

Acumoxa therapy

Select from among the following points:

Repletion patterns

Main points: *Zhong Ji* (CV-3), *Pang Guang Shu* (BL-28), *Qi Hai* (CV-6), *Yin Ling Quan* (SP-9), and *San Yin Jiao* (SP-6)

Modifications: For panting from damp toxic evil harassing the upper body,[12]

---

[12] This is probably a patient who is developing renal complications.

add *Chi Ze* (LU-5), and bleed *Shao Shang* (LU-11). For heart vexation and agitation, add *Nei Guan* (PC-6)

Vacuity patterns

Main points: *Yin Gu* (KI-10), *Shen Shu* (BL-23), *San Jiao Shu* (BL-22), *Pang Guang Shu* (BL-28), *Qi Hai* (CV-6), *Guan Yuan* (CV-4), *Zhong Ji* (CV-3), *Wei Yang* (BL-39), *Shui Dao* (ST-28), *Tai Xi* (KI-3), *Bai Hui* (GV-20), *Zu San Li* (ST-36)

Modifications: For urinary retention, add *Qi Hai* (CV-6) and *Da Ling* (PC-7). For anuria, add *San Jiao Shu* (BL-22), *Shen Shu* (BL-23), *Jing Men* (GB-25), *Yin Ling Quan* (SP-9), and moxa *Tian Shu* (ST-25) and *Qi Hai* (CV-6). For sagging sensation in the anus, add *Ci Liao* (BL-32).

External treatments

Sitz bath formulas (Chen and Jiang, 2000)[13]

Daily warm sitz baths in either plain water or a medicinal solution is generally recommended for both prevention and treatment of BPH. One may either boil the prescribed internal formula a third time and use the resulting medicinal brew as the sitz bath formula, or use a specifically designated prescription.

1. Bathe in plain hot water for 30 minutes 2–3 times per day. This is used for all types of BPH, however, it should be avoided by men who have impaired fertility because when the testicles are heated spermatogenesis and sperm vitality are impaired.

2. For damp-heat patterns, use as a hot sitz bath for 30 minutes once per day using the medicinals below. Decoct the medicinals in enough water to yield 1500–2000 ml of medicinal solution.
   Ye Ju Hua (Chrysanthemi Indici Flos), 30g
   Ku Shen (Sophorae Flavescentis Radix), 30g
   Ma Chi Xian (Portulacae Herba), 30g
   Bai Jiang Cao (Patriniae Herba), 30g
   Yan Hu Suo (Corydalis Rhizoma), 15g
   Dang Gui (Angelicae Sinensis Radix), 12g
   Bing Lang (Arecae Semen), 10g

3. For damp-heat patterns, use as a hot sitz bath solution for 30 minutes once per day. Decoct the following medicinals in enough water to yield 1500–2000 ml of medicinal solution:
   Pu Gong Ying (Taraxaci Herba), 30g
   Bai Zhi (Angelicae Dahuricae Radix), 30g
   Da Huang (Rhei Radix et Rhizoma), 30g
   Gan Cao (Glycyrrhizae Radix), 10g

---

[13] Note that these are the same formulas as provided for prostatitis.

Bi Xie (Dioscoreae Hypoglaucae seu Semptemlobae Rhizoma), 30g

Umbilical compress therapy for urinary block

Da Suan (Allii Sativi Bulbus), 3 cloves
Shan Zhi Zi (Gardeniae Fructus), 3 pieces
Mang Xiao (Natrii Sulfas), 3g.

Instructions: First grind the *Shan Zhi Zi* into powder and mix with the *Da Suan* and *Mang Xiao* to make a paste the consistency of soft mud. Place the paste into the patient's umbilicus and cover with a taped gauze bandage. Remove the medicinals once the patient has urinated. Beyond that, the length of time to retain the paste in the umbilicus is not specified. Monitor the patient carefully for signs of dermatological reactions including blistering, and be alert for signs of secondary infection if the skin has been broken (Tan and Tao, 1999).

Hot medicinal compress therapy for urinary block (Tan and Tao, 1999)

1. Place 250g of dry stir-fried warm table salt in a cloth bag. Apply to the lesser abdomen. Reheat and reuse as necessary.

2. Saute 250g of fresh chopped scallion in wine and place in cloth bag. Apply to the umbilicus and lesser abdominal region repeatedly until urination occurs.

Preventive measures and lifestyle modification

1. Avoid sitting or bicycling for long periods of time, and avoid delaying urination

Sitting for long periods of time compresses the perineal region and the urethra, and can therefore worsen bladder outlet obstruction. In terms of Chinese medicine, sitting for long periods can worsen qi stagnation and blood stasis, and further obstruct triple burner qi transformation. Cyclists should use bicycle seats with a "prostate-relief zone," which can decrease pressure on the perineum. Holding one's urine for unnecessarily long periods of time can also obstruct triple burner qi transformation and inhibit urinary flow, and encourage the collection of dampness, phlegm, and blood stasis.

2. Follow a clear-bland (*qing dan*) diet

In general, these patients should a follow a clear-bland diet and must especially moderate or eliminate their intake of greasy-fried, spicy-hot, and sweet foods, as well as alcohol. All of these foods engender dampness and heat and can impair splenic movement and transformation. Further, according to Fan (2004), alcohol is especially injurious to the prostate, and men should diligently avoid having sex while under the influence of alcohol.

3. Engage in moderate and regular exercise

In order to strengthen the body and to encourage the free movement of qi, blood, and fluids, regular moderate physical exercise is recommended for all patients with BPH. On the other hand, overexertion should be strictly avoided because it carries the risk of over-dissipating qi and leading to triple burner qi transformation failure; this could encourage the development of urinary block.

4. Avoid wearing tight undergarments

When underwear is too tightly bound around a man's anterior yin region, all the local qi, blood, and fluids are less able to move. This encourages the development of and/or worsens preexisting dampness, phlegm, qi stagnation, and blood stasis. When men choose to wear undergarments, they should choose "boxer style" shorts rather than more tightly-fitting "briefs."[14] In my own experience, one should also avoid wearing undergarments made from synthetic, nonbreathable fabrics; wearing these fabrics seems to encourage the development of dampness and heat in the anterior yin region. Hence, cotton underwear is preferred to nylon.

5. Pace sexual life

Avoid having sex while under the influence of alcohol. Avoid excessive sexual activity because it can damage the kidney yin, yang, and essence. On the other hand, regular and moderate sexual activity helps to maintain the flow of qi, blood, and fluids in the anterior yin. Ejaculation can help to drain the prostate and prevent or reduce accumulation and stagnation. Seminal retention practices are generally not recommended for patients with BPH.

6. Take hot baths regularly

Bathing in hot water regularly encourages the smooth movement of qi, blood, and fluids in the anterior yin region.[15] This simple practice is also quite helpful in relieving and preventing the symptoms of hemorrhoids, which very frequently present in men with BPH who have the pattern of spleen qi vacuity and center qi fall.

Experiential formulas

Supplementing and moving qi, and freeing and disinhibiting the waterways

Deng (1998) reports favorable results for BPH with his formula called *Qian Lie Xian Pei Da Fang* (Prostatic Enlargement Formula), which is organized around the treatment principles of supplementing and moving qi, as well as freeing and disinhibiting the waterways. The ingredients are:

Huang Qi (Astragali Radix), 30g
Li Zhi He (Litchi Semen), 10g
Ju He (Citri Reticulatae Semen), 10g
Wang Bu Liu Xing (Vaccariae Semen), 12g

---

[14] This is discussed further in Book 2, Chapter 8 on Male Infertility.

[15] The exception here is that men who are experiencing infertility should avoid this practice because when the testes are unduly heated, the formation and vitality of sperm are impaired.

Hua Shi (Talcum), 20g
Mu Tong (Akebiae Trifoliatae Caulis), 10g
Fu Ling (Poria), 15g
Chuan Shan Jia (Manitis Squama), 15g
Gan Cao (Glycyrrhizae Radix), 5g
Liang Tou Jian (Anemones Raddeanae Rhizoma),[16] 10g
Yu Mi Xu (Mays Stylus), 30g

Modifications: For patients with frequent urination, urinary urgency, and rough painful urination, add *Zhen Zhu Cao* (Phyllanthi Urinariae Herba cum Radice),[17] 15g, and *Xiao Ye Feng Wei Cao* (Pteris Multifida),[18] 15g. For bloody strangury, add *Bai Mao Gen* (Imperatae Rhizoma), 30g, *San Ye Ren Zi Cao* (Anteron Filiforme),[19] 30g, and *Dan Dou Chi* (Sojae Semen Praeparatum), 10g.

Dispelling stasis and freeing the network vessels, boosting qi and freeing stasis

Liang (1999) provides a formula called *Tong Long Tang* (Dribbling Freeing Decoction) for the treatment of BPH due to qi vacuity and stasis-obstruction. The ingredients of this formula collectively function to dispel stasis and free the network vessels, and to boost qi and free stasis.

Wang Bu Liu Xing (Vaccariae Semen), 15g
Yin Yang Huo (Epimedii Herba), 15g
Niu Xi (Achyranthis Bidentatae Radix), 15g
Huang Qi (Astragali Radix), 60g
Chuan Shan Jia (Manitis Squama), 10g
Sheng Da Huang (Rhei Radix et Rhizoma Crudi), 10g

Modifications: For patients with yang vacuity, add *Shu Fu Zi* (Aconiti Radix Lateralis Conquita) and *Rou Gui* (Cinnamomi Cortex) to warm the yang and transform qi. For damp-heat add *Zhi Mu* (Anemarrhenae Rhizoma), *Huang Bai* (Phellodendri Cortex), *Che Qian Zi* (Plantaginis Semen), *Mu Tong* (Akebiae Trifoliatae Caulis), and *Bai Hua She She Cao* (Oldenlandiae Diffusae Herba) to clear and disinhibit damp-heat. For more severe blood stasis obstructing the network vessels, add *Wu Gong* (Scolopendra), *Hu Po* (Succinum) powder, and *Tao Ren* (Persicae Semen) to quicken blood, transform stasis, and free the urinary orifice. In order to disperse phlegm and dissipate binds, add *Shan Ci Gu* (Cremastrae seu Pleiones Pseudobulbus).

---

[16] *Liang Tou Jian* is acrid, hot, and toxic; it dispels wind dampness and disperses abscesses and swelling.
[17] *Zhen Zhu Cao* is sweet and slightly bitter; it clears heat and disinhibits dampness, brightens the eyes, and disperses stagnation.
[18] *Xiao Ye Feng Wei Cao* is bland, slightly bitter, and cool; it clears heat and disinhibits dampness, and cools blood and resolves toxin.
[19] *San Ye Ren Zi Cao* is acrid and cool; it dissipates stasis and stops bleeding, and rectifies qi and resolves toxin.

Boosting qi and upbearing the clear, and disinhibiting water and freeing blockage

To treat BPH in aged men due to qi vacuity and downward fall, Cha (1996) reports on a formula called *Xuan Dao Tong Bi Tang* (Diffusing and Abducting Blockage-Freeing Decoction). The functions of this formula are to boost qi and upbear the clear, and to disinhibit water and free blockage. The ingredients are:

Huang Qi (Astragali Radix), 15g
Che Qian Zi (Plantaginis Semen), 30g
Gan Cao (Glycyrrhizae Radix), 20g
Sheng Ma (Cimicifugae Rhizoma), 7.5g
Niu Xi (Achyranthis Bidentatae Radix), 25g
Yin Yang Huo (Epimedii Herba), 15g
Hua Shi (Talcum), 25g

Modifications: For patients with bound stool, add *Rou Cong Rong* (Cistanches Herba), 20g. For pain in the urethra, add *Pu Gong Ying* (Taraxaci Herba), 25g, and *Mu Tong* (Akebiae Trifoliatae Caulis), 10g. For coughing and panting, add *Xing Ren* (Armeniacae Semen), 5g, and *Xi Xin* (Asari Herba), 5g.

Coursing the liver, transforming phlegm and dispelling stasis

Yin (1996) uses *Shu Gan San Jie Tang* (Liver-Coursing Bind-Dissipating Decoction) to treat BPH due to liver depression, phlegm stasis and congelation and stagnation. The ingredients are:

Chai Hu (Bupleuri Radix), 9g
Niu Xi (Achyranthis Bidentatae Radix), 9g
Dang Gui (Angelicae Sinensis Radix), 9g
Chi Shao (Paeoniae Radix Rubra), 9g
Dan Shen (Salviae Miltiorrhizae Radix), 9g
Mu Li (Ostreae Concha), 20g
Hai Zao (Sargassum), 12g
Kun Bu (Laminariae/Eckloniae Thallus), 12g
Hai Fu Shi (Costaziae Os/Pumex), 12g
Xuan Shen (Scrophulariae Radix), 12g
Zhe Bei Mu (Fritillariae Thunbergii Bulbus), 9g
Xia Ku Cao (Prunellae Spica), 12g
Shen Jing Zi (Latin unknown),[20] 5 grains

Warming and supplementing spleen and kidney yang

Liang (1996) uses a formula called *Liang Shi Qian Lie Xian Tang* (Master Liang's Prostate Decoction) to treat BPH in aged men due to spleen and kidney yang vacuity and insecurity of kidney qi, especially when there is nocturia and urinary incontinence. The ingredients are:

Yi Zhi Ren (Alpiniae Oxyphyllae Fructus), 30g

---

[20] *Shen Jing Zi* is the kidney stones of either goats, dogs, or cows. It is reported to be empirically effective for BPH.

Dang Shen (Codonopsis Radix), 30g
Bai Zhu (Atractylodis Macrocephalae Rhizoma), 30g
Huang Qi (Astragali Radix), 30g
Shan Yao (Dioscoreae Rhizoma), 30g
Sang Piao Xiao (Mantidis Ootheca), 15g
Shan Zhu Yu (Corni Fructus), 15g
Du Zhong (Eucommiae Cortex), 15g
Xu Duan (Dipsaci Radix), 15g
Suan Zao Ren (Ziziphi Spinosi Semen), 15g
Wu Wei Zi (Schisandrae Fructus), 15g
Duan Long Gu (Mastodi Ossis Fossilia Calcinata), 20g
Duan Mu Li (Ostreae Concha Calcinata), 20g

Supplementing the kidneys

As reported in Tan and Tao (1999), Shen Qu-Qiao suggests that this condition is mainly due to kidney vacuity, but that it also involves the spleen and lung. In his opinion—although other patterns usually complicate the basic vacuity pattern (such as damp-heat, blood stasis, and qi stagnation)—the main pattern to treat is the root kidney vacuity. He recommends two self-composed formulas—one for kidney yang vacuity and one for kidney yin vacuity. For kidney yang vacuity, he uses *Bu Shen Li Niao Tang* (Kidney-Supplementing Urine-Disinhibiting Decoction). Though no specific dosages are provided, the ingredients of this formula are:

Dang Shen (Codonopsis Radix)
Huang Qi (Astragali Radix)
Jie Geng (Platycodonis Radix)
Wu Yao (Linderae Radix)
Shan Yao (Dioscoreae Rhizoma)
Fu Pen Zi (Rubi Fructus)
Fu Ling (Poria)
Ze Xie (Alismatis Rhizoma)
Mu Dan Pi (Moutan Cortex)

For kidney yin vacuity, he uses *Yang Yin Li Niao Tang* (Yin-Nourishing Urine-Disinhibiting Decoction). The ingredients of this formula are:

Tai Zi Shen (Pseudostellariae Radix)
Mai Men Dong (Ophiopogonis Radix)
Shi Hu (Dendrobii Herba)
Wu Yao (Linderae Radix)
Shan Yao (Dioscoreae Rhizoma)
Fu Pen Zi (Rubi Fructus)
Fu Ling (Poria)
Ze Xie (Alismatis Rhizoma)
Mu Dan Pi (Moutan Cortex)
Zhi Mu (Anemarrhenae Rhizoma)
Huang Bai (Phellodendri Cortex)
Che Qian Zi (Plantaginis Semen)

Representative Chinese Research

Kidney vacuity, blood stasis, and damp-heat

Generally speaking, the three most common patterns presenting in men with BPH are kidney vacuity, blood stasis, and damp-heat. Hua (1986) reported on 150 cases and found that among his patients, there were 58 patients with kidney yin vacuity, 25 cases with kidney yang vacuity, 49 cases with vanquished essence and stasis obstruction, and 18 cases of lower burner damp-heat. The formulas he used were *Zhi Bai Di Huang Wan* (Anemarrhena, Phellodendron, and Rehmannia Pill), *Ji Sheng Shen Qi Wan* (Life Saver Kidney Qi Pill), *Huo Xue Tong Jing Wan* (Blood-Quickening Essence-Freeing Pill), and *Ba Zheng San* (Eight Corrections Powder). *Huo Xue Tong Jing Wan* is a self-composed formula containing:

Dang Gui (Angelicae Sinensis Radix)
He Shou Wu (Polygoni Multiflori Radix)
Ji Xue Teng (Spatholobi Caulis)
Chuan Niu Xi (Cyathulae Radix)
Yi Mu Cao (Leonuri Herba)
Huang Jiu (Vinum Aureum)

Results: Of the 150 cases investigated, 75 cases were cured, 62 cases were treated effectively, and 9 cases had a mild effect; this constituted a total amelioration rate of 98% (reported in Tan and Tao, 1999).

Integrated Chinese-Western medicine

Huang *et al.* (1994) reported on the treatment of 103 patients with BPH and urinary retention who were deemed unfit for surgical treatment. Instead, they were treated with either a combination of Progesterone and Chinese medicinals or with Progesterone alone. The medicinals used were:

Sang Bai Pi (Mori Cortex)
Jie Geng (Platycodonis Radix)
Qian Hu (Peucedani Radix)
Huang Qi (Astragali Radix)
Mai Men Dong (Ophiopogonis Radix)
Sheng Di Huang (Rehmanniae Radix Exsiccata seu Recens)
Che Qian Zi (Plantaginis Semen)
Ai Di Cha (Ardisia Japonica Herba)
Yi Mu Cao (Leonuri Herba)
Chi Xiao Dou (Phaseoli Semen)
Wang Bu Liu Xing (Vaccariae Semen)

Results: The group treated with combined Progesterone and Chinese medicinals consisted of 87 patients; among them, 19 cases showed marked results, 58 cases showed some results, and 10 cases showed no results. Among the 16 patients who were treated with Progesterone alone, 2 showed marked results, 9 showed some results, 4 showed no results. The authors' concluded that the use of combined Chinese-Western medicine for such patients showed better results than Western medicine alone.

External application of Chinese medicinals

Peng *et al.* (1993) used an external application of *Huo Xue Tong Lin Tang* (Blood-Quickening Strangury-Freeing Decoction) with direct current iontherapy to treat 50 cases of BPH. The ingredients of the formula were:

Zao Jiao Ci (Gleditsiae Spina)
Jin Yin Hua (Lonicerae Flos)
Huang Bai (Phellodendri Cortex)
Tu Bie Chong (Eupolyphaga seu Steliophaga)
Xia Ku Cao (Prunellae Spica)
Chuan Shan Jia (Manitis Squama)
San Leng (Sparganii Rhizoma)
E Zhu (Curcumae Rhizoma)

Results: Among the 50 cases, 32 showed marked improvement, 15 showed some effects, and 3 cases showed no results. The prostate was examined by transrectal ultrasound both before and after treatment and was markedly reduced in an unspecified number of cases.

Representative Case Studies

Noninteraction of the heart and kidneys

Zhu (1982) reported on Shi Jin Mo's successful treatment of a 66 year-old male with an eight-year history of urinary difficulty. He was previously diagnosed with BPH at a Western medical facility and was urged to have surgery. The patient had great hopes for Chinese medical care, and so came to see Master Shi. The symptoms at the initial visit were: frequent urination and very difficult urination and; episodic retention of urine, which at times was serious enough to pose the risk of renal complications and hence required periodic urinary catheterization. His tongue fur was normal and the pulse was soggy rapid.

Dr. Shi's diagnosis was noninteraction of the heart and kidney and lack of mutual control between water and fire. These patterns resulted in an ability to upbear the clear yang and downbear the turbid yin. Hence, he adopted the treatment principle of upbearing yang, disinhibiting urine, and harmonizing water and fire. He prescribed the following medicinals during the first visit:

Zhi Ma Huang (Ephedrae Herba cum Liquido Fricta), 3g
Gui Zhi (Cinnamomi Ramulus), 5g
Huang Bai (Phellodendri Cortex), 6g
Wu Zhu Yu (Evodiae Fructus), 2g
Yu Nao Shi (Pseudosciaenae Otolithum), 25g
Hua Shi (Talcum), 25g
Zhi Mu (Anemarrhenae Rhizoma), 6g
Hai Jin Sha (Lygodii Spora), 10g
Hai Fu Shi (Costaziae Os/Pumex), 10g
Wu Yao (Linderae Radix), 6g
Zhi Gan Cao (Glycyrrhizae Radix cum Liquido Fricta), 3g
Fu Ling (Poria), 10g

Chi Xiao Dou (Phaseoli Semen), 10g
Che Qian Cao (Plantaginis Herba), 20g
Xi Shuai (Gryllulus),[21] 7 pieces

The patient reported an improvement in his symptoms after taking two packets of medicinals; his urine was not dribbling and micturition was smoother overall, but the frequency had not diminished. Dr. Shi concluded that the patient needed to take the medicine regularly at a dosage of three packets per week. No further follow-up data was provided. He prescribed the following medicinals:

Zhi Ma Huang (Ephedrae Herba cum Liquido Fricta), 3g
Gui Zhi (Cinnamomi Ramulus), 5g
Zhi Mu (Anemarrhenae Rhizoma), 6g
Huang Bai (Phellodendri Cortex), 6g
Hai Jin Sha (Lygodii Spora), 6g
Hai Fu Shi (Costaziae Os/Pumex), 6g
Yu Nao Shi (Pseudosciaenae Otolithum), 25g
Hua Shi (Talcum), 25g
Fu Ling (Poria), 10g
Chi Xiao Dou (Phaseoli Semen), 20g
Dong Gua Zi (Benincasae Semen), 12g
Dong Kui Zi (Malvae Semen), 12g
Che Qian Cao (Plantaginis Herba), 10g
Han Lian Cao (Ecliptae Herba), 10g
Wu Zhu Yu (Evodiae Fructus), 5g
Chuan Lian Zi (Toosendan Fructus), 6g
Wu Yao (Linderae Radix), 6g
Zhi Gan Cao (Glycyrrhizae Radix cum Liquido Fricta), 3g
Lou Gu (Gryllotalpa),[22] 1 piece
Xi Shuai (Gryllulus), 7 pieces

Qi stagnation and phlegm congelation obstructing the urinary pathway

Yin (1996) reported a case of BPH accompanying hypertension in a 78 year-old man. His chief complaint was dribbling urination that had persisted for several years. One year prior to the first visit, he had experienced an acute episode of urinary retention and sought Western medical care at a hospital; it was at that time that the diagnosis of BPH was established. At that time, he was not considered to be a good candidate for prostate surgery; hence, he was catheterized and advised to seek care with Chinese medicine. Even though he had seen several different doctors and had taken several different formulas, he still had yet to experience relief. Further, owing to his indwelling urinary catheter, he had experienced several episodes of urinary tract infections. At the time of the first visit, his body appeared emaciated, his essence-spirit was

---

[21] *Xi Shuai* (Gryllulus) is acrid, salty, and warm, and disinhibits urine.
[22] *Lou Gu* (Gryllotalpa) is salty and cold; it disinhibits urine and frees the stool.

debilitated, his tongue fur was slimy yellow, and pulse was stringlike and felt forceful upon deep palpation.

Dr. Yin's diagnosis was qi stagnation and phlegm congelation obstructing the urinary pathway. Hence, he adopted the strategy of rectifying qi and quickening blood, and transforming phlegm and dissipating binds. He prescribed the following medicinals to be taken with a little bit of *Long Yan Rou* (Longan Arillus):

> *Chai Hu* (Bupleuri Radix), 10g
> *Niu Xi* (Achyranthis Bidentatae Radix), 10g
> *Sheng Mu Li* (Ostreae Concha Cruda), 30g, predecocted
> *Dan Shen* (Salviae Miltiorrhizae Radix), 15g
> *Dang Gui* (Angelicae Sinensis Radix), 15g
> *Chi Shao Yao* (Paeoniae Radix Rubra), 15g
> *Hai Fu Shi* (Costaziae Os/Pumex), 15g, predecocted
> *Hai Zao* (Sargassum), 15g
> *Kun Bu* (Laminariae/Eckloniae Thallus), 15g
> *Xia Ku Cao* (Prunellae Spica), 15g
> *Xuan Shen* (Scrophulariae Radix), 15g
> *Chuan Bei Mu* (Fritillariae Cirrhosae Bulbus), 3g, powder
> *Shen Jing Zi* (Latin unavailable),[23] 5 grains

At the second visit, the patient reported decreased symptoms after taking two packets of medicine, and the catheter was removed after the fifth packet. Treatment was continued further for a total of ten packets, and all his symptoms disappeared. Repeated follow-up inquiries were made to the patient, and he reported no relapses.

Kidney yin vacuity with heat and qi stagnation and blood stasis

In Chen and Jiang (2000), Chen Bo-Xian reported a case of BPH in a 70 year-old man for whom he used the treatment principle of enriching yin and clearing heat, diffusing qi and transforming stasis, and disinhibiting the urinary orifice and freeing blockage. The patient had a six-year history of prostate hyperplasia with dribbling and unsmooth urination. One week prior to the initial visit, he suddenly developed urinary block. He was catheterized at an outpatient facility and had been unable to urinate on his own since then. Further, he also had pain in the lumbus, vexation and agitation, and distention and tenseness of the lesser abdomen, but his appetite and bowel movements were normal. His facial complexion was dark, stagnant, and lusterless, the tongue was red with a slightly thin yellow slimy fur, and the pulse was stringlike fine rapid. The diagnosis was insufficiency of kidney yin with stasis obstructing the urinary pathway. Dr. Chen prescribed the following medicinals:

> *Sheng Di Huang* (Rehmanniae Radix Exsiccata seu Recens), 18g
> *Dang Gui* (Angelicae Sinensis Radix), 9g
> *Chi Shao Yao* (Paeoniae Radix Rubra), 9g

---

[23] See note 19 on page 194.

Mu Dan Pi (Moutan Cortex), 9g
Mu Tong (Akebiae Trifoliatae Caulis), 9g
Dan Zhu Ye (Lophatheri Herba), 9g
Ze Xie (Alismatis Rhizoma), 9g
Che Qian Zi (Plantaginis Semen), 9g
Xing Ren (Armeniacae Semen), 9g
Nu Zhen Zi (Ligustri Lucidi Fructus), 9g
Han Lian Cao (Ecliptae Herba), 9g
Wang Bu Liu Xing (Vaccariae Semen), 9g
Ze Lan (Lycopi Herba), 9g
Hu Po (Succinum), 3g, powdered and taken mixed with the strained
    decoction, in two divided doses
Gan Cao (Glycyrrhizae Radix), 3g

At the second visit, the patient reported that after having taken three packets of medicine, his urination became more able to flow on its own, but there was still dribbling and the flow of urine was still unsmooth; in addition, he reported pain within his penis when he urinated. After taking another six packets, however, his urine was flowing normally. He reported having bilateral leg pain and occasional cramping in the legs. Dr. Chen added *Niu Xi* (Achyranthis Bidentatae Radix), 9g, and *Bai Shao* (Paeoniae Radix Alba), 15g, and after three packets, he recovered completely from the acute symptoms. The case study gives no indication about the long-term status of the patient.

Qi vacuity with turbid dampness brewing in the interior

In Xing (1991), we find a case of BPH in a slightly younger man—a 58 year-old worker with center burner qi vacuity. The patient reported that he was generally healthy, but that six months ago he had experienced sudden onset of lower abdominal discomfort, which then progressed to urinary difficulty. He stated that it took him ten minutes of effort while attempting to urinate before any urine would flow. Also, in the recent three weeks, urination had required great effort, the quantity of urine was scanty, and it would come out only in dribbles; accompanying this was a sensation of distention and oppression in the lower abdomen.

At the initial visit, Dr. Xing noted that the patient was relatively overweight, his essence-spirit was devitalized, and he had an anguished facial expression. The digital rectal exam revealed a walnut-sized prostate. The pulse was deep moderate and the tongue was red and lacked fur. The diagnosis was qi vacuity with exuberance of yin, and turbid dampness brewing in the interior. The prescription was as follows:

Huang Qi (Astragali Radix), 30g
Ze Xie (Alismatis Rhizoma), 12g
Yi Yi Ren (Coicis Semen), 12g
Chi Shao (Paeoniae Radix Rubra), 12g
Mu Dan Pi (Moutan Cortex), 10g
Chao Bai Zhu (Atractylodis Macrocephalae Rhizoma Frictum), 10g

Tao Ren (Persicae Semen), 10g
Fu Ling (Poria), 10g
Xiang Fu (Cyperi Rhizoma), 10g
Hong Hua (Carthami Flos), 10g
Bian Xu (Polygoni Avicularis Herba), 6g
Gan Cao Shao (Glycyrrhizae Radix Tenuis), 6g
Rou Gui (Cinnamomi Cortex), 3g

After taking three packets of medicine, the patient reported that the quantity of urine had increased, that the level of difficulty he experienced during urination had decreased, and that the slight dribbling urine had changed to a sluggish trickle (*i.e.*, the flow rate had apparently improved). Further, he stated that the lower abdominal discomfort had decreased. Dr. Xing noted that the pulse had increased in force somewhat, and that the evil water qi that had been brewing in the interior was beginning to move. Feeling strengthened in his resolve that the initial prescription had hit the mark, and that *Huang Qi* was especially responsible for the positive result, he doubled its dosage. His modified prescription was:

Huang Qi (Astragali Radix), 60g
Shan Yao (Dioscoreae Rhizoma), 15g
Ze Xie (Alismatis Rhizoma), 12g
Da Fu Pi (Arecae Pericarpium), 12g
Sheng Di Huang (Rehmanniae Radix Exsiccata seu Recens), 12g
Chao Bai Zhu (Atractylodis Macrocephalae Rhizoma Frictum), 10g
Fu Ling (Poria), 10g
Chi Shao Yao (Paeoniae Radix Rubra), 10g
Tao Ren (Persicae Semen), 10g
San Leng (Sparganii Rhizoma), 10g
Qian Niu Zi (Pharbitidis Semen), 6g, powdered
Rou Gui (Cinnamomi Cortex), 3g

At the third visit—after taking five packets of the second prescription—his urination was smooth, the lesser abdominal discomfort was relieved, and his essence-spirit was clear and strengthened. He continued to take this formula in pill form for an unspecified period to maintain the results and to prevent relapse. No follow-up digital rectal examination was provided.

Blood stasis obstructing the urinary pathway

Zhang (1984) treated an 84 year-old farmer for the blood stasis obstruction pattern of BPH. The patient went to the hospital complaining of dribbling and blocked urination, and had been diagnosed with BPH. He was catheterized, received bladder puncture, and given antibiotics and diuretics. By the second day of treatment, his condition had not improved very much, so he was referred for Chinese medical care. At that time, his tongue was red and lacked fur, and his pulse was stringlike fine rapid.

Based on the fact that this patient had a history of copious urine and terminal dribbling—which was presumably due to insecurity of kidney qi—the patient was diagnosed with advanced kidney vacuity with nontransformation of qi and placed on a prescription to supplement the kidney, boost qi, and disinhibit urine; the prescription was a modification of *Zi Shen Tong Guan Wan* (Kidney-Enriching Gate-Opening Pill) with *Ze Xie* (Alismatis Rhizoma) and *Niu Xi* (Achyranthis Bidentatae Radix). Despite taking the prescription, his urination had not improved, and he still required bladder puncture for voiding. Upon re-evaluation, his pulse was still noted to be stringlike fine rapid, and the tongue was still red and lacked fur, and it was noted that there was abdominal pain refusing pressure.

Dr. Zhang diagnosed contention and binding of blood and heat, stasis obstruction in the urinary pathway, and failure of upbearing and downbearing of right qi. The treatment principle was to clear heat and eliminate stasis, and to use attacking precipitants. The prescription consisted of the following ingredients:

Da Huang (Rhei Radix et Rhizoma), 12g, add at end
Wu Gong (Scolopendra), 1 piece
Gui Zhi (Cinnamomi Ramulus), 6g
Zhe Chong (Eupolyphaga seu Steleophaga), 6g
Hong Hua (Carthami Flos), 9g
Huang Bai (Phellodendri Cortex), 10g
Niu Xi (Achyranthis Bidentatae Radix), 10g
Zhi Mu (Anemarrhenae Rhizoma), 10g
Xian Di Long (Lumbricus Vivus), 40g

After taking one packet of this new prescription, there was slight dribbling urine, but it was accompanied by urinary urgency and pain. Since his urine was still unsmooth and dribbling after one packet of this prescription, the following changes were made: *Gui Zhi* was removed, and *Sheng Di Huang* (Rehmanniae Radix Exsiccata seu Recens), 15g, *Gan Cao Shao* (Glycyrrhizae Radix Tenuis), 6g, *Nu Zhen Zi* (Ligustri Lucidi Fructus), 10g, were added to strengthen the ability of the prescription to enrich yin and clear heat.

After the second packet, the urinary frequency, urgency, and scorching pain had greatly reduced, the flow of his urine had become smooth, and his bowel movements were normal. He was advised to take *Zhi Bai Di Huang Wan* (Anemarrhena, Phellodendron, and Rehmannia Pill) regularly and to avoid eating spicy-hot, and greasy foods. After being released from the hospital and following this regimen for six months, he remained symptom-free.

Prostate Cancer

Western Medicine

Prostate cancer is one of the most common forms of malignancy in male patents. According to Fauci et al (1998), it is the third most common cause of death among men over the age of 55 in the United States. There are global differences in the death rates of prostatic carcinoma, with about 14 deaths per 100,000 men per year in the United States, 22 per 100,000 in Sweden, yet only 2 per 100,000 in Japan. It is interesting to note that although the occurrence rates in Japanese men living in Japan are lower than those of men in the United States, Japanese immigrants to the United States develop the disease at a similar rate as other men in the country. This suggests that some dietary or other environmental factor exerts its influence on these men while they are living in the United States, increasing their rates of prostate cancer, and tends to de-emphasize genetic make-up as a predisposing factor. For an unknown reason, the incidence of prostate cancer among African-American men in the United States is the highest in the nation.

As men age, their risk of prostate cancer increases, and the median age at diagnosis is 72 (Beers *et al.*, 2006). Autopsy studies report that 15–60% of men aged 60–90 have prostate cancer. The fact that many of these cases go undiagnosed while the patient is living gives testament to the fact that prostate cancer is frequently asymptomatic, and is often slow-growing and not aggressive. Aggressive disease does occur, however, and clinicians should remain alert for it.

Diagnosis

Fauci et al (1998) report that in the past, over 80% of cases already had advanced local or metastatic disease by the time they presented to their physicians, suggesting either that these men were asymptomatic, or for some reason delayed seeking help for their symptoms. Although prostatic cancer may be asymptomatic, there are certain signs to look for in clinical practice. These include symptoms of bladder outlet obstruction such as dysuria, difficulty in voiding, increased urinary frequency, terminal dribbling, and possibly even complete urinary retention in advanced disease. Back or hip pain, a possible sign of bone metastasis, and hematuria are generally signs of advanced disease. Although the digital rectal examination (DRE) may show the characteristic findings of hardness, nodulation, and an otherwise irregular surface (especially over the lateral lobes of the prostate), it may also be normal in many cases.

• PSA

Serum Prostate Specific Antigen (PSA) is elevated in 25%–90% of men with the disease, although its relevance as a screening and diagnostic marker for prostate cancer is debated. The controversy centers around the reality that PSA is moderately elevated in some men with Benign Prostatic Hyperplasia (BPH), and in men with a recent history of prostatitis. Fauci et al (1998) report that refinements of the PSA test are under investigation, and that some surgeons are beginning to apply them in the evaluation of their patients.

THE GLEASON SCORE

Named after its developer—pathologist Donald F. Gleason—the Gleason score is a scale of histologic grading used by oncologists to help determine the severity and prognosis of prostate cancer and hence to aid in the clinical decision-making process. The Gleason score is determined by a pathologist by analyzing and scoring (with a grade ranging from 2 to 10) the prostate biopsy according to the specific criteria listed below:

> **Grade 1-** The cancerous prostate closely resembles normal prostate tissue. The glands are small, well-formed, and closely packed.
>
> **Grade 2-** The tissue still has well-formed glands, but they are larger and have more tissue between them.
>
> **Grade 3-** The tissue still has recognizable glands, but the cells are darker. At high magnification, some of these cells have left the glands and are beginning to invade the surrounding tissue.
>
> **Grade 4-** The tissue has few recognizable glands. Many cells are invading the surrounding tissue.
>
> **Grade 5-** The tissue does not have recognizable glands. There are often just sheets of cells throughout the surrounding tissue.

The Gleason score is calculated in two steps. The primary grade rates the tumor pattern exhibited throughout more than 50% of the tumor tissue, and the secondary grade rates the tumor pattern exhibited in less than 50% but more than 5% of the tumor tissue. The primary grade and the secondary grade are added together to yield the final Gleason score. For example, if a patient's primary grade is 2 and the secondary grade is 4, his Gleason score is 6. A final grade of 2 is associated with the best prognosis and a grade of 10 is associated with the worst prognosis.

• *Prostate cancer staging*

As with other cancers, a staging system is used to rate the severity of prostate cancer and is used to aid in clinical decision-making. The most common staging method consists of 4 stages determined by the following criteria:

Stage I: Cancer cells are detected incidentally in a small section of prostate tissue during another procedure such as a transurethral resection of the prostate (TURP), the abnormal cells closely resemble normal cells, and the prostate feels normal on digital rectal examination (DRE).

Stage II: A larger area of the prostate is involved than in stage I, and a prostatic nodule located within the prostate can be palpated with DRE.

Stage III: The tumor has protruded through the prostatic capsule and can be palpated on the prostatic surface with DRE.

Stage IV: The tumor has spread to nearby organs and surrounding lymph nodes.

• *Clinical decision-making*

According to Thompson (2002), current clinical decision-making for prostate cancer patients generally takes the form of first referring the patient for transrectal prostate biopsy under sonogram (TRUS) when he has either a positive DRE and serum PSA greater than 2.5 ng/mL, positive DRE and normal serum PSA, or negative DRE and serum PSA greater than 2.5 ng/mL. This referral pattern is the most conservative and carries the least risk of missing the diagnosis and of delaying treatment, though it might result in some unnecessary biopsies.

Although transrectal ultrasound of the prostate (TRUS) can establish the degree of encroachment of prostate cancer on surrounding tissues, and can therefore help in the staging process, it is not considered to be independently diagnostic for the disease, and it is rather more often used as a means of guiding the surgeon's biopsy needle.

Treatment

The treatment of prostate cancer is determined by weighing several factors together including the serum PSA levels, the histologic grading (using the Gleason score), staging and assessment of metastatic disease (usually using the four-stage model), the patient's age, overall medical history, and life expectancy. The decision-making process for patients and their physicians is fairly complex and involves considering various treatment options ranging in degree of aggressiveness from watchful waiting to radical prostatectomy and orchiectomy. In general, however, there are three main treatments for prostate cancer: watchful waiting; radiotherapy and; prostatectomy.

• *Watchful waiting*

Watchful waiting—which is generally used for asymptomatic patients over the age of 70 who have other medical conditions that might otherwise lead to death—consists of annual (if not more frequent) PSA measurement, DRE, and symptomatic monitoring. If the patient's condition remains stable, no other interventions are unnecessary. If the physician detects by one or more of these methods of assessment an escalation of the disease, then more active treatment options are adopted at that time.

• Radiotherapy

Radiotherapy, generally used for patients who have more significant disease and who are younger than 70 years of age, consists of either implantation of radioactive "seeds" directly into the prostate (brachytherapy), or of the application of external beam radiotherapy to the prostate. Radiotherapy may control the disease well in many cases, but carries a high risk (approximately 50%) of erectile dysfunction, and causes obstructive and irritative urinary symptoms in a significant portion of patients.

• Surgery

Radical prostatectomy, although curative for the disease when it is confined to the prostate carries a high risk of erectile dysfunction and urinary incontinence, even with advances in "nerve-sparing" surgical techniques. For known or suspected lymphatic metastases, lymphadenectomy is also performed.

• Hormonal therapy

Androgen deprivation hormonal therapy is also available and takes the form of either internal administration of luteinizing hormone-releasing hormone (LHRH) agonists such as leuprolide or is accomplished through castration. Cytotoxic chemotherapeutic agents are also used, but are generally reserved for advanced tumors and for metastatic involvement.

Western Complementary Therapy

A number of supplements, diets, and herbal combinations have been suggested as preventatives or treatments for prostate cancer. From among those that have been evaluated in research studies, a few have emerged as having some potential for prostate cancer prevention. These include vitamin D supplementation, vitamin E supplementation (Beta Carotene Cancer Prevention Study Group, 1994), a low-fat diet (Giovannucci *et al.*, 1993), Selenium supplementation (Clark *et al.*, 1998), and soy product ingestion (Messina *et al.*, 1994).

The PC-SPES controversy

PC-SPES, purported to be an "herbal" product was found in a recent study reported in the *Journal of the National Cancer Institute* in 2002 to be highly variable in composition, and samples were tainted with pharmaceutical substances such as Warfarin, diethylstilbestrol (DES), synthetic estrogens, and indomethacin. (Sovak *et al.*, 2002). Thus, the therapeutic value attributed to the herbal ingredients of PC-SPES are under further investigation at this point and may be attributed to the synthetic estrogens, to a synergistic effect of the drugs and herbs together, or to an individual or synergistic herbal effect. Though the exact mechanisms of action and composition of PC-SPES remains elusive, some studies suggest that it compares favorably to standard hormonal treatment of prostate cancer in patients with advanced metastatic disease. Research is ongoing (DiPaola *et al.*, 1998).

According to the National Cancer Institute, the herbal ingredients of PC-SPES are:
> *Ju Hua* (Chrysanthemi Flos)
> *Gan Cao* (Glycyrrhiza Radix)
> *Dong Ling Cao* (Rabdosia Rubescens)
> *San Qi* (Notoginseng Radix)
> *Huang Qin* (Scutellaria Radix)
> *Ling Zhi* (Ganoderma)
> *Ban Lan Gen* (Isatis Radix)
> *Saw Palmetto* (Serenoa Recens)

Chinese Medicine

Disease discrimination

As we have seen, patients with symptomatic prostate cancer often experience bladder outlet obstruction accompanied by symptoms such as difficulty in voiding, increased urinary frequency, terminal dribbling, and urinary retention. Further, some men also experience hematospermia and hematuria. Based on these signs, the most appropriate Chinese disease categories to consider when reframing prostate cancer into Chinese medicine are dribbling urinary block (*long bi*), strangury (*lin zheng*),[1] hematospermia (*xue jing*), and hematuria (*xue niao*).

Hematospermia is a condition in which blood is evident in the ejaculate. While the reader will recall that there are three main causes of bleeding in Chinese medicine (heat; stasis of blood and; qi vacuity), clinically speaking hematospermia is usually caused by heat harassing the essence chamber and damaging its network vessels; as a result, heat forces the blood within the essence chamber to move recklessly outside its normal pathway. It then mixes with the semen and is evident when ejaculation occurs. Bloody urine obviously refers to a condition in which there is blood mixed with one's urine. In summary, as dribbling urinary block, strangury, hematuria and hematospermia reflect the clinical signs of patients with prostate cancer, it is under these headings that Chinese medical clinicians find useful information—reframed using Chinese medical logic—on the disease causes, pathomechanisms, and treatments of prostate cancer.

It is important to note, however, that prostate cancer is a Western disease

---

[1] For a more complete discussion of dribbling urinary block and strangury, see Prostatitis: Book 2, Chapter 1.

category and that modern Chinese andrologists always approach this disease with an integrative diagnostic and therapeutic approach. In terms of diagnosis, they rely on modern medical technology; in terms of treatment, they always use medicinals that are known to have antitumor action, often in combination with surgery, radiation, and chemotherapy, depending on the same criteria that Western oncologists use.

Disease causes and pathomechanisms

There are four main disease causes commonly cited as factors in the development of prostate cancer. They usually exist in combinations of 2–4, but listed separately they are: 1) stirring of ministerial fire in the interior due to liver and kidney yin vacuity; 2) overindulgence in rich, sweet, fatty, and greasy foods, as well as spicy-hot foods and alcohol; 3) long-term avoidance of or inability to ejaculate and; 4) generalized weakness due to either constitutional vacuity or to serious or enduring illness.

As men age, their liver and kidney yin is gradually depleted. This natural process is accelerated when we engage in activities that further exhaust yin such as excessive sexual activity and overuse of certain stimulating recreational drugs.[2] As a result of exhaustion of liver and kidney yin-humor, ministerial fire becomes hyperactive, behaves as if it is evil heat, and scorches and decocts healthy fluids and tissue in the prostate. As this process evolves, phlegm congeals and binds in the prostate and forms hard nodules. This pathomechanism also explains the development of prostate stones.

In Chinese medicine, it is well-established that overindulgence in rich and "thick-flavored" foods such as those listed above engender damp-heat. How the related pathomechanisms play out more specifically in the development of prostate cancer can be explained by the fact that these foods lead to the development of damp-heat in the center burner which then pours downward into the lower burner. As damp-heat pours downward into the lower burner and settles in the essence chamber, it becomes depressed there. Depressed heat and dampness engenders damp-heat toxin and becomes bound and depressed in the essence chamber.

Although modern Chinese practitioners of andrology identify excessive sexual activity as a cause of disease, on the other hand, they generally frown on seminal retention practices. The logic behind this is that by not ejaculating, one creates a condition of depression in the essence chamber. As the free flow of qi and blood in the anterior yin region affects and is affected by free coursing of

---

[2] Although not reflected in standard Chinese medical texts, I feel it is necessary to point out from clinical practice that for modern Western patients, excessive use of excitatory stimulating drugs such as crystal methamphetamine and cocaine appears to rapidly exhaust yin-humor. This logic might be extended to the overuse of other substances such as the increasingly popular "energy drinks," and even yang-supplementing medicinals, though I have yet to make this clear correlation clinically.

liver qi, long-term retention of semen carries the risk of causing liver channel depression. This encourages the development of vanquished essence[3] and qi stagnation and blood stasis in the essence chamber. If allowed to develop unchecked, over time stagnation and stasis bind together with vanquished essence and lead to the formation of prostate cancer.

Generalized weakness following an enduring or serious illness or due to constitutional vacuity also plays an important role in the development of prostate cancer. Reframing this in nourishing life[4] terminology, any vacuity of right qi (*zheng qi*) allows evil qi to enter the body from the exterior and also allows evil qi to form in the interior. In the case of prostate cancer, weakness of right qi allows the development of evil heat and dampness and of stasis and stagnation in the prostate. This sets the stage for long-term depression and mutual binding of these evils in the prostate and hence leads to prostate cancer.

Pattern discrimination

Theoretically speaking, the early stages of prostate cancer are dominated by repletion patterns such as qi stagnation and blood stasis. However, as the disease evils progress and as right qi declines, patterns of vacuity such as insufficiency of kidney yin and qi and blood vacuity present themselves more clearly. This does not mean that the repletion patterns disappear or convert into pure vacuity patterns, but that they continue to be present and are then further complicated by vacuity. Hence, it is a combined vacuity-repletion pattern that we usually see in clinical practice. Since it is well-established that prostate cancer is often asymptomatic in the early stages and is therefore often advanced at the time of the initial diagnosis, by the time the patient seeks out the care of a physician of Chinese medicine, these combined-vacuity repletion patterns are the rule rather than the exception.

I. Qi stagnation and blood stasis

Signs: Soreness and pain of the lesser abdomen, testes, and lumbar area, vexation and agitation and irascibility, fine urine stream, dribbling urination, dark tongue body with possible stasis macules and white tongue fur, wiry slippery, wiry tight, or wiry rough pulse. Digital rectal exam of the prostate may produce pain on pressure, and may reveal an uneven surface and a normal-sized but nodular gland that is as hard as stone.

Treatment principles: Break stasis and dissipate binds, fight cancer and disperse swelling

---

[3] Vanquished essence (*bai jing*) refers to semen that has become lifeless after being subjected to evils such as dampness and heat or to conditions such as blood stasis, and obstructs within the essence chamber.

[4] The nourishing life (*yang sheng*) tradition within Chinese medicine refers to the heterogenous body of ideas and practices concerned with maintaining health and preventing illness, and hence also with promoting longevity.

Guiding formula: Modified *Di Dang Tang* (Dead-On Decoction)

Ingredients:
    Tao Ren (Persicae Semen), 10g
    Da Huang (Rhei Radix et Rhizoma), 6g
    Zhi Zi (Gardeniae Grandiflorae Fructus), 6g
    Shui Zhi (Hirudo), 3g
    Meng Chong (Tabanus), 3g
    Hai Zao (Sargassum), 10g
    Kun Bu (Laminariae/Eckloniae Thallus), 10g
    Bie Jia (Trionycis Carapax), 15g, predecocted
    Hong Hua (Carthami Flos), 10g
    Chuan Shan Jia (Manitis Squama), 10g
    Bai Hua She She Cao (Oldenlandiae Diffusae Herba), 30g
    Ban Zhi Lian (Scutellariae Barbatae Herba), 30g
    San Leng (Sparganii Rhizoma) 10g
    E Zhu (Curcumae Rhizoma), 10g
    Niu Xi (Achyranthis Bidentatae Radix), 10g

2. Damp-heat pouring downward with damp depression and toxin

Signs: Unsmooth urination, urinary frequency and urgency, painful urination, yellow or reddish urine, bitter oral taste and bound stool, red tongue with thick slimy yellow fur, wiry slippery rapid pulse. Digital rectal exam of the prostate reveals a nodular and swollen or lumpy prostate.

Treatment principles: Clear heat and resolve toxicity, disinhibit urination and free strangury

Guiding formula: Modified *Ba Zheng San* (Eight Corrections Powder)

Ingredients:
    Bian Xu (Polygoni Avicularis Herba), 12g
    Qu Mai (Dianthi Herba), 12g
    Mu Tong (Akebiae Trifoliatae Caulis), 10g
    Hua Shi (Talcum), 10g
    Che Qian Zi (Plantaginis Semen), 15g
    Da Huang (Rhei Radix et Rhizoma), 6g
    Shan Zhi Zi (Gardeniae Fructus), 10g
    Ban Zhi Lian (Scutellariae Barbatae Herba), 30g
    Bai Hua She She Cao (Oldenlandiae Diffusae Herba), 30g
    Dong Kui Zi (Malvae Semen), 15g
    E Zhu (Curcumae Rhizoma), 10g
    San Leng (Sparganii Rhizoma), 10g
    Wang Bu Liu Xing (Vaccariae Semen), 15g
    Chuan Shan Jia (Manitis Squama), 15g
    Tu Fu Ling (Smilacis Glabrae Rhizoma), 15g

3. Liver and kidney yin vacuity with hyperactive ministerial fire

Signs: Dribbling and unsmooth urination or urinary block, yellow urine, reddish urine, or hematuria, dizzy head and tinnitus, limpness and soreness of the lumbus and knees, vexation and heat in the five hearts, dry mouth and throat, premature ejaculation and seminal emission, red tongue with thin fur or scanty fur, fine rapid pulse. Digital rectal exam may reveal a slightly swollen and lumpy prostate.

Treatment principles: Enrich liver and kidney yin, clear vacuity fire

Guiding formula: Modified *Zhi Bai Di Huang Wan* (Anemarrhena, Phellodendron, and Rehmannia Pill)

Ingredients:
    Zhi Mu (Anemarrhenae Rhizoma), 12g
    Huang Bai (Phellodendri Cortex), 12g
    Shan Zhu Yu (Corni Fructus), 12g
    Sheng Di Huang (Rehmanniae Radix Exsiccata seu Recens), 12g
    Fu Ling (Poria), 15g
    Ze Xie (Alismatis Rhizoma), 15g
    Mu Dan Pi (Moutan Cortex), 10g
    Zhi Zi (Gardeniae Fructus), 10g
    Bai Hua She She Cao (Oldenlandiae Diffusae Herba), 30g
    Ban Zhi Lian (Scutellariae Barbatae Herba), 30g
    Ban Bian Lian (Lobeliae Chinensis Herba), 30g
    Bie Jia (Trionycis Carapax), 15g, predecocted
    Sheng Gan Cao (Glycyrrhizae Radix Cruda), 6g

4. Qi and blood vacuity[5]

Signs: Insidious onset of symptoms, unsmooth urination and urinary block, shortness of breath and lassitude of spirit, emaciation, poor appetite, puffy swelling of the lower extremities, soreness and pain of the lumbus and knees, pale tongue with scanty fur, fine weak pulse. Digital rectal exam of the prostate reveals a swollen, enlarged, and hard prostate.

Treatment principles: Supplement and boost qi and blood, quicken the blood and dissipate stasis

Guiding formula: Modified *Shi Quan Da Bu Tang* (Perfect Major Supplementation Decoction)

---

[5] According to Guo *et al.* (1999), this pattern is common among men after prostate surgery.

Ren Shen (Ginseng Radix), 10g
Bai Zhu (Atractylodis Macrocephalae Rhizoma), 12g
Fu Ling (Poria), 12g
Gan Cao (Glycyrrhizae Radix), 6g
Shu Di Huang (Rehmanniae Radix Praeparata), 12g
Bai Shao (Paeoniae Radix Alba), 10g
Dang Gui (Angelicae Sinensis Radix), 10g
Chuan Xiong (Chuanxiong Rhizoma), 10g
Rou Gui (Cinnamomi Cortex), 10g
Chuan Shan Jia (Manitis Squama), 30g
Bie Jia (Trionycis Carapax), 30g
Sheng Huang Qi (Astragali seu Hedysari Radix Cruda), 30g
Tao Ren (Persicae Semen), 10g
Hong Hua (Carthami Flos), 10g
Niu Xi (Achyranthis Bidentatae Radix), 10g

Acumoxa therapy

Main points: *Hui Yin* (CV-1), *Ci Liao* (BL-32), *San Yin Jiao* (SP-6), *Li Gou* (LV-5), *Da Dun* (LV-1), *Zhong Ji* (CV-3), *Shui Dao* (ST-28)

For blood stasis patterns, add *Xue Hai* (SP-10), *Di Ji* (SP-8), *Qi Chong* (ST-30), *Ge Shu* (BL-17), *Shang Ju Xu* (ST-37), and *Xia Ju Xu* (ST-39)

For damp-heat brewing and binding in the essence chamber, add *Jie Xi* (ST-41), *Tai Chong* (LV-3), *Ji Mai* (LV-12), *Fu Liu* (KI-7), and *Zhi Bian* (BL-54)

For liver and kidney yin vacuity with hyperactive ministerial fire, add *Gan Shu* (BL-18), *Shen Shu* (BL-23), *Xing Jian* (LV-2), *Zhao Hai* (KI-6), and *Ran Gu* (KI-2)

For qi and blood vacuity, add *Zu San Li* (ST-36), *Zhong Wan* (CV-12), *Qi Hai* (CV-6), *Shan Zhong* (CV-17), *Pi Shu* (BL-20), *Wei Shu* (BL-21), *Ge Shu* (BL-17), and *Tai Xi* (KI-3)

Experiential formulas (Zhang, Wang, and Gao, 2001)

Quickening blood and transforming stasis, supplementing and securing kidney qi, clearing heat and draining dampness

This formula is recommended for the early stage of prostate cancer when the urinary outlet obstruction symptoms are relatively mild, but when there are signs of blood stasis including a dark tongue that may have stasis macules. It quickens blood and transforms stasis, supplements and secures kidney qi, and clears heat and drains dampness. The ingredients are:
Da Huang (Rhei Radix et Rhizoma), 10g
Dang Gui (Angelicae Sinensis Radix), 10g
Tao Ren (Persicae Semen), 10g
Di Bie Chong (Eupopolyphaga), 10g
Gou Qi Zi (Lycii Fructus), 10g

Tu Si Zi (Cuscutae Semen), 15g
Wu Wei Zi (Schisandrae Fructus), 5g
Che Qian Zi (Plantaginis Semen), 15g
Sha Yuan Zi (Astragali Complanati Semen), 10g
Chuan Niu Xi (Cyathulae Radix), 15g

Supplementing spleen and kidney qi, nourishing blood, clearing heat and drying dampness, and clearing heat and resolving the exterior

There is no specific pattern discrimination provided for this formula in the source text, though from the ingredients it appears to supplement spleen and kidney qi, nourish blood, clear heat and dry dampness, and resolve toxicity. The ingredients are as follows:

Sheng Huang Qi (Astragali seu Hedysari Radix Cruda), 15g
Dang Shen (Codonopsis Radix), 12g
Yin Yang Huo (Epimedii Herba), 12g
Rou Cong Rong (Cistanches Herba), 6g
Ba Ji Tian (Morindae Officinalis Radix), 6g
Gou Qi Zi (Lycii Fructus), 12g
He Shou Wu (Polygoni Multiflori Radix), 12g
Chuan Shan Jia (Manitis Squama), 15g
Niu Xi (Achyranthis Bidentatae Radix), 12g
Da Huang (Rhei Radix et Rhizoma), 6g
Huang Bai (Phellodendri Cortex), 10g
Zhi Mu (Anemarrhenae Rhizoma), 6g
Tu Fu Ling (Smilacis Glabrae Rhizoma), 15g
Qi Ye Yi Zhi Hua (Paris Chinensis Rhizoma),[6] 12g
Bai Hua She She Cao (Oldenlandiae Diffusae Herba), 15g
Bai Shao (Paeoniae Radix Alba), 12g
Zhi Gan Cao (Glycyrrhizae Radix cum Liquido Fricta), 6g

Clearing heat and drying dampness, and clearing heat and resolving toxicity

Mu Tong (Akebiae Trifoliatae Caulis), 10g
Qu Mai (Dianthi Herba), 10g
Hua Shi (Talcum), 15g
Gan Cao (Glycyrrhizae Radix), 5g
Che Qian Zi (Plantaginis Semen), 10g
Bian Xu (Polygoni Avicularis Herba), 10g
Bai Jiang Cao (Patriniae Herba), 15g
Bai Hua She She Cao (Oldenlandiae Diffusae Herba), 30g
Chuan Shan Jia (Manitis Squama), 12g
Bai Mao Gen (Imperatae Rhizoma), 30g
Tu Fu Ling (Smilacis Glabrae Rhizoma), 30g

---

[6] *Qi Ye Yi Zhi Hua* (Paris Chinensis Rhizoma) clears heat and resolves toxicity, disperses swelling, and stops pain.

Chi Shao (Paeoniae Radix Rubra), 15g
Huang Bai (Phellodendri Cortex), 10g
Yi Yi Ren (Coicis Semen), 15g

Quickening blood and transforming stasis

When a blood stasis pattern predominates, the following formula is recommended:

Dang Gui (Angelicae Sinensis Radix), 15g
Chi Shao (Paeoniae Radix Rubra), 15g
Tao Ren (Persicae Semen), 10g
Hong Hua (Carthami Flos), 10g
Wu Ling Zhi (Trogopteri Faeces), 10g
Wu Yao (Linderae Radix), 10g
Wang Bu Liu Xing (Vaccariae Semen), 10g
Yan Hu Suo (Corydalis Rhizoma), 10g
Chuan Shan Jia (Manitis Squama), 10g
Dan Shen (Salviae Miltiorrhizae Radix), 10g
Bai Jiang Cao (Patriniae Herba), 10g
Qu Mai (Dianthi Herba), 10g
Ma Bian Cao (Verbenae Herba),[7] 10g
Ze Xie (Alismatis Rhizoma), 15g
Shi Jian Chuan (Salviae Chinensis Herba),[8] 30g

This formula is recommended for prostate cancer with pain from bone metastasis:

Di Bie Chong (Eupopolyphaga), 10g
Bai Hua She (Bungarus seu Agkistrodon), 10g
Dang Gui (Angelicae Sinensis Radix), 10g
Xu Chang Qing (Cynanchi Paniculati Radix),[9] 10g
Lu Feng Fang (Vespae Nidus), 6g
Zhi Gan Cao (Glycyrrhizae Radix cum Liquido Fricta), 6g
Wu Gong (Scolopendra), 3g
Dang Shen (Codonopsis Radix), 12g
Huang Qi (Astragali Radix), 12g
Shu Di Huang (Rehmanniae Radix Praeparata), 15g
Ji Xue Teng (Spatholobi Caulis), 15g
Ru Xiang (Olibanum), 9g
Mo Yao (Myrrha), 9g

---

[7] *Ma Bian Cao* (Verbenae Herba) quickens blood and disperses abdominal masses, clears heat and resolves toxicity, and disinhibits urination.

[8] *Shi Jian Chuan* (Salviae Chinensis Herba) clears heat and resolves toxicity and quickens blood and stops pain.

[9] *Xu Chang Qing* (Cynanchi Paniculati Radix) eliminates wind and stops pain and quickens blood and disperses swelling.

Quickening blood and transforming stasis and softening hardness and dissipating binds with salty medicinals

The strategy of using salty medicinals that soften hardness along with blood-quickening medicinals is frequently used in formulas for prostate cancer. As an example, see the following formula:

Hai Zao (Sargassum), 30g

Kun Bu (Laminariae/Eckloniae Thallus), 30g

San Leng (Sparganii Rhizoma), 15g

E Zhu (Curcumae Rhizoma), 10g

Dang Gui (Angelicae Sinensis Radix), 15g

Chi Shao Yao (Paeoniae Radix Rubra), 15g

Mu Dan Pi (Moutan Cortex), 30g

Chi Fu Ling (Poria Rubra), 30g

Supplementing qi and yin

When there is dual vacuity of qi and yin, the following formula should be considered:

Huang Qi (Astragali Radix), 15g

Chuan Shan Jia (Manitis Squama), 15g

Bai Hua She She Cao (Oldenlandiae Diffusae Herba), 15g

Tu Fu Ling (Smilacis Glabrae Rhizoma), 15g

Dang Shen (Codonopsis Radix), 12g

Yin Yang Huo (Epimedii Herba), 12g

Gou Qi Zi (Lycii Fructus), 12g

He Shou Wu (Polygoni Multiflori Radix), 12g

Niu Xi (Achyranthis Bidentatae Radix), 12g

Qi Ye Yi Zhi Hua (Paridis Rhizoma), 12g

Bai Shao (Paeoniae Radix Alba), 12g

Rou Cong Rong (Cistanches Herba), 6g

Ba Ji Tian (Morindae Officinalis Radix), 6g

Da Huang (Rhei Radix et Rhizoma), 6g

Da Huang (Anemarrhenae Rhizoma), 6g

Zhi Gan Cao (Glycyrrhizae Radix cum Liquido Fricta), 6g

Using Chinese medicine for treating side effects of radiotherapy and chemotherapy for prostate cancer

Because I have not found the data to support such a claim, I do not suggest in this chapter that Chinese medicine should be used as a primary treatment for prostate cancer. From the scant resources available to me at the time of writing this chapter, prostate cancer appears to largely fall within the realm of the oncologist in Chinese medical circles as it does among Western doctors. In modern China, using Chinese medicine in the treatment of cancer is generally within the purview of doctors who practice "Integrated Chinese-Western Medicine (*zhong xi yi jie he*)." These are doctors who are dually trained in Western and Chinese medicine and are interested in the use of Chinese medicine along with Western medicine for a variety of diseases spanning a number of specialties. In the realm of oncology, this usually means using Chinese medicine as an adjunctive therapy to "support the right [qi] (*fu zheng*)," and to deal with any side effects of surgery, radiation, or chemotherapy.

During a clinical internship at the Guang Zhou Municipal Hospital of Chinese Medicine in 1988, I had the opportunity to study with Dr. Zhang Fei-Xian, who was chief of the oncology department. From Dr. Zhang's experience, according to Chinese medicine radiation behaves like a heat evil, and the most common side effects of radiotherapy are discriminated into the following Chinese medical patterns: 1) heat toxin; 2) yin-blood damage; 3) dual vacuity of qi and blood and; 4) detriment and damage to liver and kidney yin-essence. The pathomechanism in all of these patterns is heat evil damaging all aspects of right qi, including, yin, blood, essence, fluids, qi, and blood. In the case of heat toxin, heat becomes depressed locally and then engenders heat toxin.

Although the question of how to treat side effects of cancer chemotherapy and radiation is beyond the scope of this text and can be found in Chinese medical oncology texts, I do want to offer Dr. Zhang's protocols for treating radiocystitis, which is a local problem that may result from irradiation of the prostate. The most common pattern is one of damp-heat toxin. This formula is only applicable when the signs and symptoms support such a diagnosis.

Radiocystitis formula

Modified *Ba Zheng San* (Eight Corrections Powder):
    Sheng Di Huang (Rehmanniae Radix Exsiccata seu Recens), 15g
    Dan Zhu Ye (Lophatheri Herba), 10g
    Mu Tong (Akebiae Trifoliatae Caulis), 10g
    Bi Xie (Dioscoreae Hypoglaucae seu Semptemlobae Rhizoma), 10g
    Che Qian Cao (Plantaginis Herba), 15g
    Chi Shao (Paeoniae Radix Rubra), 10g
    Da Ji (Cirsii Japonici Herba seu Radix), 10g
    Xiao Ji (Cirsii Herba), 10g
    Tu Fu Ling (Smilacis Glabrae Rhizoma), 15g
    Qu Mai (Dianthi Herba), 12g
    Huang Bai (Phellodendri Cortex), 12g
    Ce Bai Ye (Platycladi Cacumen), 10g
    Bian Xu (Polygoni Avicularis Herba), 12g
    Ban Zhi Lian (Scutellariae Barbatae Herba), 12g
    Ze Xie (Alismatis Rhizoma), 12g
    Zhi Mu (Anemarrhenae Rhizoma), 10g
    Jin Yin Hua (Lonicerae Flos), 12g

External treatments

According to Huang and Bai (2004), the medicinals below can be used as an externally-applied paste to break stasis and dissipate binds, and draw out toxin and disperse tumors. It contains toxic medicinals, so it should be used and stored only with great care. I include it here because although it does contain toxic substances which are generally unnecessary to use in modern times, the life-threatening nature of prostate cancer may tilt the balance of the cost-benefit analysis toward using it. Only known farm-raised or possibly synthetic *She Xiang* should be used, or a suitable substitute can be used instead.

> *Bing Pian* (Borneolum), 10g
> *Xiong Huang* (Realgar), 10g
> *Qing Fen* (Calomelas), 20g
> *Mang Xiao* (Natrii Sulfas), 100g
> *She Xiang* (Moschus), 5g

Instructions: Stone-bake all the medicinals and grind them into a fine powder. Mix them with petroleum jelly until the mixture has the consistency of a thick plaster. Clean the perineal region thoroughly. Apply the plaster to the perineum and cover with a cotton bandage. Change the dressing every twenty-four hours, washing thoroughly in between applications, and remaining alert for any signs of localized skin irritation. Ten to fifteen applications constitutes one treatment course.

Preventive measures and lifestyle modification

1. Eat a healthful clear-bland diet

Excessive consumption of spicy-hot, greasy-fried, or sweet foods, and drinking too much alcohol promotes the formation of damp-heat in the center burner which can pour downward and become depressed in the essence chamber. Over time, depressed damp-heat can form phlegm, blood stasis, and possibly heat toxin. In some men, these factors come together and lead to prostate cancer. Therefore, to prevent and assist in the treatment of prostate cancer, it is most prudent to maintain a clear-bland diet rich in fresh vegetables and fruits, grains, and small quantities of lean meats, fish, and poultry.

2. Do not allow chronic heat or damp-heat in the lower burner to go untreated

From the perspective of Chinese medicine, any enduring heat or damp-heat in the lower burner can theoretically lead to prostate cancer. This is so because enduring heat scorches fluids and forms phlegm, decocts blood and forms blood stasis, and damages right qi and makes the essence chamber more susceptible to the collection of these and other evils. Over time, cancer could form. To avoid this scenario, it is advisable to treat damp-heat or heat in the lower burner early.

3. Maintain a positive mental outlook

Maintaining a positive mental outlook encourages the liver qi to flow freely. When liver qi flows freely, qi, blood, and fluids in the anterior yin region in general also flow freely, and one is less likely to develop depression, congelation, and stagnation. In this way, men can avoid the conditions that set the stage for the development of prostate cancer.

4. Regulate sexual life

To maintain free flow through the essence chamber, it is advisable to have regular sexual activity. However, it is not advisable to either overly restrain sexual urges (which can lead to obstruction in the essence chamber) or to be overly active sexually (which can damage the kidneys and make the essence chamber more vulnerable to attack by evils).

Erectile Dysfunction

Western Medicine

According to Fauci et al. (1998), Erectile Dysfunction (ED) is the inability to achieve or maintain an erection sufficient for satisfactory sexual performance. There are many possible causes as understood by Western medicine, but broad distinction is made between organic and psychological causes. While in the past, physicians largely assumed that most cases of ED were primarily of psychological etiology, current thinking has shifted towards a greater appreciation of organic causes as either primary or concomitant factors in its development. The incidence and severity of ED does increase with age, and is presumed to be associated with certain age-related physiological and psychological disease processes. However, ED should not necessarily be considered a normal part of the aging process, as many healthy men may retain their sexual function well into their seventies (Kasper *et al.*, 2007). Over 80% of cases of ED occur in men with atherosclerosis, diabetes, or as a side effect of medications.

Diagnosis

A physician's approach to a man with erectile dysfunction is to first determine whether the problem is due to psychogenic or organic causes, or both. One of the key points of differentiation supporting a primary psychogenic cause is the presence of spontaneous erection during sleep (called nocturnal penile tumescence [NPT]) or in the early morning. Most men with psychogenic ED will regularly experience NPT or early morning erections, whereas men with organic ED will not. This information is usually obtained through history-taking. However, when the history is unclear, NPT is sometimes measured in a sleep laboratory or with a home strain gauge monitor, though according to Fauci *et al.* (1998), false positives and negatives are fairly common.

Once the etiology is determined, the physician can proceed with either psychological, psychiatric, or medical treatment, or very often with a combination of different modalities. According to Kasper *et al.* (2007), it is important to keep in mind, however, that even when ED is due to primary organic causes, secondary psychological reactions will usually occur, and psychogenic causes can-result in physiological changes. For example, anxiety is sometimes accompanied by hyperactive sympathetic stimulation which increases penile smooth muscle tone, or other psychological disturbances can inhibit penile blood flow to the penis by inhibiting reflexogenic responses from the sacral spinal cord. (Kasper *et al.*, 2007).

Kasper *et al.* (2007) provide a very logical means of differentiating the causes of ED by organizing them under three headings: 1) failure to initiate; 2) failure to fill and; 3) failure to store. The authors are quick to point out that these three factors frequently coexist in the same patient. Failure to initiate means a failure to initiate the erectile response and can be due to psychogenic, endocrine, or neurogenic causes. Failure to fill is arteriogenic in that any disease process or drug reaction that impairs arterial blood flow to the penis will result in ED. Failure to store refers to the inability of the valves within the penile veins to constrict and prevent the blood gathered within the penis from escaping. This is a very useful model to keep in mind as we explore the causes of ED in greater detail.

• *Psychogenic causes*

There are several possible psychogenic causes of ED which operate singly or in combination including disinterest in the sexual partner, relationship discord (including anger and resentment towards the partner), anxiety, fear of sexual incompetence, and depression. Situational ED is usually due to psychogenic causes and occurs more frequently with new sexual partners or when sexual activity occurs in an environment in which the man does not feel fully relaxed.

When ED is primarily due to psychogenic factors, patient education and support, psychotherapy (including sex therapy in some cases), and psychiatric medication may be used in concert with an oral medication such as sildenafil (Viagra) or another PDE-5 inhibitor. Of course, one must bear in mind that many antidepressant agents may result in ED, which presents a clinical dilemma for the physician who may have to weigh the relative degree of suffering the patient experiences from depression against that experienced from ED. In many cases, antidepressants are used along with ED medications like sildenafil in order to achieve the therapeutic goals of treating ED and depression.

• *Organic causes*

In terms of organic causes of ED, impairment of normal blood flow to and from the penis is the most common cause. Men with atherosclerosis and hypercholesterolemia frequently experience ED for this reason. And men who have suffered any trauma to the arteries in the penile region or have other arterial diseases are also at high risk for ED. Normal erectile function requires not only sufficient blood flow into the penis, it also requires maintaining this blood within the penis. Hence, if venous blood leaks out of the penis due to organic factors such as insufficient relaxation of smooth muscle or abnormalities in the structure of the corpus cavernosa, erection will either not occur at all, or complete or partial detumescence will rapidly follow achievement of erection. While organic causes are usually responsible for this mechanism, at times psychogenic causes such as anxiety may be the culprit.

• Diabetes

Diabetes results in ED in about 35–75% of cases due to vascular as well as neurological alterations. Some of the vascular changes associated with diabetes are directly correlated with how well-managed the blood glucose is in a given patient and his age. Hence, the higher his serum glucose (and the longer it remainshigh), and the older a man is, the greater are his chances for developing ED. For this reason, diabetic men who wish to avoid ED should carefully manage their serum glucose through diet, exercise, and medications when necessary.

• Medication side effects

As mentioned previously, ED very frequently occurs as a side effect of drugs. Among the most frequently cited categories of medications we find antiandrogens (such as histamine blockers like cimetidine), antihypertensives (especially beta-blockers), anticholinergics, antidepressants (especially MAO inhibitors and tricyclic antidepressants), antipsychotics, and central nervous system depressants (such as barbituates and antianxiety agents). Among recreational drugs that may lead to ED, we find alcohol, heroin, methadone, and tobacco. When ED arises primarily as a side effect of a drug, modification in drug choices or dosage is crucial for clinical success.

• Neurogenic causes

There are many neurogenic causes of ED including spinal cord disorders, lesions of the anterior temporal lobe, and urological surgeries such as radical prostatectomy or cystectomy. Since the cavernosal nerves—which enervate the penis—run along the posterolateral surface of the prostate, if surgery is performed on the prostate or bladder without sparing these nerves, ED ensues (Fauci *et al.*, 1998).

• Endocrine causes

Endocrine disorders can lead to ED. For example, testicular failure leads to decreased androgen levels and causes ED. Contrary to popular belief, however, this is a relatively uncommon cause of ED. Hyperprolactinemia, caused by a prolactin-secreting tumor of the pituitary can be difficult to diagnose because it may not be obvious on physical examination, yet should be considered. To rule out endocrine-based ED, serum testosterone and prolactin levels are measured.

• Penile diseases

Peyronie's disease, which involves fibrotic plaque formation on the dorsum of the penis as a result of chronic inflammation, can alter the blood flow to and from the penis and hence result in ED. It can also result in abnormal curvature of the erect penis so as to make coitus difficult, painful, or even impossible. Trauma to the penis can also damage the penile arteries and veins and lead to ED. A history of priapism that has resulted in fibrotic deposition in the sinusoidal spaces of the corpora cavernosa can also lead to ED.

Treatment

Fundamentally, treatment of ED is based on the underlying cause and can be divided into several broad categories including patient education, oral medication, androgen therapy, vacuum constriction device, intraurethral or intracavernosal self-injection of Alprostadil, surgery, and sex therapy (Kasper *et al.*, 2007).

• *Patient education*

The patient and his long-term partner (should he have one) should be educated about the causes and treatments for ED. He should be encouraged to reduce ED-producing habits such as smoking, excessive alcohol intake, and recreational drug use. Further, he should be encouraged to make appropriate dietary changes (focusing on reducing saturated fat intake and increasing fiber), and to increase his aerobic capacity by exercising regularly.

• *Oral medication*

Sildenafil (Viagra), vardenafil (Levitra), and tardalafil (Cialis) are currently the main oral medications used for treating ED. They are widely prescribed for ED of various etiology including psychogenic, neurogenic, and vasculogenic. Further, they are also used for ED caused by nerve-sparing urological surgeries and according to Vardi and Nini (2007), diabetes. They mainly act by selectively inhibiting PDE-5, the phoshodiesterase isoform[1] within the penis. Side effects include headache, nasal congestion, and visual disturbance. Other agents are currently under investigation that target nitric oxide (NO) and intracellular GMP (Priviero and Leite *et al.*, 2007).

•*Androgen therapy*

As stated previously, androgen insufficiency is a relatively uncommon cause of ED. But in those cases where hypogonadism and testicular failure is the cause, androgen therapy is used.

•*Vacuum constriction device*

A nonsurgical and nondrug alternative for patients with ED is the vacuum constriction device (VCD). The VCD consists of a tube-shaped vacuum pump into which the man inserts his penis. The pump draws blood into the penis and a rubber constriction ring is used to keep the blood in the penis once the pump is removed. Once sexual intercourse is completed, the ring is removed and the penis returns to its flaccid state. It can be purchased in any major pharmacy without a prescription.

---

[1] PDE-5 (phoshodiesterase isoform) is one of many PDEs which serve to catalyze cAMP and cGMP hydrolysis. PDE-5 is normally responsible for degradation of cGMP in the corpus cavernosum. By inhibiting PDE-5, drugs such as sildenafil lead to increased levels of cGMP in the penis and hence to firmer and longer-lasting erections. PDE-5 is found in many tissues throughout the body, but is especially present in the corpus cavernosum and the retina; this accounts for both its desired effect and its potential for causing visual disturbances.

• *Intraurethral or intracavernosal injection of Alprostadil*

Alprostadil is a prostaglandin—given in the form of an intraurethral pellet or intracavernosal injection—that is vasoactive and produces an erection in over 90% of men who use it. It can be used for psychogenic, vasogenic, neurogenic and some milder cases of vasculogenic ED. Some men find it difficult to use, however, due to pain on injection and because it produces priapism and penile fibrosis in rare cases and with chronic use.

• *Surgery*

Surgical intervention of ED mainly consists of implantation of a semi-rigid or inflatable penile prosthesis. High patient satisfaction is generally reported, though, as with any surgery, complications are possible, including infection (Kasper *et al.*, 2007).

• *Sex therapy*

This form of treatment is most useful when there are interpersonal factors between the man and his partner, or when an other emotional conflict presents a barrier to normal sexual functioning, including when there is unresolved sexual abuse, performance anxiety, etc.

Western Complementary Medicine

There are many substances that have been investigated as enhancers of male sexual function and are especially used for erectile dysfunction. I limit my focus here to those that have been shown by clinical research to be effective and those that are especially popular. These include Yohimbine, Korean red ginseng, Gingko biloba, L-Arginine, and Pycnogenol.

• *Yohimbe bark*

Yohimbe bark extract is an extract of an active alkaloid from the African plant (Pausinystalia Yohimbe Pierre ex Beille Rubiaceae). Yohimbine or Yohimbine hydrochloride is a standardized extract of yohimbe bark pharmacologically characterized as an alpha-2 adrenergic receptor antagonist. It has been shown to be effective for erectile dysfunction in several human clinical trials, including for ED from selective serotonin reuptake inhibitors (SSRIs).[2] Researchers generally express a preference for using the standardized prescription form over the nonstandardized traditional bark itself, stating that the traditional form is not guaranteed to contain adequate amounts of the active ingredient yohimbine. However, as with all herbal medicines, if one purchases the product from a reputable source or uses a nonprescription standardized extract, one can be reasonably assured of effectiveness. Dosage ranges of Yohimbine hydrochloride are usually about 5mg three times a day or 1–2 hours before anticipated sexual activity.

---

[2] See Balon, 1993

• Korean red ginseng

Many studies show positive effects of Korean red ginseng for erectile dysfunction including Hong (2002) and de Andrade *et al.* (2007). The posited mode of action for erectile dysfunction is enhancement of nitric oxide in the penis. Most studies use 900–1000mg of extract three times per day.

• Gingko biloba

Some studies suggest that Gingko biloba extract may be effective in reducing erectile dysfunction (Sikora *et al.*, 1998 and Cohen and Bartlick, 1998). The mechanism of action is presumed to be related to Gingko's enhancement of nitric oxide release. The dosage in most trials showing positive effects is about 120mg two times per day.

• L-Arginine and pycnogenol

The amino acid L-Arginine is thought to play a role in the physiology of nitric oxide which enhances the erectile capability of the spongy erectile tissue within the penis. McKay (2002) reports that Arginine has been shown to be effective in the treatment of ED, especially when combined with Pycnogenol—a natural antioxidant found in pine bark. Generally, the dosage of Arginine ranged from 2–5g per day and the dosage of Pycnogenol was about 120mg per day.

Chinese Medicine

Disease discrimination

The Chinese medical disease categories that best fit erectile dysfunction are yang wilt (*yang wei*), yin wilt (*yin wei*), and sinew wilt (*jin wei*). All three of these names are used in different premodern texts with essentially the same meaning. In the case of the term yang wilt, yang refers to the yang aspect of erection and male sexuality, whereas in the case of the term yin wilt, yin refers to the anterior yin—and especially the penis as an organ located within that region. Sinew wilt invokes one of the early names for the penis in the Chinese literature—the ancestral sinew (*zong jin*). Yang wilt, yin wilt, and sinew wilt are all characterized by either an inability to achieve or maintain an erection at all, or a slight erection that is not firm enough for satisfying sexual activity. From this definition we can see that these terms fit perfectly with ED. Most modern text use the term yang wilt; hence I will follow the current trend.

Two of the earliest mentions of yang wilt in the premodern Chinese medical literature occur in the *Ling Shu* (*Magic Pivot*)[3] and *Su Wen* (*Plain Questions*).[4] For example, chapter 11 of *Ling Shu* states: "heat causes slackness and loss of use of the [ancestral] sinew; [this is] yang wilt and loss of use [of the penis]," and chapter 44 of *Su Wen*—which is devoted to various types of wilting (*wei*)

---

[3] *Ling Shu* is the second section of the *Huang Di Nei Jing* (*Yellow Emperor's Inner Canon*), which was published in the 1st century CE.
[4] *Su Wen* is the first section of *Huang Di Nei Jing*.

diseases—states: "Incessant preoccupation and thought, desiring that which one cannot have, desires and lust of the outer body [*et al.*, the penis], and overly-frequent sexual intercourse cause slackness of the ancestral sinew and lead to sinew wilting and white ooze."[5]

Among the prominent Sui and Tang dynasty texts which discuss this condition, we must include *Zhu Bing Yuan Hou Lun* (*On the Origin and Indicators of Disease*)[6] and *Wai Tai Mi Yao* (*Essential Secrets from Outside the Metropolis*).[7] It was not until the Ming dynasty, however, that the term yang wilt was fairly consistently used (rather than yin wilt or sinew wilt), for example by Zhang Jing-Yue in his famous text, *Jing-Yue Quan Shu* (*Jing-Yue's Complete Compendium*).[8]

Disease causes and pathomechanisms

The disease causes and pathomechanisms of yang wilt are categorized under three main headings: 1) affect-mind internal damage; 2) viscera-bowel weakness and debility and; 3) external contraction of evils. In clinical practice, the rule (rather than the exception) is to see a combination of these disease causes and pathomechanisms operating simultaneously and in mutually promoting scenarios. For example, affect-mind internal damage often weakens the viscera and bowels. And viscera-bowel weakness creates the circumstances in which external evils take advantage of vacuity to invade.

Affect-mind internal damage

• Affect-mind dissatisfaction leading to binding depression of liver qi
When there is binding depression of liver qi, the liver loses its free coursing function and the qi dynamic of the entire body (including the penis) is adversely affected. So, men who have a greater tendency to check their emotions and not express them, or who have a sense of dissatisfaction with their circumstances, or who hold grudges and repress their anger for long periods of time have a greater likelihood of experiencing yang wilt. The reason is that enduring depression of liver qi and resultant failure of free coursing and orderly reaching will lead to sluggish movement of liver blood and inability to fill the penis with blood adequately to experience a satisfying erection.

• Excessive anxiety and preoccupation damaging the heart and spleen
The heart governs sovereign fire and the spirit–affect and also controls ministerial fire. The spleen governs anxiety and preoccupation and is the later heaven source for the engenderment and transformation of qi and blood. When the heart and spleen are taxed by excessive worries and concerns, the spirit dynamic is distorted; this can profoundly affect a man's sexual performance. For example, when men yearn day and night for sexual gratification, or when they have dreams with sexual content and dream emissions, the

---

[5] For further discussion of the characteristics of white ooze (*bai zhuo*), see Book 1, Chapter 6 on Chinese andrological disease categories.

[6] *Zhu Bing Yuan Hou Lun* was written by Chao Yuan-Fang and published in 610.

[7] *Wai Ti Mi Yao* was written by Wang Tao and published in 752.

[8] *Jing-Yue Quan Shu* was published in 1624.

heart's sovereign fire and the spleen are both weakened. Because the heart and spleen are weakened, qi and blood are not adequately engendered and transformed, the ancestral sinew is undernourished, and yang wilt develops.

• **Fright and fear damaging the heart and kidneys**
Sudden fright damages the heart and enduring fear damages the kidneys. When the heart is damaged, it cannot govern the spirit-affect or control the physiological activities of the other viscera and bowels and—by extension—the penis. When the kidneys are damaged, kidney qi becomes chaotic and is unable to govern the anterior yin region. Heart and kidney vacuity then leads to an inability to achieve or maintain an erection and hence to yang wilt.

Viscera-bowel weakness and debility

• **Kidney yang vacuity and debility of ministerial fire**
Ministerial fire is the source of warmth and power for all the physiological activities of the human body. Because the kidneys have a special resonance with reproduction and the anterior yin region, the penis derives its warmth and power directly from the kidney yang. So, a normal erection requires that kidney yang be in sufficient supply and sufficiently active. Factors that lead to kidney yang vacuity include the changes that occur with age, natural endowment insufficiency or constitutional yang vacuity, kidney essence-yin vacuity that is affecting kidney yang, excessive consumption of cold raw foods, and chronic diseases that damage the kidney yang-origin. Alone or in combination, these disease causes lead to debility of ministerial fire and inability to warm and power the penis adequately; hence, yang wilt results.

• **Insufficiency of kidney essence and effulgence of vacuity fire**
As the foundational yin-substance that serves as the material basis for kidney yang to attach to, kidney yin-essence must be in adequate supply for normal erectile function. When yin-essence is lacking, erection cannot be achieved or maintained because there is no structure to support the activity of yang in the penis. Further, insufficient kidney yin results in vacuity fire which scorches the ancestral sinew and deprives it of nourishment. Causes of kidney essence-yin insufficiency include natural endowment insufficiency and constitutional vacuity, as well as unrestrained indulgence in sexual activity. These disease factors damage kidney essence-yin and lead to hyperactivity of ministerial fire. When ministerial fire becomes hyperactive, it damages kidney yin and can lead either to complete yang wilt by scorching the penis and depriving it of nourishment, or to readily-obtained erections that quickly become soft because yang has no support from yin.

• **Spleen-lung dual vacuity and insufficiency of ancestral qi (*zong qi*)**
The lungs govern the qi of the entire body and the spleen is the later heaven source of engenderment and transformation of qi and blood. Together, the spleen and lungs engender ancestral qi, which upon leaving the lungs differentiates into construction (ying) qi and defensive (wei) qi. Construction qi enters the channels and network vessels by first entering the lung channel and then travels in its specific order through the entire channel system, reaching every

organ and tissue of the body. Since the lungs are where ancestral qi forms in the first place, they are considered the governor of the qi of the entire body. Since the spleen governs movement and transformation of water and grain essence, which then serves as the material foundation for the engenderment of ancestral qi by the lungs, and of blood by the collective actions of the lung and heart, the spleen is the later heaven source of engenderment and transformation of qi and blood which powers and nourishes the entire body.

Since the lung and spleen qi are dependent on each other for their formation and activity, lung and spleen qi vacuity usually occur together clinically. Causes of lung-spleen dual vacuity include enduring lung diseases such as cough, asthma, lung distention, and lung wilt, and enduring spleen-stomach diseases such as diarrhea and dysentery. As a result of these or other causes, the ancestral sinew lacks power and nourishment and yang wilt results.

Repletion evils, phlegm and blood stasis, and trauma

• Damp-heat pouring downward into the liver channel

Men who are overweight are especially prone to damp-heat because they constitutionally have a preponderance of phlegm-dampness. If they also have a predilection for greasy, spicy, fatty, and sweet foods and/or drink a large quantity of alcohol, they are even more susceptible to developing damp-heat. Of course, being overweight just increases one's chances of developing this problem; hence, thin men with such a diet and level of alcohol intake are also at risk. In either case, there is splenic movement and transformation failure and collection of dampness that becomes depressed and transforms heat. Dampness and heat bind together and pour downward from the center burner into the lower burner and brew and bind in the liver channel. Since the liver channel skirts the genitals, damp-heat in the liver channel blocks the flow of qi and blood into the penis and results in yang wilt.

In two other scenarios that also lead to damp-heat in the liver channel, excessively forceful intercourse or forcefully withholding ejaculation leads to stasis and stagnation of vanquished essence in the essence pathway and unhygienic sexual intercourse directly exposes the anterior yin region to damp-heat toxin. In the former case, accumulated vanquished essence brews and forms damp-heat which then obstructs qi and blood flow to the ancestral sinew. In the latter, unhygienic sex leads to damp-heat toxin in the liver channel and behaves in the same way.

An additional cause is damp-heat disease in which damp-heat is not completely cleared, it then pours downward into the lower burner and into the liver channel.

In all cases of yang wilt caused by damp-heat in the liver channel the pathomechanism is essentially the same, regardless of the origin of the damp-heat. When it lodges in the liver channel, it obstructs free flow of qi and blood into the penis and leads to yang wilt.

• Cold evil congealing and stagnating in the liver channel

Cold is a yin evil. As such, it mainly causes disease by damaging yang qi and congealing yin-blood. Cold can be either externally-contracted or internally-engendered from yang vacuity. Men who spend a lot of time in cold and damp environments may contract cold into their liver channel. Men with constitutional or natural endowment yang vacuity may develop internally-engendered cold which may also lodge in their liver channel. In either case, the penis may fail to become hard and hence yang wilt results because cold evil is obstructing qi and congealing blood.

• Mutual binding of phlegm and blood stasis in the ancestral sinew

In men with chronic diseases, there is usually a mutual binding of blood stasis and phlegm. The static blood that often accompanies enduring diseases was explained by Ye Tian-Shi in the Qing dynasty in the phrase: "enduring disease enters the network vessels." More specifically, enduring diseases of various viscera and bowels and channels and network vessels results in failed qi transformation throughout the body. This makes qi unable to move the blood and unable to move and transform water-damp. Blood stasis and phlegm are the natural outcomes of this pathomechanism. These two evils tend to bind together to form phlegm-stasis. If phlegm-stasis collects in the anterior yin region and especially in or around the channels and network vessels surrounding the ancestral sinew, yang wilt may result.

• Trauma damaging the thoroughfare vessel, the conception vessel, or the governing vessel

Whenever there is trauma to these channels, qi and blood flow to the anterior yin region is obstructed. Hence, erection is either compromised or does not occur at all. Causes not only include traumatic injuries to the anterior yin region, but also urological surgeries.

Pattern discrimination

Repletion patterns

1. Binding depression of liver qi

Signs: Functional yang wilt[9] accompanied by an oppressed spirit, gallbladder timidity, or irascibility, fullness, pain, and distention of the rib-side, a tendency to sigh, a dark tongue with a thin slimy tongue fur, stringlike pulse. The patient usually tends to repress his feelings and/or is under a lot of emotional pressure.

Treatment principles: Course the liver, rectify qi, and resolve depression

---

[9] This means that at times the man is able to have an erection and may experience morning erections from time to time. The term functional here is used in juxtaposition to organic, which means that actual tissue is damaged in some way rather than just not functioning properly while remaining structurally normal.

Guiding formula: Modified *Chai Hu Shu Gan San* (Bupleurum Liver-Coursing Powder)

Ingredients:
    Chai Hu (Bupleuri Radix), 9g
    Sheng Ma (Cimicifugae Rhizoma), 6g
    Xiang Fu (Cyperi Rhizoma), 9g
    Bai Shao (Paeoniae Radix Alba), 12g
    Ju Ye (Citri Reticulatae Folium), 9g
    Bai Ji Li (Tribuli Fructus), 9g
    Dang Gui (Angelicae Sinensis Radix), 12g
    Chuan Xiong (Chuanxiong Rhizoma), 9g
    Wu Gong (Scolopendra),[10] 2 pieces
    Lu Feng Fang (Vespae Nidus), 10g
    Gan Cao (Glycyrrhizae Radix), 6g

Modifications: For patients with more severe emotional depression and repression, as well as oppression in the chest, add *He Huan Hua* (Albizziae Flos), 10g, *Mei Gui Hua* (Rosae Rugosae Flos), 9g, and *Shi Chang Pu* (Acori Tatarinowii Rhizoma), 9g, to further course the liver, rectify qi, and resolve depression. For patients who also have blood stasis, add *Dan Shen* (Salviae Miltiorrhizae Radix), 15g, and *Hong Hua* (Carthami Flos), to quicken the blood and transform stasis. For concurrent kidney yang vacuity, add *Ba Ji Tian* (Morindae Radix), 15g, *Rou Cong Rong* (Cistanches Herba), 15g, and *Tu Si Zi* (Cuscutae Semen), 15g, to warm and supplement kidney yang. When binding depression of liver qi transforms heat, remove *Sheng Ma* and add *Mu Dan Pi* (Moutan Cortex), 12g, and *Zhi Zi* (Gardenia Fructus), 12g, to clear heat from the liver and cool blood. With insomnia and copious dreams, add *Ye Jiao Teng* (Polygoni Multiflori Caulis), 15g, to nourish the heart and calm the spirit.

2. Liver channel damp-heat

Signs: Slow insidious onset, either a shrunken and soft penis or slight erection that is not hard enough for satisfying sexual activity, hypertonicity of the lesser abdomen, soreness and distention in the inguinal region and the perineum, dribbling, incomplete, and unsmooth urination, possible urinary urgency, frequency, yellow turbid urine, scrotal sweating, dampness, itching, and malodor, bitter taste in the mouth and dry throat, stringlike rapid or stringlike slippery pulse, red tongue with yellow slimy fur.

Note: This pattern usually presents in men with a history of excessive alcohol intake or genitourinary tract infections or inflammation including cystitis and prostatitis.

---

[10] *Wu Gong* frees the liver network vessels and thereby helps to promote free flow of qi and blood to the penis and enhance erection. However, it is toxic. Therefore, one should begin with a low dose and the patient should generally not take it for long periods of time without periodic abstinence from ingesting it.

Treatment principles: Clear and disinhibit damp-heat, course the liver and raise that which has wilted

Guiding formula: Modified *Long Dan Xie Gan Tang* (Gentian Liver-Draining Decoction)

Ingredients:
Long Dan Cao (Gentianae Radix), 12g
Zhi Zi (Gardeniae Fructus), 9g
Huang Bai (Phellodendri Cortex), 9g
Bai Shao (Paeoniae Radix Alba), 12g
Dang Gui (Angelicae Sinensis Radix), 12g
Mu Dan Pi (Moutan Radix), 12g
Bi Xie (Dioscoreae Hypoglaucae seu Semptemlobae Rhizoma), 12g
Ze Xie (Alismatis Rhizoma), 15g
Li Zhi He (Litchi Semen), 9g
Bai Mao Gen (Imperatae Rhizoma), 15g
Wu Gong (Scolopendra),[11] 2 pieces

Modifications: If damp-heat is not severe, then reduce the dosages of *Long Dan Cao*, *Zhi Zi*, and *Huang Bai* by one-third to one-half. When urinary urgency and frequency are prominent, add *Bian Xu* (Polygoni Avicularis Herba), 12g, and *Qu Mai* (Dianthi Herba), 15g, to clear and disinhibit the waterways. For patients with pulling pain in the lesser abdomen, add *Yan Hu Suo* (Corydalis Rhizoma), 9g, *Chuan Lian Zi* (Toosendan Fructus), 9g, and *Wu Zhu Yu* (Evodia Fructus), 6g, to course the liver and rectify qi. For patients with blood in the urine, add *Ce Bai Ye* (Platycladi Cacumen), 12g, and *Sheng Di Huang* (Rehmanniae Radix Exsiccata seu Recens), 15g, to cool the blood and staunch bleeding. For patients with heaviness and aching of the lumbus due to dampness, add *Cang Zhu* (Atractylodis Rhizoma), 12g, *Yi Yi Ren* (Coicis Semen), 15g, and *Niu Xi* (Achyranthis Bidentatae Radix), 12g, to transform and drain dampness.

3. Cold evil stagnating in the liver channel

Signs: The signs usually worsen with exposure to cold and are relieved by warmth, and include shrinking and retraction of the penis and partial or complete inability to achieve an erection, cold damp scrotum, lesser abdominal hypertonicity or pulling pain in the testes, pale dark tongue with slimy white fur, and sinking wiry or sinking slow pulse.

Note: This pattern usually presents in men who either have constitutional or natural endowment yang vacuity and develop internally-engendered cold, in men who are frequently exposed to cold damp conditions in their work or recreational activities, and in men who have had enduring and recalcitrant genitourinary infections or inflammation.

[11] See previous footnote for *Wu Gong*

Treatment principles: Warm the channels and relax the liver, free the network vessels and raise that which has wilted

Guiding formula: Modified *Nuan Gan Jian* (Liver-Warming Brew)

Ingredients:
  Rou Gui (Cinnamomi Cortex), 6g
  Wu Yao (Linderae Radix), 10g
  Chen Xiang (Aquilariae Lignum Resinatum), 3g
  Wu Zhu Yu (Evodia Fructus), 3g
  Xiao Hui Xiang (Foeniculi Fructus), 6g
  Dang Gui (Angelicae Sinensis Radix), 12g
  Gou Qi Zi (Lycii Fructus), 12g
  Ju He (Citri Reticulatae Semen), 6g
  Fu Ling (Poria), 12g
  Lu Feng Fang (Vespae Nidus), 10g
  Wu Gong (Scolopendra),[12] 2 pieces
  Sheng Jiang (Zingiberis Rhizoma Recens), 3 slices

Modifications: For men with concurrent kidney yang vacuity and externally contracted cold in the liver channel, add *Fu Zi* (Aconiti Radix Lateralis Praeparata), 6g, *Gui Zhi* (Cinnamomi Ramulus), 10g, and *Ma Huang* (Ephedrae Herba), 3g, to simultaneously warm the interior and resolve the exterior, dissipate cold, and to free the yang. For men who have constitutional yin-blood insufficiency, reduce the dosage and/or decrease the number of warm dry medicinals in the prescription, and add *Sheng Di Huang* (Rehmanniae Radix Exsiccata seu Recens), 12g, and *Bai Shao* (Paeoniae Radix Alba), 15g, to enrich yin and nourish blood. These two medicinals can also be added to prevent long-term administration of the prescription from damaging yin-blood, even when there is no history of yin-blood insufficiency.

4. Blood stasis obstruction

Signs: Complete or partial lack of erection, soot-black facial complexion, purple lips, thirst without desire to drink fluids, episodic chest oppression and discomfort, dark purple tongue with stasis macules and points, and a sinking fine rough, bound, or intermittent pulse.

Note: This pattern occurs in men with a history of diabetes mellitus, heart disease, trauma, or surgery.

Treatment principles: Free the networks vessels and raise that which has wilted

Guiding formula: Modified *Xue Fu Zhu Yu Tang* (House of Blood Stasis-Expelling Decoction)

---

[12] See footnote 10, p.229 for *Wu Gong*

Ingredients:

Dang Gui (Angelicae Sinensis Radix), 12g
Chi Shao (Paeoniae Radix Rubra), 10g
Chuan Xiong (Chuanxiong Rhizoma), 6g
Tao Ren (Persicae Semen), 6g
Chai Hu (Bupleuri Radix), 6g
Zhi Ke (Aurantii Fructus), 6g
Jie Geng (Platycodi Radix), 6g
Niu Xi (Achyranthis Bidentatae Radix), 15g
Sheng Di Huang (Rehmanniae Radix Exsiccata seu Recens), 12g
Da Huang (Rhei Radix et Rhizoma), 6g
Wu Gong (Scolopendra),[13] 2 pieces
Lu Feng Fang (Vespae Nidus), 10g
Gan *Cao* (Glycyrrhizae Radix), 3g

Modifications: For men who have mutual binding of phlegm and stasis, who are overweight, and have a thick slimy tongue fur, reduce the dosage of or remove *Sheng Di Huang*, and add *Dan Nan Xing* (Arisaematis Rhizoma cum fel bovis), 10g, and *Quan Xie* (Scorpio),[14] 6g, to transform phlegm and free the network vessels. For rough painful urination, add *Hu Po* (Succinum), 2g, taken mixed with the strained decoction, to free the network vessels and open the orifice. When there is also kidney vacuity, add *Yin Yang Huo* (Epimedii Herba), 15g, *Rou Cong Rong* (Cistanches Herba), 12g, and *Xu Duan* (Dipsaci Radix), 15g, to supplement the kidneys and invigorate yang. For men with spleen qi vacuity, add *Ren Shen* (Ginseng Radix), 12g, and *Huang Qi* (Astragali Radix), 15g, to supplement the spleen and boost qi. For severe and enduring blood stasis, add *Meng Chong* (Tabanus), 6g, and *Shui Zhi* (Hirudo), 6g, to break the blood and transform stasis.

Vacuity patterns

1. Heart-spleen dual vacuity

Signs: initially, there is low libido which gradually progresses to include softness and limpness of the penis and erections that lack strength or to complete lack of erection, physical fatigue and lassitude of spirit, insomnia and copious dreaming, poor memory, gallbladder timidity and a tendency to have many doubts, palpitations and spontaneous sweating, reduced food intake, loose stools, lusterless facial complexion, pale tender tongue with tooth marks and a thin white fur, fine weak pulse or moderate weak pulse.

Note: This pattern is generally seen among men with consumption of qi and blood from enduring diseases and general weakness, from using their mental capacity excessively in their work (such as professors, writers, researchers, scientists, etc.), and from excessive worry and preoccupation.

---

[13] See footnote 10, p. 229 on *Wu Gong*.

[14] *Quan Xie* is toxic. It should be used in low doses at first and should not be taken for long periods of time without periodic abstinence from ingesting it.

Treatment principles: Supplement spleen qi, nourish the heart and calm the spirit, raise that which has wilted

Guiding formula: Modified *Gui Pi Tang* (Spleen-Returning Decoction)

Ingredients:
>*Ren Shen* (Ginseng Radix), 12g
>*Huang Qi* (Astragali Radix), 15g
>*Bai Zhu* (Atractylodis Macrocephalae Rhizoma), 15g
>*Fu Shen* (Poria cum Pini Radice), 15g
>*Chen Pi* (Citri Reticulatae Pericarpium), 6g
>*Mu Xiang* (Aucklandiae Radix), 9g
>*Suan Zao Ren* (Ziziphi Spinosi Semen), 15g
>*Yuan Zhi* (Polygalae Radix), 10g
>*Long Yan Rou* (Longan Arillus), 6g
>*Sheng Jiang* (Zingiberis Rhizoma Recens), 3 slices
>*Da Zao* (Jujubae Fructus), 6 pieces
>*Zhi Gan Cao* (Glycyrrhizae Radix cum Liquido Fricta), 6g

Modifications: For patients with more fatigue, increase the dosage of *Ren Shen* to 15g, and *Huang Qi* to 30–60g to further supplement and boost the spleen and heart qi. For patients with abdominal distention, flatus, and reduced food intake, remove *Dang Gui*,[15] and add *Mai Ya* (Hordei Fructus Germinatus), 15g, and *Shan Zha* (Crataegi Fructus), 10g, to dissolve and abduct stagnated food. For patients with prominence of loose stools, add *Shan Yao* (Dioscoreae Rhizoma), 15g, and *Lian Zi* (Nelumbinis Semen), 12g, to further supplement spleen qi and to secure and bind the stools. With signs of center qi fall such as prominent abdominal distention and hemorrhoids, add *Chai Hu* (Bupleuri Radix), 6g, and *Sheng Ma* (Cimicifugae Rhizoma), 6g, to upbear the yang and raise the fallen. When spleen vacuity affects the kidneys, add *Ba Ji Tian* (Morinda Radix), 15g, *Tu Si Zi* (Cuscutae Semen), 15g, and *Bu Gu Zhi* (Psoraleae Fructus), 10g, to supplement kidney yang.

2. Life gate fire debility

Signs: Complete or partial lack of erection, somber white facial complexion, dizziness of the head and eyes, tinnitus, listlessness of essence-spirit, soreness and limpness of the lumbus and knees, coldness of the lesser abdomen, fear of the cold and cold limbs, nocturia with long clear urination, urinary frequency and dribbling, inhibited urination, pale tender tongue with tooth marks, thin white fur, sinking fine weak pulse.

Note: This pattern generally occurs in men with constitutional vacuity or natural endowment insufficiency, in older men, and in men who are suffering from enduring illnesses.

---

[15] In my clinical experience, I find that a significant percentage of American patients frequently develop flatus and abdominal distention from taking *Dang Gui*.

Treatment principles: Warm the life gate fire and invigorate yang, raise that which has wilted

Guiding formulas: Modified *Zan Yu Dan* (Procreation Elixir) and *You Gui Wan* (Right-Restoring Pill)

Ingredients:
> *Fu Zi* (Aconiti Radix Lateralis Praeparata), 6g
> *Rou Gui* (Cinnamomi Cortex), 6g
> *Yin Yang Huo* (Epimedii Herba), 15g
> *Bai Ji Tian* (Morindae Radix), 15g
> *Shu Di Huang* (Rehmanniae Radix Praeparata), 15g
> *Shan Yao* (Dioscoreae Rhizoma), 15g
> *Shan Zhu Yu* (Corni Fructus), 10g
> *Dang Gui* (Angelicae Sinensis Radix), 12g
> *Gou Qi Zi* (Lycii Fructus), 12g
> *Jiu Cai Zi* (Allii Tuberosi Folium), 10g
> *Rou Cong Rong* (Cistanches Herba), 10g
> *Bai Zhu* (Atractylodis Macrocephalae Rhizoma), 12g
> *Lu Jiao Jiao* (Cervi Cornus Gelatinum), 6g, dissolved into the
>   strained decoction
> *Zhi Gan Cao* (Glycyrrhizae Radix cum Liquido Fricta), 6g

Modifications: For men with loose stools from fire not engendering earth, remove *Shu Di Huang* and *Rou Cong Rong*, increase the dosage of *Bai Zhu* to 15g, and add *Ren Shen* (Ginseng Radix), 12g, and *Fu Ling* (Poria), 12g, to supplement and fortify the spleen. For men with vacuity of the governing vessel who have more prominent soreness and limpness of the lumbus and knees, add *Du Zhong* (Eucommiae Cortex), 15g, and *Gou Ji* (Cibotii Rhizoma), 15g, to further supplement the kidneys and strengthen the sinews and bones.

3. Kidney yin vacuity with effulgent fire

Signs: Hyperactive libido with ability to have an erection, but the erection is not firm enough and rapidly wilts, insomnia and copious dreaming and a tendency to have dream emissions, exhaustion of essence-spirit, heat of the five hearts, soreness and limpness of lumbus and knees, dizzy head and tinnitus, dry mouth with inability to drink copious amounts of fluids, scanty reddish urine, tender red tongue with a thin yellow fur, and a fine rapid pulse.

Note: This pattern is most common among men who have natural endowment insufficiency or constitutional vacuity of kidney yin-essence, or who have had excessive sexual activity.

Treatment principles: Enrich yin and downbear fire, replenish essence and boost marrow, raise that which has wilted

Guiding formulas: Modified *Zhi Bai Di Huang Wan* (Anemarrhena, Phellodendron, and Rehmannia Pill) plus *Zuo Gui Wan* (Left-Restoring [Kidney Yin] Pill)

Ingredients:
    Zhi Mu (Anemarrhenae Rhizoma), 6g
    Huang Bai (Phellodendri Cortex), 6g
    Sheng Di Huang (Rehmanniae Radix Exsiccata seu Recens), 15g
    Shan Yao (Dioscoreae Rhizoma), 15g
    Shan Zhu Yu (Corni Fructus), 12g
    Mu Dan Pi (Moutan Cortex), 6g
    Fu Ling (Poria), 6g
    Ze Xie (Alismatis Rhizoma), 10g
    Gui Ban (Testudinis Carapax et Plastrum), 10g, predecocted
    Bie Jia (Trionycis Carapax), 10g, predecocted

Modifications: For men with prominence of insomnia and copious dreaming, add *Dan Shen* (Salviae Miltiorrhizae Radix), 15g, *Suan Zao Ren* (Ziziphi Spinosi Semen), 15g, and *Ye Jiao Teng* (Polygoni Multiflori Caulis), 12g, to nourish heart blood and calm the spirit. For dream emissions, add *Sha Yuan Zi* (Astragali Complanati Semen), 9g, *Jin Ying Zi* (Rosae Laevigatae Fructus), 10g, and *Lian Xu* (Nelumbinis Stamen), 10g, to secure essence. When there is dual vacuity of yin and yang, add *Yin Yang Huo* (Epimedii Herba), 10g, and *Rou Cong Rong* (Cistanches Herba), 12g, to gently warm and supplement yang. For men who also have liver fire flaming upward, add *Zhi Zi* (Gardeniae Fructus), 10g, and *Mu Li* (Ostreae Concha), 15g, to calm the liver and drain fire.

4. Fright and fear damaging the heart and kidneys

Signs: Soreness of the lumbus and knees, frequent urination, dream emissions, palpitations and susceptibility to fright, gallbladder timidity and a tendency to have many doubts, insomnia and copious dreaming, distracted essence-spirit, pale tongue with thin white fur, fine weak pulse, possible fine stringlike pulse, or possible stirred bean-like pulse (*dong mai*).

Note: This pattern usually occurs in men who have complete or partial lack of erection and who have a history of traumatic and fearful experiences such as those encountered in combat, or who have been victims of violence, torture, or other forms of abuse.

Treatment principles: Boost the kidneys and quiet the spirit, raise that which has wilted

Guiding formulas: Modified *Xuan Zhi Tang* (Mind-Diffusing Decoction) plus *Yuan Zhi Wan* (Polygalae Pill)

Ingredients:
    Shu Di Huang (Rehmanniae Radix Praeparata), 15g
    Bai Ji Tian (Morindae Radix), 15g

Yi Zhi Ren (Alpiniae Oxyphyllae Fructus), 10g
Wu Wei Zi (Schisandrae Fructus), 10g
Ren Shen (Ginseng Radix), 15g
Dang Gui (Angelicae Sinensis Radix), 12g
Bai Zhu (Atractylodis Macrocephalae Rhizoma), 12g
Shan Yao (Dioscoreae Rhizoma), 15g
Fu Shen (Poria cum Pini Radice), 15g
Suan Zao Ren (Ziziphi Spinosi Semen), 15g
Yuan Zhi (Polygalae Radix), 10g
Chai Hu (Bupleuri Radix), 6g
Sheng Ma (Cimicifugae Rhizoma), 6g
Shi Chang Pu (Acori Tatarinowii Rhizoma), 6g
Long Chi (Mastodi Dentis Fossilia), 15g, predecocted

Modifications: For men with constitutional or natural endowment insufficiency of kidney essence, add *Shan Zhu Yu* (Corni Fructus), 12g, and *Gou Qi Zi* (Lycii Fructus), 15g, to supplement the kidneys and replenish essence. With hyperactivity of heart fire, add *Lian Zi Xin* (Nelumbinis Plumula), 6g, and *Huang Lian* (Coptidis Rhizoma), 6g, to clear and drain sovereign fire (heart fire).

Acumoxa therapy

Main points: *Guan Yuan* (CV-4), *Zhong Ji* (CV-3), *Shen Shu* (BL-23), *Ci Liao* (BL-32), *San Yin Jiao* (SP-6), *Tai Xi* (KI-3), *Zu San Li* (ST-36), *Chang Qiang* (GV-1), *Hui Yin* (CV-1)

Repletion patterns

For liver binding depression of liver qi, add *Tai Chong* (LV-3), *He Gu* (LI-4), and *Gan Shu* (BL-18)

For liver channel damp-heat, add *Li Gou* (LV-5), *Qu Quan* (LV-8), *Yin Ling Quan* (SP-9), *Feng Long* (ST-40), *Dan Shu* (BL-19), and *Pang Guang Shu* (BL-28)

For cold in the liver channel, add moxibustion to the lesser abdominal area and to *Zhong Ji* (CV-3), *Guan Yuan* (CV-4), *Li Gou* (LV-5), *Qu Quan* (LV-8), and *Tai Chong* (LV-3)

For blood stasis obstruction, add *San Yin Jiao* (SP-6), *Ge Shu* (BL-17), *Xue Hai* (SP-10), *Shang Ju Xu* (ST-37), *Xia Ju Xu* (ST-39), and *Da Zhu* (BL-11)[16]

Vacuity patterns

For heart-spleen dual vacuity, add *Pi Shu* (BL-20), *Wei Shu* (BL-21), *Qi Hai* (CV-6), *Zhong Wan* (CV-12), *Shan Zhong* (CV-17), *Shen Men* (HT-7), and *Nei Guan* (PC-6)

---

[16] ST-37, ST-39, and BL-11 are points corresponding to the sea of blood and can be used for all blood disorders.

For life gate fire debility, add moxibustion on *Shen Shu* (BL-23) and *Guan Yuan* (CV-4), and also needle and/or moxa *Ming Men* (GV-4)

For kidney yin vacuity with effulgent fire, add *Ran Gu* (KI-2) and *Zhao Hai* (KI-6)

For fright and fear damaging the heart and kidneys, add *Xin Shu* (BL-15), *Shen Men* (HT-7), *Nei Guan* (PC-6), and *Bai Hui* (GV-20)

Experiential herbal formulas of famous physicians

Coursing the liver and rectifying qi

Wang Qi's *Tiao Gan Zhen Wei Tang* (Liver-Regulating Wilt-Rousing Decoction)[17] treats yang wilt from liver depression. It consists of:

Bai Ji Li (Tribuli Fructus)
Chai Hu (Bupleuri Radix)
Zhi Shi (Aurantii Fructus Immaturis)
Bai Shao (Paeoniae Radix Alba)
Dang Gui (Angelicae Sinensis Radix)
Niu Xi (Achyranthis Radix)
Wu Gong (Scolopendra)

Modifications: For binding depression of liver qi, add *Yu Jin* (Curcumae Radix), *Xiang Fu* (Cyperi Rhizoma), and *Jiu Xiang Chong* (Aspongopus). For liver qi rising in counterflow, add *Shi Jue Ming* (Haliotidis Concha), *Mu Li* (Ostreae Concha), and *Ling Yang Jiao* (Saigae Tataricae Cornu).[18] For damp-heat in the liver channel, add *Long Dan Cao* (Gentianae Radix), *Ze Xie* (Alismatis Rhizoma), *Che Qian Zi* (Plantaginis Semen), and *She Chuang Zi* (Cnidii Fructus). For blood stasis blocking the network vessels, add *Shui Zhi* (Hirudo), *Di Long* (Pheretima), *Chi Shao* (Paeoniae Radix Rubra), and *Lu Lu Tong* (Liquidambaris Fructus). For phlegm-stasis blocking the network vessels, add *Bai Jiang Can* (Bombyx Batryticatus) and *Lu Feng Fang* (Vespae Nidus). For life gate fire debility, add *Tu Si Zi* (Cuscutae Semen), *Rou Cong Rong* (Cistanches Herba), *Yin Yang Huo* (Epimedii Herba), and *Zi Shao Hua* (Spongilla). For liver and kidney yin vacuity, add *Sheng Di Huang* (Rehmanniae Radix Exsiccata seu Recens), *Shan Zhu Yu* (Corni Fructus), and *Gou Qi Zi* (Lycii Fructus). For cold stagnating in the liver channel, add *Wu Zhu Yu* (Evodia Fructus), *Ding Xiang* (Caryophylli Flos), and *Rou Gui* (Cinnamomi Cortex). For fright and fear damaging the kidneys, add *Yuan Zhi* (Polygalae Radix), *Shi Chang Pu* (Acori Tatarinowii Rhizoma), *Fu Shen* (Poria cum Pini Radice), and *Hu Po* (Succinum). For liver blood vacuity, add *Shu Di Huang* (Rehmanniae Radix Praeparata), and *Zi He Che* (Hominis Placenta). For spleen and stomach qi vacuity, add *Huang Qi* (Astragali Radix) and *Dang Shen* (Codonopsis Radix).

---

[17] Reported in Wang (2003). Wang Qi is a well-known doctor of Chinese andrology. In his writings, he is very verbal about the centrality of liver pathology in yang wilt.
[18] Care should be taken only to use *Ling Yang Jiao* from farmed sources.

Warming and supplementing kidney yang

Chen Shu-Sen's *Bu Shen Zhuang Yang Wan* (Kidney-Supplementing Yang-Invigorating Decoction) treats yang wilt from kidney yang vacuity. (Chen, 1989). It consists of:

> *Ren Shen* (Ginseng Radix), 30g
> *Yin Yang Huo* (Epimedii Herba), 30g
> *Rou Cong Rong* (Cistanches Herba), 30g
> *Gou Qi Zi* (Lycii Fructus), 30g

Instructions: The medicinals are ground into a powder, infused with honey and formed into 2g pills. One pill should be taken 2–3 times per day. Alternatively, the medicinals can be soaked in alcohol for two weeks and taken in 5–10 ml doses 2–3 times per day.

Modifications: For premature ejaculation, add *Wu Wei Zi* (Schizandra Fructus), 50g.

Supplementing qi, blood, yin and yang

Qin *et al.* (1989) report on Qin Bo-Wei's *Zan Hua Xue Yu Dan* (Transformation-Fostering Hair Elixir) treats yang wilt from qi, blood, yin, and yang vacuity. It consists of:

> *Xue Yu Tan* (Crinis Carbonisatus)
> *Shu Di Huang* (Rehmanniae Radix Praeparata)
> *Gou Qi Zi* (Lycii Fructus)
> *Dang Gui* (Angelicae Sinensis Radix)
> *Lu Jiao Jiao* (Cervi Cornus Gelatinum)
> *Tu Si Zi* (Cuscutae Semen)
> *Du Zhong* (Eucommiae Cortex)
> *Bai Ji Tian* (Morindae Officinalis Radix)
> *Xiao Hui Xiang* (Foeniculi Fructus)
> *Fu Ling* (Poria)
> *Rou Cong Rong* (Cistanches Herba)
> *Hu Tao Rou* (Juglandis Semen)
> *He Shou Wu* (Polygoni Multiflori Radix)
> *Ren Shen* (Ginseng Radix)

External treatments

According to Guo *et al.* (1999), the following formula was listed in *She Sheng Mi Pou* (*Penetrating the Secrets of Life Cultivation*),[19] and is recommended to be used as a paste applied topically to the penis:

> *She Chuang Zi* (Cnidii Fructus)
> *Yuan Zhi* (Polygalae Radix)
> *Lu Feng Fang* (Vespae Nidus)
> *Xi Xin* (Asari Herba)
> *Di Long* (Pheretima)

---

[19] Publication date unavailable.

Note: Dosages and duration of use is not specified. Care should be taken to not leave the paste on for too long to avoid any possible skin irritation from *Xi Xin*.

Guo *et al.* (1999) also reported *Lu Fang Qi Wei Fang* (Hornet's Nest Wilt-Raising Formula) from *Qian Jin Yao Fang* (*A Thousand Gold Pieces Emergency Formulary*)[20] as a topical treatment for erectile dysfunction. It consists of *Lu Feng Fang* (Vespus Nidus), roasted to ash, and applied directly to the penis during the night as a paste.

Preventive measures and lifestyle modification

1. Maintain physical conditioning

In order for a man to have a satisfying sexual life, he must maintain good physical conditioning. In terms of Chinese medicine, this guarantees free flow of qi and blood to the anterior yin region. In Western medicine, good aerobic capacity supports cardiopulmonary function and thus vascular health. There are many different methods of *qi gong* that specifically support male sexual function. One should seek out a qualified teacher in order to learn such methods. However, other forms of exercise also support male sexual health including regular walking, jogging, yoga, etc. Men should be encouraged to choose a form of exercise that best suits them, yields good results and minimizes injury, and that they can maintain for life.

2. Maintain psychological wellness

In order for the ancestral sinew to become erect and to maintain its firmness, the spirit-mind must be relaxed. Men should be encouraged to express their feelings and not to repress them so that their liver and heart qi will flow freely and hence qi and blood to the penis will also flow freely.

General lifestyle modifications

1. Avoid smoking

In terms of Chinese medicine, smoking cigarettes scorches and damages qi and blood and leads to qi vacuity and blood stasis. In western medicine, it is a well-known cause of erectile dysfunction.

2. Avoid excessive alcohol intake

While a small amount of alcohol might improve the movement of qi and blood, excessive alcohol consumption leads to the formation of damp-heat in the center burner which pours downward into the liver channel. Once there, it obstructs qi and blood. As a result, the ancestral sinew does not receive adequate qi and blood in order to become and remain erect. This leads to yang wilt.

3. Eat a balanced, light, and clear diet

Eating a balanced, light, and clear diet consists of eating lots of fresh vegeta-

---

[20] *Qian Jin Yao Fang* was written by Sun Si-Miao in the 7th century, during the Tang dynasty.

bles and fruits, legumes, whole grains, small amounts of lean meats and seafood, and avoiding excessive amounts of fats, sweets, and spicy-hot foods. A light diet enhances the flow of qi and blood to the penis by nourishing the viscera and bowels and the anterior yin region, and by avoiding the accumulation of dampness, phlegm, and heat. On the contrary, fats and sweets encourage the collection of dampness, phlegm, and heat in the anterior yin. Eating spicy-hot foods in moderation—especially in colder climates and by men with constitutional yang vacuity—can be beneficial by warming the anterior yin region. Excessive consumption of spicy-hot foods, however, can scorch and damage yin, and lead to the formation of evil heat in the interior. Over time and if severe, this heat can consume kidney yin-essence and lead to yang wilt.

In addition to eating a generally healthful diet, it is wise for men to periodically eat foods that are especially known to supplement kidney essence and enhance male sexual health. These include oysters, sea cucumber, abalone, shitake mushrooms, shrimp, scallops, walnuts, chestnuts, Chinese chives, venison, lamb, goat, and turtle.

Representative Chinese Research

Treatment with Chinese medicinals

Yang wilt treated according to pattern discrimination

Xuan (1994) reported on 595 cases of yang wilt discriminated into three patterns—yin vacuity with blood stasis and heat, qi and yin dual vacuity, and liver depression. The formula for yin vacuity with blood stasis and heat was a modification of *Yang Kang Tang* (Yang-Restoring Decoction) and contained the following medicinals:

Sheng Di Huang (Rehmanniae Radix Exsiccata seu Recens), 10g
Shu Di Huang (Rehmanniae Radix Praeparata), 10g
Shan Zhu Yu (Corni Fructus), 10g
Ze Xie (Alismatis Rhizoma), 10g
Ze Lan (Lycopi Herba), 10g
Mu Dan Pi (Moutan Cortex), 10g
Dan Shen (Salviae Miltiorrhizae Radix), 10g
Xu Duan (Dipsaci Radix), 10g
Gou Qi Zi (Lycii Fructus), 10g
He Shou Wu (Polygoni Multiflori Radix), 10g
Bie Jia (Trionycis Carapax), 10g
Fu Ling (Poria), 15g
Tu Si Zi (Cuscutae Semen), 15g
Yin Yang Huo (Epimedii Herba), 15g
Bu Gu Zhi (Psoraleae Fructus), 15g
Che Qian Zi (Plantaginis Semen), 15g
Huang Bai (Phellodendri Cortex), 15g
Mu Li (Ostreae Concha), 30g

The formula for qi and yin dual vacuity was based on *Sheng Mai San* (Pulse-Engendering Powder) and contained the following medicinals:

Ren Shen (Ginseng Radix), 10g
Huang Qi (Astragali Radix), 10g
Mai Men Dong (Ophiopogonis Radix), 10g
Wu Wei Zi (Shizandrae Fructus), 10g
Fu Shen (Poria cum Pini Radice), 10g
Bai Zhu (Atractylodis Macrocephalae Rhizoma), 10g
Zhi Ke (Aurantii Fructus), 10g
Gou Qi Zi (Lycii Fructus), 10g
Lu Rong (Cervi Cornu Pantotrichum), 2g, powdered and taken with the strained decoction
Bu Gu Zhi (Psoralae Fructus), 15g
Xian Mao (Curculiginis Rhizoma), 15g
Bie Jia (Trionycis Carapax), 15g
Rou Cong Rong (Cistanches Herba), 15g
Sheng Di Huang (Rehmanniae Radix Exsiccata seu Recens), 15g
Tu Si Zi (Cuscutae Semen), 15g
Yin Yang Huo (Epimedi Herba), 15g

For the liver depression pattern, the following medicinals were used as a modification of *Xiao Chai Hu Tang* (Minor Bupleurum Decoction):

Chai Hu (Bupleuri Radix), 10g
Ren Shen (Ginseng Radix), 10g
Sheng Ma (Cimicifugae Rhizoma), 10g
Huang Qin (Scutellariae Radix), 10g
Ban Xia (Pinelliae Rhizoma), 10g
Chen Pi (Citri Reticulatae Pericarpium), 10g
He Shou Wu (Polygoni Multiflori Radix), 10g
Gou Qi Zi (Lycii Fructus), 10g
Xiang Yuan (Citri Fructus), 10g
Zhi Ke (Aurantii Fructus), 10g
Suan Zao Ren (Ziziphi Spinosi Semen), 10g
Dan Shen (Salviae Miltiorrhizae Radix), 10g
Dang Gui (Angelicae Sinensis Radix), 10g

Results: The treatment course ranged from 1–6 months and the outcome was reported as follows: 1) complete cure in 77 cases (13%); 2) obvious results in 119 cases (20%) and; 3) good results in 224 cases (41%). The total amelioration rate was 75%.

Yang wilt and blood stasis

Tao (1994) reported on 50 cases of yang wilt treated with a pill formula containing *Shui Zhi* (Hirudo), *Wu Gong* (Scolopendra), and *Ji Nei Jin* (Galli Gigeriae Endothelium Corneum) combined with a specific formula based on pattern discrimination. For qi vacuity and blood stasis, a modification of *Bu Zhong Yi Qi*

Tang (Center-Supplementing Qi-Boosting Decoction) was used. For qi stagnation and blood stasis, a modification of *Xiao Yao San* (Free Wanderer Powder) was used. For phlegm-dampness with blood stasis, he used *Dao Tan Tang* (Phlegm-Abducting Decoction) plus *Huang Lian* (Coptidis Rhizoma), *Shi Chang Pu* (Acori Tatarinowii Rhizoma), *Bai Ji Li* (Tribuli Fructus). If the tongue fur was thick slimy and there were no heat signs, *Ping Wei San* (Stomach-Calming Powder) and *Er Chen Tang* (Two Matured Ingredients Decoction) plus *Bai Zhi* (Angelicae Dahuricae Radix) and *Shi Chang Pu* (Acori Tatarinowii Rhizoma) were used.

Results: Three months comprised one treatment course. After two treatment courses, the results were reported as follows: 14 cases had obvious results, 22 cases had some results, and 14 cases had no results.

Yang wilt and the liver

Qian (1990) studied the results of primarily treating the liver for 100 cases of yang wilt. The base formula consisted of:
> *Chai Hu* (Bupleuri Radix), 5g
> *Dang Gui* (Angelicae Sinensis Radix), 10g
> *Chi Shao* (Paeoniae Radix Rubra), 10g
> *Bai Shao* (Paeoniae Radix Alba), 10g
> *Chuan Xiong* (Chuanxiong Rhizoma), 10g

Modifications: When there is also blood stasis, add *Hong Hua* (Carthami Flos) and *Tao Ren* (Persicae Semen). When there is also damp-heat, add *Huang Bai* (Phellodendri Cortex) and *Ze Xie* (Alismatis Rhizoma). When there is also kidney yang vacuity, add *Yin Yang Huo* (Epimedii Herba) and *Lu Jiao* (Cervi Cornu). When there is also kidney yin vacuity, add *Shu Di Huang* (Rehmanniae Radix Praeparata) and *Gou Qi Zi* (Lycii Fructus).

Results: The treatment course lasted from 10–90 days. Seventy-one cases were completely cured, 23 cases had good results, and 6 cases had no results, for an overall amelioration rate of 94%.

Self-composed formula for yang wilt

Yin *et al.* (1995) reported on the treatment of 274 cases of yang wilt with a self-composed formula called *Zhi Wei Tang* (Wilt-Treating Decoction). The ingredients of the formula were:
> *Shan Zhu Yu* (Corni Fructus), 30g
> *Gou Qi Zi* (Lycii Fructus), 30g
> *Tu Si Zi* (Cuscutae Semen), 30g
> *Sha Yuan Ji Li* (Astragali Complanati Semen), 30g
> *Xian Mao* (Curculiginis Rhizoma), 25g
> *She Chuang Zi* (Cnidii Fructus), 25g
> *Yin Yang Huo* (Epimedii Herba), 25g
> *Ba Ji Tian* (Morinda Radix), 25g
> *Dang Gui* (Angelicae Sinensis Radix), 20g
> *Shu Di Huang* (Rehmanniae Radix Praeparata), 20g

Hu Lu Ba (Trigonellae Semen), 15g
Rou Gui (Cinnamomi Cortex), 10–15g

Modifications: For patients with heart-spleen dual vacuity, add *Dang Shen* (Codonopsis Radix) and *Huang Qi* (Astragali Radix). For fright and fear damaging the heart and kidneys, add *Long Gu* (Mastodi Ossis Fossilia), *Yuan Zhi* (Polygalae Radix), and *Mu Li* (Ostreae Concha). For patients with liver depression, add *Chai Hu* (Bupleuri Radix) and *Xiang Fu* (Cyperi Rhizoma). The medicinals were decocted in water and one packet was used as one day's dose. fifteen packets comprised one treatment course.

Results: Two hundred twenty-six cases were cured (85%), 40 cases had good results (14.5%), and 8 cases had no result (3%). The total amelioration rate was 97%.

Yang wilt and damp-heat

Cao *et al.* (1990) investigated the use of *Long Dan Di Long Qi Wei Tang* (Gentian and Earthworm Wilt-Raising Decoction) for 64 cases of damp-heat yang wilt. The base formula consisted of:
    Long Dan Cao (Gentianae Radix), 15g
    Dang Gui (Angelicae Sinensis Radix), 15g
    Zhi Da Huang (Rhei Radix et Rhizoma Preparata), 12g
    Sheng Di Huang (Rehmanniae Radix Exsiccata seu Recens), 12g
    Ze Xie (Alismatis Rhizoma), 12g
    She Chuang Zi (Cnidii Fructus), 12g
    Di Long (Pheretima), 20g
    Chai Hu (Bupleuri Radix), 9g
    Che Qian Zi (Plantagninis Semen), 18g
    Mu Tong (Akebiae Trifoliatae Caulis), 10g
    Fu Ling (Poria), 30g
    Wu Gong (Scolopendra), 5 pieces

Modifications: For patients who also have liver depression, add *He Huan Pi* (Albizzia Cortex) and increase the dosage of *Chai Hu*. For spleen vacuity, add *Dang Shen* (Codonopsis Radix), *Cang Zhu* (Atractylodis Rhizoma), and *Bai Zhu* (Atractylodis Macrocephalae Rhizoma). For patients with seminal emission, add *Lian Xu* (Nelumbinis Stamen). For unquiet heart-spirit, add *Zhi Yuan Zhi* (Polygalae Radix cum Liquido Fricta). The investigators prescribed one packet per day and 20 days comprised one treatment course.

Results: Fifty-one cases were cured, 4 cases had obvious results, 4 cases had some results, and 5 cases had no result. Forty-seven of the cases that were cured were followed for a two-year period and only 9 experienced a recurrence.

Treatment with acumoxa therapy

Ju Yang Xue (Yang-Raising Point) for yang wilt

Ren *et al.* (1991) used *Ju Yang Xue* to treat 258 cases of yang wilt. *Ju Yang Xue* is located at the midpoint between *Zhi Bian* (BL-54) and *Huan Tiao* (GB-

30). The investigators needled it to a depth of 5 *cun* towards the pubic bone until the patient felt numbness, distention, and pulling pain at the root of the penis. The needle was then retained for 30 minutes and manipulated every 10 minutes with even supplementation and even drainage.

Modifications: For men with kidney yang vacuity, add *Guan Yuan* (CV-4), *Ming Men* (GV-4), *Shen Shu* (BL-23), and *San Yin Jiao* (SP-6); needle all the points with supplementation and apply 7 cones of moxa to *Shen Shu* after removing the needles. For heart-spleen dual vacuity, add *Shen Shu* (BL-15), *Nei Guan* (PC-6), *Zhong Wan* (CV-12), *Zu San Li* (ST-36), *Shen Shu* (BL-23), and *San Yin Jiao* (SP-6); needle all the points with supplementation. For heart and kidney yin vacuity, add *Zhong Ji* (CV-3), *Ci Liao* (BL-32), *San Yin Jiao* (SP-6), *Da Ling* (PC-7), *Shen Men* (HT-7), and *Fu Liu* (KI-7); needle *Da Ling*, *Shen Men*, and *Fu Liu* with draining, and the rest of the points with supplementation.

Results: All patients were treated once per day for 12 days, which comprised one treatment course. 87 cases were cured, 157 had some results, and 14 cases had no results. The cure rate was 33.7%, and the total amelioration rate was 94.6%.

Electro-acupuncture for yang wilt

Liu (1993) used electro-acupuncture to treat 82 cases of yang wilt. Two main groups of acumoxa points were used: 1) *Guan Yuan* (CV-4), *Zhong Ji* (CV-3), *Gui Lai* (ST-29), *Zu San Li* (ST-36), and *San Yin Jiao* (SP-6) and; 2) *Shen Shu* (BL-23), *Ci Liao* (BL-32), *Xia Liao* (BL-34), and *Tai Xi* (KI-3).

Modifications: For patients with damp-heat pouring downward, add *Hui Yin* (CV-1). For low libido, add *Yin Lian* (LV-11) and *Bai Hui* (GV-20). For insomnia, add *Nei Guan* (PC-6) and *Shen Men* (HT-7). For liver depression, add *Xing Jian* (LV-2) and *Tai Chong* (LV-3). The two groups of points were used on alternate days. After the needles were inserted, electro-stimulation was applied to the main points so that the patient experienced the needling sensation into the penis and testes, and this was maintained for 30 minutes. All added points were needled with the goal of attaining a local sensation of soreness and distention, but were not used with electric stimulation. 10 treatments comprised one treatment course.

Results: Forty-six cases were cured, 26 cases had good results, and 10 cases had no results. The total amelioration rate was 87.8%.

Acupuncture based on pattern discrimination

He (1989) used acumoxa therapy to treat 76 cases of yang wilt. The patient population ranged in age from 26–57 years, and had yang wilt for anywhere from 3 months to 25 years, none had any structural abnormalities of their genitals, and all had used Chinese medicine or Western medicine without any effects in the past. The main acumoxa points used in the study were *Shen Shu* (BL-23), *Guan Yuan* (CV-4), and *San Yin Jiao* (SP-6); all were used with the supplementing method.

Modifications: For patients with kidney yang vacuity, *Ming Men* (GV-4) and *Zu San Li* (ST-36) were added; after these points were needled, moxa was also applied to them. For liver depression and qi stagnation, *Tai Chong* (LV-3) was added (with draining), and *Tai Xi* (KI-3) was added (with supplementation). For damp-heat pouring downward, *Ci Liao* (BL-32), *Qi Chong* (ST-30), *Yin Ling Quan* (SP-9), and *Xing Jian* (LV-2) were added; all of these points were used with drainage. The needles were retained for 30 minutes, one treatment was given per day, and 10 treatments comprised one treatment course. Forty-nine cases were cured, 19 cases had obvious results, and 8 cases had no result. The overall amelioration rate was 89.4%.

Yang wilt due to kidney qi vacuity

In *Dang Dai Zhong Guo Zhen Jiu Lin Zheng Jing Yao* (*Essentials of Modern Clinical Acumoxa* [*Therapy*]), there was a case reported about a 36 year-old male with yang wilt.[21] For more than ten years, the patient had suffered from dizzy head and tinnitus, palpitations and shortness of breath, soreness and limpness of the lumbus and knees, insomnia with copious dreaming, and gradually worsening premature ejaculation. In recent years, he had begun to experience yang wilt, and despite having sought treatment from various doctors, it had yet to be treated successfully. His facial complexion was soot-black, he had exhaustion of essence-spirit, a lack of spirit in his eyes, and he had a faint low voice. The pulse was sinking fine and forceless, the tongue fur was thin white, and the tongue was pale. The diagnosis was kidney qi vacuity-detriment and treatment required supplementing the kidneys.

The following acumoxa points were chosen: *Shen Shu* (BL-23), *Huan Zhong Shang Xue* (an empirical point located 2.5 *cun* above *Huan Zhong* [In the Round]),[22] needled to a depth of 4 *cun* with the needling sensation extending to the anterior yin region; *Shen Shu* (BL-23), needled with supplementation. The patient was treated for an unspecified number of treatments for one month and the yang wilt was relieved.

Representative Case Studies

Yang wilt due to dual vacuity of yin and yang

Xiao Jun-Yi reported a case study of yang wilt in Dong (1990). The patient was 31 years old and had been experiencing yang wilt for more than three years. In an attempt to treat himself, and at the advice of friends and family, he had taken many yang-supplementing medicinals including *Ren Shen* (Ginseng Radix) and *Lu Rong* (Cervi Cornu Pantotrichum) without any salubrious effect. Doctor Xiao took the patient's history and examined him and reported the following findings: emaciation, general poor health, somber yellow facial complexion, dizzy head which at times was so severe that he was unable to get

---

[21] Reported in Shi *et al.* (2001).
[22] *Huan Zhong* is located at the midpoint between *Huan Tiao* (GB-30) and *Yao Shu* (GV-2).

out of bed, cold limbs (despite the fact that he had repeatedly taken ginseng and velvet deer horn), satisfactory appetite, dry mouth without desire to drink, one bowel movement every two days, pale red tongue with thin white fur, and a fine stringlike pulse.

Dr. Xiao felt strongly that this was a case of detriment to yang affecting (*yin yang sun ji yin*) and dual vacuity of yin and yang. From his experience, he knew that in such cases one should not use too many warming and drying medicinals, but rather one should evenly supplement both yin and yang, enrich yin to assist yang, and supplement blood and engender essence. He prescribed the following formula:

Sha Shen (Adenophorae seu Glehniae Radix), 12g
Tian Men Dong (Asparagi Radix), 15g
Sheng Di Huang (Rehmanniae Radix Exsiccata seu Recens), 20g
Shu Di Huang (Rehmanniae Radix Praeparata), 20g
He Shou Wu (Polygoni Multiflori Radix), 20g
Gou Qi Zi (Lycii Fructus), 12g
Bu Gu Zhi (Psoraleae Fructus), 12g
Tu Si Zi (Cuscutae Semen), 15g
Fu Pen Zi (Rubi Fructus), 15g
Yin Yang Huo (Epimedii Herba), 15g
Rou Cong Rong (Cistanches Herba), 12g

The patient fully recovered his erectile function after taking forty packets of the prescription.

In his commentary about the case, Dr. Xiao emphatically stated that in his clinical experience, "Many blame yang wilt on yang vacuity and debilitation of life gate fire and are therefore eager to use warm supplementation to treat it." He warned, "When treating yang wilt do not be biased towards warm supplementation but [rather] evenly supplement both yin and yang." To further support his argument, he invoked Zhang Jing-Yue who said: "[To] effectively supplement yin, [one] must seek yin within yang; [to] effectively supplement yang, [one] must seek yang within yin" (Dong, 1990, p. 431).

Yang wilt due to kidney qi vacuity and vacuous yang floating astray

In Dong (1990), Dr. Zhao Fen reported a case of yang wilt in a 36 year-old male. The patient had been married for five years and had yet to father a child. He complained of sometimes having complete erectile dysfunction and sometimes having a partial erection that was not hard enough for intercourse. On the occasions when did get an erection that was rather firm, he would ejaculate at the slightest touch. He also reported a scanty quantity of ejaculate. Additional signs included: dizzy head; weight loss despite having a good appetite, and little sleep with copious dreaming, a sinking fine pulse, and a pale red tongue with thin fur. His blood pressure was 120/74 mmHg and there were no structural abnormalities of his reproductive organs. Further, he reported a history of masturbation before he was married. The diagnosis was kidney qi vacuity and vacuous yang floating astray. The treatment principle was to warm the kidneys and support yang, assisted by subduing and downbearing.

Dr. Zhao prescribed the formula below and the patient saw noticeable results after taking twenty-two packets. After taking it consistently for one year, the patient's wife became pregnant and they had a healthy baby.

> *Tu Si Zi* (Cuscutae Semen), 15g
> *Dang Shen* (Codonopsis Radix), 15g
> *Chao Du Zhong* (Eucommiae Cortex Frictus), 15g
> *Gou Qi Zi* (Lycii Fructus), 15g
> *Shan Yao* (Dioscoreae Rhizoma), 15g
> *Xu Duan* (Dipsaci Radix), 15g
> *Wu Wei Zi* (Schisandrae Fructus), 9g
> *Mai Ya* (Hordei Fructus Germinatus), 30g
> *Gu Ya* (Setariae Fructus Germinatus), 30g
> *Zi Shi Ying* (Fluoritum), 30g
> *Che Qian Zi* (Plantaginis Semen), 9g
> *Chi Shao* (Paeoniae Radix Rubra), 9g
> *Zi He Che* (Hominis Placenta), 9g

In his commentary about his prescription, Dr Zhao pointed out that he used a modification of *Wu Zi Yan Zong Wan* (Five-Seed Progeny Pill). Further, he revealed that the reason he was using *Dang Shen*, *Shan Yao*, *Mai Ya*, and *Gu Ya* was to supplement later heaven in order to engender early heaven. In other words, by supplementing the spleen and stomach, one supplements the kidneys indirectly since early and later heaven mutually transform into one another. Additionally, he cited the importance of using one or two medicinals that "breathe out" stagnation within a supplementing formula; and that in this case, he used *Chi Shao* for this purpose. Finally, he explained that *Zi Shi Ying* warms the kidneys and leads fire back to its source, and that *Zi He Che* is a medicinal with an affinity to flesh and blood and was therefore necessary in this case to enrich essence-blood.

Yang wilt due to damp-heat pouring downward and liver depression transforming fire

Cheng Guo-Rong reported a case of yang wilt in a 28 year-old male in Dong (1990). The patient had been married for 4 years and still had not fathered a child. He complained of the disappearance of his sex drive and of having frequent dream emissions. He was also unable to get an erection and hence was incapable of having sexual intercourse. Other symptoms included: poor quality sleep, a fair appetite, dry mouth, bitter taste, and thirst, dry bound stools, and short voidings of reddish urine. There was also tidal reddening of the face, red tongue with dry yellow fur, and a fine stringlike pulse which was sinking in the cubit (*chi*) position.

Dr. Cheng made a diagnosis of yang wilt due to damp-heat pouring downward and to liver depression transforming fire and used a modification of *Long Dan*

Xie Gan Tang (Gentian Liver-Draining Decoction) to course the liver and resolve depression, and to clear heat and drain fire. The prescription was as follows:

    Chai Hu (Bupleuri Radix), 6g
    Long Dan Cao (Gentianae Radix), 6g
    Huang Qin (Scutellariae Radix), 6g
    Shan Zhi Zi (Gardeniae Fructus), 6g
    Ze Xie (Alismatis Rhizoma), 6g
    Sheng Di Huang (Rehmanniae Radix Exsiccata seu Recens), 15g
    Che Qian Zi (Plantaginis Semen), 15g
    Mu Tong (Akebiae Trifoliatae Caulis), 4.5g
    Gan Cao (Glycyrrhizae Radix), 3g

After taking 6 packets of this prescription his sleep gradually became more peaceful, his micturition and bowel movements became regular, and his tongue also normalized. Dr. Cheng modified the prescription by removing *Mu Tong* (Akebiae Trifoliatae Caulis) and by adding *Mu Dan Pi* (Moutan Cortex), *Yi Yi Ren* (Coicis Semen), and *Fu Ling* (Poria), and prescribed ten more packets. After taking these ten packets, Dr Cheng detected that the patient's liver was coursing much more freely based on the changes he observed in his overall signs and symptoms, including in his pulse and tongue. However, the patient did not report any major improvement in his erectile function, and he now reported soreness, limpness, and lack of strength of the lumbus and knees and the pulse changed to sinking fine. Dr. Cheng now felt that he should switch the emphasis of treatment to supplementing spleen and kidney vacuity. The new prescription was as follows:

    Dang Shen (Codonopsis Radix), 15g
    Huang Qi (Astragali Radix), 15g
    Sheng Di Huang (Rehmanniae Radix Exsiccata seu Recens), 15g
    Bai Shao (Paeoniae Radix Alba), 15g
    Rou Cong Rong (Cistanches Herba), 15g
    He Shou Wu (Polygoni Multiflori Radix), 15g
    Gou Qi Zi (Lycii Fructus), 15g
    Dang Gui (Angelicae Sinensis Radix), 6g
    Chuan Xiong (Chuanxiong Rhizoma), 6g
    Mu Dan Pi (Moutan Cortex), 6g
    Yin Yang Huo (Epimedii Herba), 6g
    Ba Ji Tian (Morindae Officinalis Radix), 6g

After taking this formula for two weeks, his sexual function gradually became more normal, but he still felt like his erections did not stay firm long enough and he sometimes experienced premature ejaculation. *Suo Yang* (Cynomorii Herba), *Shan Zhu Yu* (Corni Fructus), *Jiu Cai Zi* (Allii Tuberosi Semen), and *Jin Ying Zi* (Rosae Laevigatae Fructus) were added to further supplement kidney yang and to secure and bind kidney essence. After one more month of treatment, the patient felt much better and his wife gave birth the following year.

In the commentary about the case, Dr. Cheng revealed that the strategy of first coursing the liver and clearing and draining damp-heat was necessary before being able to supplement the spleen and kidneys. Apparently, other doctors had tried to supplement this patient's kidney qi without first doing this, and had failed. This represented the strategy (not the only possible strategy of course) of first draining repletion before supplementing vacuity in vacuity-repletion combination diseases.

Yang wilt due to damp-heat obstruction

In Dong (1990), Zhao Shao-Qin reported a case of yang wilt in a 24 year-old male due to obstruction by damp-heat. The patient had been married three months prior to the initial visit and shortly thereafter had begun to suffer from yang wilt. Additionally, he had been fatigued for over six months, sometimes to the point of falling asleep at work. Thinking that he suffered from kidney vacuity, he took many supplementing medicinals including *Ren Shen* (Ginseng Radix) and *Huang Qi* (Astragali Radix), high dosages of yang-warming medicinals such as *Rou Gui* (Cinnamomi Cortex) and *Fu Zi* (Aconiti Radix Lateralis Praeparata), and essence-enriching medicinals such as *Lu Rong* (Cervi Cornu Pantotrichum) and *Gui Ban* (Testudinis Carapax et Plastrum). The lack of positive effect from any of these medicines greatly depressed him and he sought solace in alcohol.

Dr. Zhao examined him and reported that he was overweight, his face was bright, shiny, and red, the tongue fur was slimy and very thick, and the tongue body was red. The pulse was soft slippery, on light pressure was soft rapid, and on heavy pressure was stringlike rapid tense. As a result of these findings, Dr. Zhao concluded that this was a case of yang wilt caused by damp-heat obstruction. He prescribed two packets of the following prescription:

> *Chai Hu* (Bupleuri Radix), 6g
> *Zi Su Geng* (Perillae Caulis), 10g
> *Du Huo* (Angelicae Pubescentis Radix), 5g
> *Cao Dou Kou* (Alpiniae Katsumadai Semen), 5g
> *Che Qian Zi* (Plantaginis Semen), 10g
> *Shan Zhi Zi* (Gardeniae Fructus), 6g
> *Huang Qin* (Scutellariae Radix), 10g
> *Long Dan Cao* (Gentianae Radix), 10g
> *Da Huang* (Rhei Radix et Rhizoma) 10g, add at end

After taking the two packets of medicine, the patient returned five days later and reported some relief from the yang wilt and a decrease in fatigue. The pulse on his left wrist was stringlike slippery and soft rapid on light pressure, and the strength was relatively moderate. Although the pulse at the right wrist was still soft slippery in the bar (*guan*) and cubit (*chi*) positions, the rapid tense quality had greatly decreased. The tongue fur was gradually transforming and the tongue body color was quite light. According to Dr. Zhao, these facts showed that the accumulation of damp-heat was gradually being transformed and that the triple burner qi dynamic was gradually becoming free. After taking the prescription, the patient had three bowel movements, which demonstrated that the heat in the bowels was definitely reducing. The treatment principle for the next prescription was to clear and transform damp-heat, quicken the blood and open the network vessels, and to relax the sinews. Three packets of the following prescription were prescribed:

Chai Hu (Bupleuri Radix), 6g

Huang Qin (Scutellariae Radix), 10g

Ze Lan (Lycopi Herba), 10g

Jiang Huang (Curcumae Longae Rhizoma), 6g

Chan Tui (Cicadae Periostracum), 6g

Gou Teng (Uncariae Ramulus cum Uncis), 10g

Chuan Lian Zi (Toosendan Fructus), 10g

Fang Feng (Saposhnikoviae Radix), 6g

Xing Ren (Armeniacae Semen), 10g

Da Huang (Rhei Radix et Rhizoma), 2g, powdered and taken mixed with the strained decoction

Long Dan Cao (Gentianae Radix), 4g, powdered and taken mixed with the strained decoction

After taking the medicine, the patient no longer suffered from yang wilt. To consolidate the positive effect, Dr. Zhang also advised him to exercise regularly, and to avoid drinking alcohol and eating sweet, greasy, and fried foods.

In his commentary for the case, Dr. Zhao points out that it is a definite error to assume all cases of yang wilt are due to qi, yin, or yang vacuity, and that the main issues in this case were depression and brewing of damp-heat and gastrointestinal accumulation and stagnation. This patient's predilection for alcohol also caused damp-heat to brew and become depressed in the liver channel and to distress the anterior yin region.

Premature Ejaculation (PE)

Western Medicine

The American Urological Association reports that 27–34% of men experience premature ejaculation (PE). According to Goldman and Ausiello (2004), the Diagnostic and Statistical Manual of Mental Disorders VI defines premature ejaculation as follows: "Persistent or recurrent ejaculation with minimal sexual stimulation that (1) occurs before, upon, or shortly after penetration and before the person wishes; (2) is associated with marked distress or interpersonal difficulty; and (3) is not a direct effect of substance abuse such as opiate withdrawal." Currently, PE is not considered to be caused by a specific organic disease, but rather by sexual inexperience, anxiety, and by other psychological causes. Increasingly, however, the consensus is shifting in the direction toward PE as a neurobiologically-based condition. Also, some men with benign prostatic hyperplasia (BPH) or chronic prostatitis of various types report PE at a higher incidence than the general population (Screponi *et al.*, 2001). Further, as it is physiological for men to ejaculate within two minutes of intromission, most men need to learn orgastic control by experience in order to increase their intravaginal ejaculatory latency time (IELT), thus enhancing the pleasure they and their partners experience during sexual intercourse.

The psychological effects of PE on both the men who suffer from it and their partners cannot be overestimated. Most studies show that men with PE rate their overall sexual satisfaction lower than normal males, and their general satisfaction with life is usually also lower (Rowland *et al.*, 2007). Low self-esteem, anxiety, shame, and feelings of inferiority are also common (Sotomayer, 2005).

Treatment

Before the advent of selective serotonin reuptake inhibitors (SSRIs)—increasingly the treatment of choice for PE—the therapeutic options for PE included behavioral therapy, sex therapy, and penile constriction rings ("cock rings").

• SSRI treatment

The SSRIs were accidentally discovered as a treatment for PE when males undergoing antidepressant therapy began to exhibit delays in IELT. Since then, they have been widely investigated as a treatments for PE, but are still prescribed "off label." Many studies show that ongoing use is more effective for PE than on-demand use. Some men with ED and PE do not find them effective, however, because they decrease the rigidity of their already compromised erections, making their ED worse. The search for a very specific low-dose on-demand SSRI for PE is ongoing.

• Behavioral therapy

Behavioral therapy generally consists of the use of systematic desensitization techniques (the "stop and start technique") that gradually teach men greater and greater awareness of the sensations of imminent orgasm. Hence, men learn to recognize sensations of early arousal and imminent orgasm so they can alter their behavior during sexual intercourse by slowing down the frequency and depth of their intravaginal thrusting or by stopping for 20–30 seconds. These practices are performed either by the man alone or together with his partner and gradually result in greater orgastic control and improved sexual satisfaction for the majority of men and couples that practice them. Currently, these behavioral methods and sex therapy are still used, but increasingly, SSRIs are prescribed instead of or in combination with these methods.

• Penile constriction rings

Penile constriction rings are commercially available in some pharmacies and in adult entertainment shops. Some men find them somewhat effective for delaying ejaculation and post-ejaculatory detumescence. The research reports that they are not generally very effective for PE; they are more effective (when combined with a vacuum constriction device) for PE associated with ED (Hosseini, 2007 and Levin, 2002).

• New pharmaceutical options

New pharmaceutical strategies for PE are currently under investigation. For example, El-Nashar and Shamloul (2007) found that in patients with PE associated with chronic bacterial prostatitis, antibiotic therapy increased intravaginal ejaculatory latency time. Further, Salonia et al. (2002) found that paroxetine (Paxil) was more effective for PE when given together with on-demand sildenafil (Viagra). Finally, Salem et al (2007) found that tramadol hydrochloride—a nonnarcotic analgesic and antiinflammatory agent—is effective as an on-demand treatment for PE.

Western Complementary Medicine

Given the high incidence of PE in the general population, it is surprising that there are not more complementary medicines aimed at treating it. Presumably, as in the case of some Western pharmaceutical medications, there is some cross-over use between complementary medicines for ED and PE. Hence, the same substances used for ED—Yohimbine, Korean red ginseng, Gingko biloba, and Arginine—might have some promise as complementary modalities for PE.[1]

An interesting new avenue for exploration of PE has recently been proposed by several researchers who have discovered decreased magnesium levels in the seminal plasma of men with PE. Omu *et al.* (2001) propose that "Decreased levels of magnesium gives rise to vasoconstriction from increased thromboxane levels, increased endothelial intracellular Ca2+, and decreased nitric oxide. This may lead to premature emission and ejaculation processes. Magnesium is probably involved in semen transport." None of the papers I surveyed suggested a magnesium-based therapeutic strategy, but perhaps magnesium supplementation should be considered as a potential treatment for PE.

Chinese Medicine

Disease discrimination

The basic definition of premature ejaculation in Chinese medicine is very similar to Western medicine. It is characterized by either rapid ejaculation soon after the initiation of sexual intercourse, or even before intromission occurs. One of the earliest mentions of a pathomechanism behind premature ejaculation occurred in *Zhu Bing Yuan Hou Lun* (*On the Origin and Indicators of Disease*),[2] which states: "[When there is] kidney qi vacuity and weakness, essence spills [out]."

However, it was not until the Qing dynasty that the term premature ejaculation (*zao xie*) gradually acquired widespread use. For example, *Bian Zheng Lu* (*Record of Pattern Identification*)[3] stated, "[When] a man has extreme seminal efflux, as soon as he arrives at a woman's gate [*i.e.*, the vaginal meatus], semen is discharged," and *Shen Shi Zeng Sheng Shu* (*Shen's Life-Respecting Text*) described this condition saying, "Without intercourse, [there is] sudden discharge, or with intercourse, abruptly, there is sudden discharge." Also in the Qing dynasty, Ye Tian-Shi, in *Mi Ben Zhong Zi Jin Dan* (*The Secret Root of Golden Elixir Seed Planting*),[4] offered, "Men whose jade stalk foreskin is soft and tender, and [who] suffer [from a] small [penis], [and have] unbearable itching—every time they have intercourse, yang essence has already [been] discharged before yin essence has flowed [*i.e.*, before a woman has become aroused and her vagina is lubricated]. This is called chicken essence." Gradually, the term premature ejaculation became more common and is universally used in modern Chinese andrological literature.

---

[1] For more information on these treatments, see Book 2, Chapter 4 on erectile dysfunction.

[2] *Zhu Bing Yuan Hou Lun* was written by Chao Yuan-Fang and published in 610 CE, during the Sui dynasty.

[3] *Bian Zheng Lu* was written by Chen Shi-Duo and published in 1687, during the Qing dynasty.

[4] *Mi Ben Zhong Zi Jin Dan* was written by Ye Tian-Shi and published during the Qing dynasty.

Disease causes and pathomechanisms

Generally speaking, premature ejaculation is primarily viewed as a disease of the heart, liver, and kidneys in Chinese medicine. To illustrate this perspective, it is useful to consider the following passage from Zhu Dan-Xi:[5] "The kidney governs blockage and storage, and the liver governs coursing and discharge. Both of these viscera posses ministerial fire, and tie with the heart above." Dan-Xi explained further that the physiological storage and discharge of essence depends on close coordination among these three viscera, and that sovereign fire within the heart (especially when disturbed by desire) can overly excite ministerial fire within the liver and kidneys, and that this can result in premature ejaculation.

Further, we must also consider the role of the spleen—as the later heaven source for the engenderment and transformation of qi and blood—in premature ejaculation. Later heaven and early heaven mutually transform. This means that kidney qi—which has the primary role of sealing and storing essence within the kidneys and essence chamber by maintaining the integrity of the essence gate (jing guan)—is dependent on spleen qi for support. So, when spleen qi is vacuous, it eventually affects the kidneys by making kidney qi vacuous and thereby unable to govern the sealing and storage of semen. Hence, premature ejaculation results.

In summary, the primary disease causes and pathomechanisms for premature ejaculation are liver channel damp-heat, yin vacuity and hyperactivity of yang, insecurity of kidney qi, and heart-spleen dual vacuity. We will explore them in greater detail in the following section. Clinically, there is quite often kidney vacuity combined with one or more of the other patterns discussed below.

• Liver channel damp-heat

The main causes of liver channel damp-heat include constitutional irascibility, emotional repression and depression, and prolonged and excessive intake of greasy, fatty, and spicy foods. When these emotions persist over a long period of time, binding depression of liver qi transforms fire. Dietary irregularities such as these damage the spleen and lead to internally-engendered damp-heat which pours downward from the center burner into the lower burner and into the liver channel. Because the liver channel qi is depressed along with the qi of the liver viscus, damp-heat lodges in the liver channel and brews and binds there. Since the liver channel skirts the genitals, the penis, essence chamber, and essence gate are all adversely affected in this scenario. Because the liver possesses ministerial fire, and is therefore physiologically warm by nature, depressed fire within the liver channel harasses the essence gate and overly excites it to the point of making it unable to withstand the additional warmth and excitation provided by sexual stimulation. Thus, ministerial fire stirs ex-

---

[5] Zhu Dan-Xi was one of the four great masters of the Jin-Yuan dynasty. He lived and worked from 1281–1358.

cessively and causes the liver to course and discharge excessively, and premature ejaculation results. It is important to mention that this pattern can occur without the dampness, in which case we refer to it as binding depression of liver qi with depressed fire.

•Yin vacuity with hyperactivity of yang

This pattern occurs in men with constitutional yin vacuity, in men who overwork and/or have engaged in excessive sexual activity, and in men who started sexual activity at a young age (including masturbation). In all of these cases, either by natural endowment or due to behaviors and habits, yin-essence has been damaged which leads to a lack of attachment for yang. As a result, yang becomes hyperactive and causes excessive stirring of ministerial fire and abnormal excitation; hence insecurity of the essence gate and premature ejaculation result. This pattern can present in men from the very beginning of their sexual contact, or can develop later in life in men who have never experienced it before. In the former case, constitutional yin-essence vacuity is usually the culprit; in the latter, yin vacuity has usually been acquired through excessive draining of essence.

• Noninteraction of the heart and kidney

Since the heart is ascribed to fire and the kidney is ascribed to water in five phase theory, under normal physiological circumstances, "water and fire benefit each other." While there a few meanings to this dictum, the main one we invoke here is the mutually-enriching natures of heart and kidney yin—namely that heart yin nourishes kidney yin, and kidney yin-essence in turn nourishes heart yin. When long-term worry and contemplation damage the heart-spirit and engender fire, vacuity fire scorches yin and hence heart and kidney yin both suffer damage. Vacuity fire then harasses the essence gate and causes it to open prematurely. This is the main mechanisms through which this pattern causes premature ejaculation. Closely related to yin vacuity and hyperactivity of yang previously described, this pattern may arise as its complication.

• Insecurity of kidney qi

The main causes of this pattern include natural endowment insufficiency or constitutional vacuity of kidney qi, overwork, poor diet, chronic disease that damages qi, and excessive sexual activity. The kidney governs the sealing and storage of essence. In all cases, kidney qi becomes vacuous and is therefore unable to govern the sealing and storage of essence within the essence chamber or to maintain the integrity of the essence gate; premature ejaculation results.

• Heart-spleen dual vacuity

The heart governs the spirit and the spleen governs movement and transformation of water and grain essence. The heart is the sovereign viscus and the spirit governs the physiological activity of all the other viscera and bowels. When spleen qi is vacuous, the later heaven source of qi, blood, and essence is insufficient. Hence, there is insufficient raw material for the engenderment of qi and blood, and the heart suffers from a lack of power and nourishment and is unable to direct the kidney in its action of sealing and storage of essence. Further, spleen qi vacuity leads to kidney qi vacuity, to insecurity of the essence gate, and an inability to secure essence. In clinical practice, this pattern usually presents together with insecurity of kidney qi.

Pattern discrimination

1. Liver channel damp-heat

Signs: Hyperactive libido and readily-obtained erections, rapid ejaculation after commencing sexual activity, dizzy head and eyes, bitter taste in the mouth and dry throat, yellowish-red or turbid urine, heart vexation and propensity to anger, dampness and itching of the scrotum, red tongue with slimy yellow fur, stringlike rapid or slippery rapid pulse.

Treatment principles: Clear heat and drain dampness from the liver channel

Guiding formula: Modified *Long Dan Xie Gan Tang* (Gentian Liver-Draining Decoction)

Ingredients:
   Long Dan Cao (Gentianae Radix), 12g
   Huang Qin (Scutellariae Radix), 10g
   Zhi Zi (Gardeniae Fructus), 10g
   Gou Qi Zi (Lycii Fructus), 12g
   Mu Tong (Akebiae Trifoliatae Caulis), 12g
   Che Qian Zi (Plantaginis Semen), 15g
   Dang Gui (Angelicae Sinensis Radix), 10g
   Sheng Di Huang (Rehmanniae Radix Exsiccata seu Recens), 12g
   Chai Hu (Bupleuri Radix), 10g
   Ze Xie (Alismatis Rhizoma), 12g
   Gan Cao (Glycyrrhizae Radix), 6g

Modifications: For patients with more prominent heart vexation and bitter taste in the mouth, use *Huang Lian* (Coptidis Rhizoma), 6g, instead of *Huang Qin,* to strengthen the ability of the formula to clear heart fire. For turbid strangury, add *Pu Gong Ying* (Taraxaci Herba), 15g, and *Huang Bai* (Phellodendri Cortex), 12g, to enhance the ability of the formula to clear heat and free strangury.

2. Yin vacuity with hyperactivity of yang

Signs: Vacuity vexation and insomnia, readily-obtained erections with rapid ejaculation after commencing sexual activity, frequent dream emissions, soreness and limpness of lumbus and knees, heat and vexation of the five hearts, tidal heat effusion and night sweating, small thin red tender tongue with scanty fur, fine rapid pulse.

Treatment principles: Enrich yin and subdue the yang

Guiding formulas: Modified *Zhi Bai Di Huang Wan* (Anemarrhena, Phellodendron, and Rehmannia Pill) plus *Er Zhi Wan* (Double Supreme Pill)

Ingredients:
    Sheng Di Huang (Rehmanniae Radix Exsiccata seu Recens), 15g
    Shan Zhu Yu (Corni Fructus), 12g
    Shan Yao (Dioscoreae Rhizoma), 15g
    Zhi Mu (Anemarrhenae Rhizoma), 10g
    Huang Bai (Phellodendri Cortex), 10g
    Ze Xie (Alismatis Rhizoma), 10g
    Mu Dan Pi (Moutan Cortex), 10g
    Fu Ling (Poria), 12g
    Nu Zhen Zi (Ligustri Lucidi Fructus), 15g
    Han Lian Cao (Ecliptae Herba), 12g
    Sha Yuan Ji Li (Astragali Complanati Semen), 10g
    Jin Ying Zi (Rosae Laevigatae Fructus), 15g
    Gui Ban (Testudinis Carapax et Plastrum), 15g, predecocted
    Duan Long Gu (Mastodi Ossis Fossilia Calcinata), 30g, predecocted
    Duan Mu Li (Ostreae Concha Calcinata), 30g, predecocted

Modifications: For patients with more prominent insomnia, add *Suan Zao Ren* (Ziziphi Spinosi Semen), 15g, and *Bai He* (Lilii Bulbus), 10g, to nourish the heart and calm the spirit. For more prominent night sweats, add *Di Gu Pi* (Lycii Cortex), 15g, to enhance the ability of the formula to clear vacuity heat.

3. Noninteraction of the heart and kidney

Signs: Rapid ejaculation after commencing sexual activity, dream emissions and seminal efflux, dizziness and lack of strength, palpitations and fearful throbbing, insomnia, copious dreaming, thirst and heart vexation, red facial complexion, short reddish urine with a heat sensation, red tender tongue with a redder tip, fine rapid pulse.

Treatment principles: Enrich yin and clear heat, promote heart and kidney interaction

Guiding formula: Modified *Huang Lian E Jiao Tang* (Coptis and Ass Hide Glue Decoction)

Ingredients:
    Huang Lian (Coptidis Rhizoma), 6g
    Bai Shao (Paeoniae Radix Alba), 15g
    Ji Zi Huang (Galli Vitellus), 2 yolks, stirred into the strained decoction
    E Jiao (Asini Corii Colla), 10g, dissolved into the strained decoction
    Huang Qin (Scutellariae Radix), 10g
    Qian Shi (Euryales Semen), 12g
    Jin Ying Zi (Rosae Laevigatae Fructus), 15g
    Wu Wei Zi (Schisandrae Fructus), 12g
    Yuan Zhi (Polygalae Radix), 10g

Modifications: For more prominent insomnia, add *Suan Zao Ren* (Ziziphi Spinosi Semen), 20g, *Long Gu* (Mastodi Ossis Fossilia), 15g, *Mu Li* (Ostreae Concha), 15g, and *Lian Zi Xin* (Nelumbinis Plumula), 6g, to nourish the heart and calm the spirit, to settle and calm the spirit, and to further clear hyperactive heart fire.

4. Insecurity of kidney qi

Signs: Low libido, soft erections or erectile dysfunction, seminal efflux, rapid ejaculation soon after commencing sexual activity, less intense orgasmic sensations, clear dilute semen, long clear urination, nocturia, dizzy head and eyes, cold limbs, listlessness of essence-spirit, pale tender tongue with white fur, sinking fine weak pulse.

Treatment principles: Boost the kidney and secure essence

Guiding formula: Modified *Jin Gui Shen Qi Wan* (Golden Coffer Kidney Qi Pill)

Ingredients:
> *Shu Fu Zi* (Aconiti Radix Lateralis Conquita), 6g, predecocted
> *Rou Gui* (Cinnamomi Cortex), 6g
> *Shu Di Huang* (Rehmanniae Radix Exsiccata seu Recens), 15g
> *Shan Zhu Yu* (Corni Fructus), 15g
> *Fu Ling* (Poria), 12g
> *Shan Yao* (Dioscoreae Rhizoma), 15g
> *Mu Dan Pi* (Moutan Cortex), 10g
> *Ze Xie* (Alismatis Rhizoma), 12g
> *Sang Piao Xiao* (Mantidis Ootheca), 10g
> *Jin Ying Zi* (Rosae Laevigatae Fructus), 15g
> *Wu Wei Zi* (Schisandrae Fructus), 12g

Modifications: For soreness and limpness of lumbus and knees, add *Du Zhong* (Eucommiae Cortex), 15g, *Niu Xi* (Achyranthis Bidentatae Radix), 12g, and *Ba Ji Tian* (Morindae Radix), 15g, to supplement the kidneys and strengthen the sinews and bones. For poor memory, dizziness of head, and tinnitus, add *Lu Jiao Jiao* (Cervi Cornus Gelatinum), 10g, dissolved into the strained decoction, to enrich essence with a medicinal with affinity to flesh and blood.

5. Heart-spleen dual vacuity

Signs: Rapid ejaculation soon after commencing sexual activity, fatigue and lack of strength, emaciation, lusterless facial complexion, loose stools and poor appetite, palpitations and shortness of breath, poor memory and copious dreaming, pale tender tongue with white fur, fine pulse without strength.

Treatment principles: Supplement and boost the heart and spleen

Guiding formula: Modified *Gui Pi Tang* (Spleen-Returning Decoction)

Ingredients:

Dang Shen (Codonopsis Radix), 15g
Bai Zhu (Atractylodis Macrocephalae Rhizoma), 15g
Huang Qi (Astragali Radix), 15g
Dang Gui (Angelicae Sinensis Radix), 12g
Fu Shen (Poria cum Pini Radice), 15g
Yuan Zhi (Polygalae Radix), 10g
Suan Zao Ren (Ziziphi Spinosi Semen), 15g
Mu Xiang (Aucklandiae Radix), 10g
Wu Wei Zi (Schisandrae Fructus), 12g
Jin Ying Zi (Rosae Laevigatae Fructus), 15g
Duan Long Gu (Mastodi Ossis Fossilia Calcinata), 30g, predecocted
Duan Mu Li (Ostreae Concha Calcinata), 30g, predecocted
Zhi Gan Cao (Glycyrrhizae Radix cum Liquido Fricta), 6g

Modifications: For patients with heart yin vacuity, add *Mai Men Dong* (Ophiopogonis Radix), 6g, to nourish and enrich heart yin. For more prominent blood vacuity, add *Huang Jing* (Polygonati Rhizoma), 12g, *Chuan Xiong* (Chuanxiong Rhizoma), 10g, and *Bai Shao* (Paeoniae Radix Alba), 12g, to nourish blood.

Acumoxa therapy

Main points: *Shen Shu* (BL-23), *Qi Hai* (CV-6), *Guan Yuan* (CV-4), *San Yin Jiao* (SP-6)

Repletion patterns

For damp-heat in the liver channel, add *Tai Chong* (LV-3), *Li Gou* (LV-5), *Ba Liao* (BL-31–BL-34), *Tai Xi* (KI-3), *Qiu Xu* (GB-40), and *Dan Shu* (BL-19)

Vacuity patterns

For yin vacuity with hyperactivity of yang, add *Tai Xi* (KI-3), *Zhao Hai* (KI-6), *Nei Guan* (PC-6), *Tai Chong* (LV-3), and *Shen Shu* (BL-23)

For insecurity of kidney qi, use moxa in addition to needles on *Shen Shu* (BL-23) and *Guan Yuan* (CV-4), and also needle and moxa *Zhong Ji* (CV-3) and *Ming Men* (GV-4)

For noninteraction of the heart and kidneys, add *Shen Men* (HT-7) and *Nei Guan* (PC-6)

For heart-spleen dual vacuity, add *Zu San Li* (ST-36), *Zhong Wan* (CV-12), *Pi Shu* (BL-20), *Wei Shu* (BL-21), *Xin Shu* (BL-15), and *Shen Men* (HT-7)

Experiential formulas

Insecurity of kidney qi (Gu *et al.*, 1996)

Zhao Zheng-Yuan is an old Chinese doctor that treats premature ejaculation with a self-composed formula called *Zao Xie Tang* (Premature Ejaculation Decoction). The main action of the formula is to supplement kidney yang and secure essence. However, Dr. Zhao subscribes to Zhang Jing-Yue's theory that one should seek yang within the midst of yin. Therefore, his formula consists not only of yang supplementing medicinals, but also contains many medicinals to enrich and nourish yin. The ingredients are:

    Shu Di Huang (Rehmanniae Radix Praeparata), 20g
    Gou Qi Zi (Lycii Fructus), 12g
    Shan Yao (Dioscoreae Rhizoma), 15g
    Fu Ling (Poria), 15g
    Wu Wei Zi (Schisandrae Fructus), 6g
    Yuan Zhi (Polygalae Radix), 6g
    Lu Jiao Jiao (Cervi Cornus Gelatinum), 12g, dissolved into the strained decoction
    Tu Si Zi (Cuscutae Semen), 15g
    Yin Yang Huo (Epimedii Herba), 12g
    Long Gu (Mastodi Ossis Fossilia), 30g
    Zhi Mu (Anemarrhenae Rhizoma), 12g
    Yan Huang Bai (Phellodendri Cortex Salsa), 10g
    Gan Cao (Glycyrrhizae Radix), 6g

Using a modification of *San Ren Tang* (Three Kernels Decoction) to treat premature ejaculation

Cao (1990) describes the use of a variation of *San Ren Tang* called *Gu Jing Tang* (Essence-Securing Decoction) to treat a complex pattern of premature ejaculation due to kidney yang vacuity and insecurity of kidney qi, binding depression of liver qi, and collection of dampness in the triple burner. The ingredients are:

    Yi Yi Ren (Coicis Semen), 15g
    Xing Ren (Armeniacae Semen), 12g
    Bai Dou Kou (Amomi Fructus Rotundus), 6g
    Hua Shi (Talcum), 20g
    Wu Wei Zi (Schisandrae Fructus), 6g
    Qian Shi (Euryales Semen), 15g
    Sang Piao Xiao (Mantidis Ootheca), 12g
    Dan Zhu Ye (Lophatheri Herba), 6g
    Rou Cong Rong (Cistanches Herba), 12g
    Chai Hu (Bupleuri Radix), 9g
    Xuan Shen (Scrophulariae Radix), 12g

Modifications: For yin vacuity with hyperactivity of yang, add *Nu Zhen Zi* (Ligustri Lucidi Fructus) and *Han Lian Cao* (Ecliptae Herba). For more prominent insecurity of kidney qi, add *Suo Yang* (Cynomorii Herba) and *Jin Ying Zi* (Rosae Laevigatae Fructus). For patients with liver channel damp-heat, add *Long Dan Cao* (Gentianae Radix) and *Shan Zhi Zi* (Gardeniae Fructus).

Insufficiency of kidney yin and hyperactivity of ministerial fire

Shi (1992) reports on Chen Shu-Sen's experience treating premature ejaculation due to kidney yin vacuity and hyperactivity of ministerial fire with a self-composed formula called *Zhi Bai San Zi Tang* (Anemarrhena Phellodendron Three Seed Decoction). The ingredients are:

Zhi Mu (Anemarrhenae Rhizoma), 10g
Huang Bai (Phellodendri Cortex), 10g
Wu Wei Zi (Schisandrae Fructus), 6g
Jin Ying Zi (Rosae Laevigatae Fructus), 10g
Gou Qi Zi (Lycii Fructus), 10g

Modifications: For patients with insomnia, add *Lian Zi Xin* (Nelumbinis Plumula), 2g, *Suan Zao Ren* (Ziziphi Spinosi Semen), 10g, to clear the heart and calm the spirit. For exhaustion of essence-spirit, add *Ren Shen Xu* (Ginseng Radix Tenuis), 6g, to supplement qi and raise [*i.e.*, uplift] the spirit.

Insecurity of kidney qi and insufficiency of kidney essence

Chen (2002) cites the use of *Tian Jing Gu Xie Wan* (Essence-Replenishing Discharge-Securing Pill) for the treatment of an unspecified number of cases of premature ejaculation due to insecurity of kidney qi and insufficiency of kidney essence. The ingredients are:

Shan Yao (Dioscoreae Rhizoma), 60g
Gou Qi Zi (Lycii Fructus), 90g
Fu Pen Zi (Rubi Fructus), 90g
Shan Zhu Yu (Corni Fructus), 90g
Jin Ying Zi (Rosae Laevigatae Fructus), 90g
Qian Shi (Euryales Semen), 90g
Sang Shen Zi (Mori Fructus), 90g
Nu Zhen Zi (Ligustri Lucidi Fructus), 90g
Rou Cong Rong (Cistanches Herba), 100g
Shu He Shou Wu (Polygoni Multiflori Radix Preparata), 120g
Dang Shen (Codonopsis Radix), 90g
Bai Zhu (Atractylodis Macrocephalae Rhizoma), 60g
Zhi Huang Qi (Astragali Radix cum Liquido Fricta), 60g
Rou Gui (Cinnamomi Cortex), 30g
Lu Rong (Cervi Cornu Pantotrichum), 30g
Hai Ma (Hippocampus),[6] 30g
Gui Ban Jiao (Testudinis Carapacis et Plastri Gelatinum), 100g

Instructions: The medicinals should be ground into fine powder and suffused with honey into pills. Ten grams of pills should be taken two times per day— once in the morning and once in the evening with warm salted water. One month comprises one treatment course.

External treatments (Chen and Jiang, 2000)

Herbal penile desensitization formulas

The main goal of these three formulas is to desensitize the penis to increase intravaginal ejaculatory latency time. The patient should be instructed to stay alert for signs of penile or urethral irritation and discontinue use if they occur.

---

[6] *Hai Ma* is a threatened species and should not be used. One can simply omit it from this formula and expect similar results.

1. Make a very fine powder of equal parts of the medicinals listed below. Mix with cool water and make a paste the consistency of rice gruel. Apply to the head of the penis about one-half hour before intercourse and wash off before intromission.

   Ying Su Ke (Papaveris Pericarpium)[7]
   He Zi (Chebulae Fructus)
   Duan Long Gu (Mastodi Ossis Fossilia Calcinata)

2. Soak 20g each of *Ding Xiang* (Caryophylli Flos) and *Xi Xin* (Asari Herba) in 100 ml. of 95% alcohol for 15 days. Strain and reserve. Use the liquid to wash the penis for 1.5–3 minutes per day and about one-half hour before intercourse. Ten days comprises one treatment course.

3. Decoct 10g each of *She Chuang Zi* (Cnidii Fructus), *Di Gu Pi* (Lycii Cortex), and *Shi Liu Pi* (Granati Pericarpium). Strain, cool sufficiently to reduce burn risk and use the resulting solution to steam and wash the genital region (especially the head of the penis) for at least 10 minutes. Do this immediately before intercourse.

Preventive measures and lifestyle modification

1. Maintain psychological wellness

Since premature ejaculation is associated with considerable emotional stress, having an understanding partner is crucial to limiting the negative essence-spirit effects of the problem as treatment progresses. While premature ejaculation persists, men should satisfy their partners through means other than intercourse. For female partners, men should use direct clitoral stimulation orally and/or manually before, during, or after intercourse so that their partners are sexually satisfied. As in all satisfying sexual relationships, close communication and expression of likes and dislikes encourages greater sexual satisfaction.

2. Maintain physical wellness

By maintaining physical conditioning, one keeps qi, blood, and fluids flowing smoothly and maintains the securing and binding ability of qi. Hence, the emotional stress associated with PE is reduced, dampness, phlegm, and blood stasis are prevented and encouraged to move if they have already accumulated, and kidney qi is strengthened. One may seek out a qualified *qi gong* practitioner, as there are many forms of *qi gong* that are specifically geared towards supplementing the kidneys.

3. Use condoms during sexual intercourse

The use of condoms during sexual intercourse—and especially condoms containing a desensitizing agent on the inside of the condom—can be helpful for

---

[7] *Ying Su Ke* is the husk of the opium poppy and is strictly controlled by narcotics laws in many countries.

men with PE. The advantage they have over traditional penile desensitizing lubricants formerly applied to the outside of the penis prior to intercourse is that they do not affect the partner's sensitivity. In severe cases, these condoms can be used temporarily while waiting for the effects of the treatment to take effect, or along with treatment for men who find them helpful. The danger, however, is that by wearing them a man may develop a dependence and be delayed in developing tolerance of the penile sensations associated with sexual stimulation.

4. Eat a balanced, light, and clear diet

Eating a balanced, light, and clear diet consists of eating lots of fresh vegetables and fruits, legumes, whole grains, small amounts of lean meats and seafood, and avoiding excessive amounts of fats, sweets, and spicy-hot foods. A light diet enhances the flow of qi and blood to the penis by nourishing the viscera and bowels and the anterior yin region, and by avoiding the accumulation of dampness, phlegm, and heat. On the contrary, fats and sweets encourage the collection of dampness, phlegm, and heat in the anterior yin. Eating spicy-hot foods in moderation—especially in colder climates and by men with constitutional yang vacuity—can be beneficial by warming the anterior yin region. Excessive consumption of spicy-hot foods, however, can scorch and damage yin, and lead to the formation of evil heat in the interior. Over time and if severe, this heat can consume kidney yin-essence and lead to premature ejaculation from hyperactivity of yang.

In addition to eating a generally healthful diet, it is wise for men with premature ejaculation from kidney vacuity to periodically eat foods that are especially known to supplement kidney essence and enhance male sexual health. These include oysters, sea cucumber, abalone, shitake mushrooms, shrimp, scallops, walnuts, chestnuts, Chinese chives, venison, lamb, goat, and turtle. For men with kidney essence vacuity, bone marrow soup stock and oxtail soup is quite useful. For men with premature ejaculation from liver channel damp-heat, avoiding alcohol is of special importance. For those with heart-spleen dual vacuity, using a decoction of *Huang Qi* (Astragali Radix) (at a concentration of about 30g per 50g of rice) as the cooking solution for rice is an easy and effective way to build spleen qi.

Representative Chinese Research

An empirical formula to treat premature ejaculation

Liu (1990) reported on the use of an empirical formula called *Qing Chun Le Er Hao* (Youthful Vigor and Joy #2) to treat 159 cases of premature ejaculation. The ingredients are:

> *Dan Shen* (Salviae Miltiorrhizae Radix)
> *Wu Gong* (Scolopendra)
> *Hong Ren Shen* (Ginseng Radix Rubra)
> *Chi Shao* (Paeoniae Radix Rubra)
> *Yang Qi Shi* (Actinolitum)
> *Ye Jiao Teng* (Polygoni Multiflori Caulis)

Shi Hu (Dendrobii Herba)
Suo Yang (Cynomorii Herba)
Gan Cao (Glycyrrhizae Radix)

The formula was ground into powder and divided into 30 portions, one packet comprising 15 days dosage. Each subject in the study took between 2–4 packets of the formula (30–45 days dosage).

Results: One-hundred and forty cases were cured, (88.05%), 17 cases made some positive progress (10.69%), and 2 cases had no result (1.26%).

Modified *Huang Lian E Jiao Tang* (Coptis and Ass Hide Glue Decoction) for treating yang wilt and premature ejaculation

Ji (1994) used a variation of *Huang Lian E Jiao Tang* to treat 80 men with yang wilt and premature ejaculation. The base formula consisted of the following medicinals:
Huang Lian (Coptidis Rhizoma), 5g
Bai Shao (Paeoniae Radix Alba), 15g
Lian Zi (Nelumbinis Semen), 15g
Yuan Zhi (Polygalae Radix), 15g
Fu Ling (Poria), 15g
Huang Bai (Phellodendri Cortex), 10g
Sang Piao Xiao (Mantidis Ootheca), 10g
Wu Wei Zi (Schisandrae Fructus), 10g
Bai Zi Ren (Platycladi Semen), 10g
E Jiao (Asini Corii Colla), 10g, dissolved into the strained decoction
Ji Zi Huang (Galli Vitellus), 1 yolk, stirred into the strained decoction

Modifications: For men with hyperactivity and effulgence of heart fire, *Shan Zhi Zi* (Gardeniae Fructus) was added; for effulgent ministerial fire, *Long Dan Cao* (Gentianae Radix) was added. For kidney yang vacuity *Tu Si Zi* (Cuscutae Semen) and *Jiu Cai Zi* (Allii Tuberosi Folium) were added. For men with more prominent yang wilt, *Suo Yang* (Cynomorii Herba) and *Yin Yang Huo* (Epimedii Herba) were added. For men with prominent premature ejaculation, *Long Gu* (Mastodi Ossis Fossilia), *Mu Li* (Ostreae Concha), and *Qian Shi* (Euryales Semen) were added.

During the treatment course, all the subjects were asked to avoid eating spicy hot food, daikon radish, and mung beans, and to avoid any sexual activity. The treatment period ranged from 14–60 days.

Results: Thirty-six cases were cured, 40 cases had good results, and 4 cases had no results.

Long Dan Xie Xin Tang (Gentian Heart-Draining Decoction) for treating premature ejaculation

Xiao (1998) modified *Long Dan Xie Xin Tang* according to pattern discrimination to treat 60 cases of premature ejaculation. The formula consists of the following medicinals:

> *Long Dan Cao* (Gentianae Radix), 10g
> *Shan Zhi Zi* (Gardeniae Fructus), 10g
> *Huang Qin* (Scutellariae Radix), 10g
> *Huang Bai* (Phellodendri Cortex), 10g
> *Mu Dan Pi* (Moutan Cortex), 10g
> *Chi Shao* (Paeoniae Radix Rubra), 10g
> *Chuan Niu Xi* (Cyathulae Radix), 10g
> *Che Qian Zi* (Plantaginis Semen), 10g
> *Chai Hu* (Bupleuri Radix), 8g
> *Sheng Di Huang* (Rehmanniae Radix Exsiccata seu Recens), 15g
> *Gan Cao* (Glycyrrhizae Radix), 6g

Modifications: For concurrent urinary tract infection, *Mu Dan Pi* and *Chi Shao* were reduced, and *Bai Jiang Cao* (Patriniae Herba) and *Bai Hua She She Cao* (Oldenlandiae Diffusae Herba) were added. For anxiety, fear, and flusteredness, *Mu Dan Pi* and *Chi Shao* were removed, and *Suan Zao Ren* (Ziziphi Spinosi Semen) and *Long Chi* (Mastodi Dentis Fossilia) were added. For reduced libido, *Sheng Di Huang, Mu Dan Pi,* and *Chi Shao* were reduced, and *Yin Yang Huo* (Epimedii Herba), *Tu Si Zi* (Cuscutae Semen), and *Bu Gu Zhi* (Psoraleae Fructus) were added. For hyperactive libido, *Huang Bai* (Phellodendri Cortex) and *Niu Xi* (Achyranthis Bidentatae Radix) were added.

Results: In this study, 5 days comprised one treatment course and most patients completed from 1–3 treatment courses. Twenty-three cases were cured, 30 cases had good results, and 6 cases had no results.

Modified *Zhen Gan Xi Feng Tang* (Liver-Settling Wind-Extinguishing Decoction) for premature ejaculation

Zhang, Song, and Gao (2003) used a modification of *Zhen Gan Xi Feng Tang* to treat 45 cases of premature ejaculation. The ingredients of the base formula were as follows:

> *Huai Niu Xi* (Achyranthis Bidentatae Radix), 30g
> *Dai Zhe Shi* (Haematitum), 30g
> *Long Gu* (Mastodi Ossis Fossilia), 30g
> *Mu Li* (Ostreae Concha), 30g
> *Tian Men Dong* (Asparagi Radix), 9g
> *Zhi Gui Ban* (Testudinis Carapax et Plastrum cum Liquido Fricti), 15g
> *Xuan Shen* (Scrophulariae Radix), 15g
> *Wu Wei Zi* (Schisandrae Fructus), 9g
> *Wu Gong* (Scolopendra), 3 pieces
> *Gan Cao* (Glycyrrhizae Radix), 9g

Modifications: If accompanied by liver channel damp-heat, *Long Dan Cao* (Gentianae Radix) and *Ze Xie* (Alismatis Rhizoma) were added. For patients with yin vacuity and effulgent fire, *Zhi Mu* (Anemarrhenae Rhizoma) and

Huang Bai (Phellodendri Cortex) were added. For insecurity of kidney qi, *Shan Yao* (Dioscoreae Rhizoma), *Shan Zhu Yu* (Corni Fructus), and *Shu Di Huang* (Rehmanniae Radix Praeparata) were added.

Results: One month comprised one treatment course. Twenty-six cases were cured (were able to maintain intravaginal erection without ejaculation for at least two minutes), 15 cases had some effect (able to maintain intravaginal erection without ejaculation for at least 0.5 minutes, and 4 cases had no effect at all. The overall amelioration rate was 91.1%.

Using Modified *Gu Jing Zhi Xie Tang* (Essence-Securing Emission-Ending Decoction) to treat premature ejaculation

Wang (1996) used a modification, varied according to pattern, of *Gu Jing Zhi Xie Tang* to treat 56 cases of premature ejaculation. The ingredients of the formula were:

Cao Jue Ming (Cassiae Semen), 12g
Lian Xu (Nelumbinis Stamen), 15g
Shu Di Huang (Rehmanniae Radix Praeparata), 15g
Yu Biao (Piscis Vesica Aeris Colla),[8] 9g, mixed with the strained decoction
Chao Huang Bai (Phellodendri Cortex Frictus), 10g
Zhi Mu (Anemarrhenae Rhizoma), 10g
Tian Men Dong (Asparagi Radix), 10g
Sha Ren (Amomi Fructus), 10g
Long Gu (Mastodi Ossis Fossilia), 30g
Mu Li (Ostreae Concha), 30g
Gan Cao (Glycyrrhizae Radix), 6g

Modifications: For men with liver channel damp-heat, *Long Dan Cao* (Gentianae Radix), *Che Qian Zi* (Plantaginis Semen), and *Ku Shen* (Sophorae Flavescentis Radix) were added. For heart yin vacuity and effulgent fire, *Chao Suan Zao Ren* (Ziziphi Spinosi Semen Frictus), *Zhi Yuan Zhi* (Polygalae Radix cum Liquido Fricta), *Huang Lian* (Coptidis Rhizoma), and *Rou Gui* (Cinnamomi Cortex) were added. For heart-spleen dual vacuity, *Huang Bai* and *Zhi Mu* were removed, and *Huang Qi* (Astragali Radix), *Bai Zhu* (Atractylodis Macrocephalae Rhizoma), and *Shan Yao* (Dioscoreae Rhizoma) were added. For insecurity of kidney qi, *Huang Bai* and *Zhi Mu* were removed, and *Shu Fu Zi* (Aconiti Radix Lateralis Conquita), *Rou Gui* (Cinnamomi Cortex), *Jin Ying Zi* (Rosae Laevigatae Fructus), and *Sang Piao Xiao* (Mantidis Ootheca) were added.

Results: Of the 56 cases treated, 41 experienced definite results (defined by an intravaginal latency period of over 2 minutes on more than 60% of their

---

[8] The function of *Yu Biao Jiao* in this formula is to supplement the kidney and enrich essence. It specifically treats seminal emission and premature ejaculation.

attempts at intercourse), 11 cases had good results (defined by an intravaginal latency period of more than one minute on 40–60% of their attempts at intercourse, and 4 cases had no results (mainly defined as having no improvement in their intravaginal ejaculatory latency time).

External treatment

Xiao (1988) used a steam wash with *Wu Bei Zi* (Galla Chinensis) to treat 5 cases of premature ejaculation. Twenty grams of *Wu Bei Zi* was decocted and used as a steam wash for the penis for several minutes and then the penis was submerged in the warm decoction for 5–10 minutes every night for 15–20 days, which comprised one treatment course.

Results: Generally speaking, the subjects completed 1–2 treatment courses. All subjects were advised to avoid sexual intercourse during treatment. Of the 5 subjects, 2 only used this treatment for their premature ejaculation. The remaining 3 subjects also had either seminal emission or yang wilt and hence also took an internally-administered (unspecified) pattern-based herbal prescription along with the external formula. All 5 cases had satisfying results.

Sheng Jing Ling Yao Jiu (Essence-Engendering Efficacious Medicinal Wine) for premature ejaculation

Zhang *et al.* (1996) reported on the clinical efficacy of treating premature ejaculation and yang wilt using a medicinal wine made with the following ingredients:

Hong Ren Shen (Ginseng Radix Rubra), 15g
Lu Rong (Cervi Cornu Pantotrichum), 15g
Jiu Cai Zi (Allii Tuberosi Folium), 25g
Ge Jie (Gecko), 1 pair
Yin Yang Huo (Epimedii Herba), 25g
Ba Ji Tian (Morindae Officinalis Radix), 25g
Sheng Huang Qi (Astragali seu Hedysari Radix Cruda), 50g
Rou Gui (Cinnamomi Cortex), 10g
Bai Jiu (Granorum Spiritus Incolor), 400 ml[9] of 60% alcohol

Preparation method: The medicinals were soaked in the alcohol for an unspecified period of time (though usually a few weeks to a few months is adequate), and then the subjects took 10–20 ml two to three times per day until finished (about 20–40 days).

Results: Of the 725 cases treated, the authors claimed that a cure was obtained in 680 cases, that good results were obtained in 25 cases, and that no effect was obtained in 20 cases.

---

[9] Vodka may be used in place of Chinese *Bai Jiu*.

Acumoxa therapy

Zhang *et al.* (1985) treated 212 cases of premature ejaculation with acumoxa therapy. The following points were needled: *Qu Gu* (CV-2), *Ci Liao* (BL-32), *Yin Lian* (LV-11), *Zu San Li* (ST-36), and *Nei Guan* (PC-6). Further, moxa was applied to the following points: *Da Dun* (LV-1), *Shen Que* (CV-8).

Results: Among the 212 cases treated, 61 cases were cured, 14 cases had obvious effects, and 8 cases had some improvement. The overall amelioration rate was 86.32%.

Representative Case Studies

Dual vacuity of yin and yang

Chen and Jiang (2000) reported on a case of premature ejaculation in a 32 year-old male successfully treated by the famous modern Chinese doctor Shi Jin-Mo. The patient had been married at a young age and shortly thereafter had started to feel generalized weakness and generalized body soreness, poor memory, and seminal emission and premature ejaculation. The tongue fur was thin white and his pulse was fine and weak. Dr. Shi's diagnosis was dual vacuity of yin and yang and the treatment principle was to supplement yang and benefit yin. He prescribed 10 packets of the following prescription:

    Xu Duan (Dipsaci Radix), 10g
    Shu Di Huang (Rehmanniae Radix Praeparata), 10g
    Du Zhong (Eucommiae Cortex), 10g
    Lu Jiao Jiao (Cervi Cornus Gelatinum), 10g, dissolved into the strained
        decoction
    Zi He Che (Hominis Placenta), 10g
    Sha Ren (Amomi Fructus), 5g
    Yi Zhi Ren (Alpiniae Oxyphyllae Fructus), 5g
    Bu Gu Zhi (Psoraleae Fructus), 10g
    Shan Zhu Yu (Corni Fructus), 10g
    Gou Ji (Cibotii Rhizoma), 15g
    Gou Qi Zi (Lycii Fructus), 15g
    Chao Shan Yao (Dioscoreae Rhizoma Frictus), 25g
    Zhi Gan Cao (Glycyrrhizae Radix cum Liquido Fricta), 5g
    Wu Bei Zi (Galla Chinensis), 5g
    Wu Wei Zi (Schisandrae Fructus), 5g

During the course of treatment with this formula, he had no seminal emission or premature ejaculation, and his body felt stronger. Dr. Shi prescribed another 10 packets of the prescription, but added the following medicinals:

    Yan Huang Bai (Phellodendri Cortex Salsa), 6g
    Long Gu (Mastodi Ossis Fossilia), 10g
    Mu Li (Ostreae Concha), 10g

After taking these ten packets, the patient returned for another visit and reported continued good results. In all, he had not had any seminal emission since beginning treatment 20 days ago, and also reported good results with the premature ejaculation. As a means of consolidating and continuing treatment, Dr. Shi prescribed the following medicinals, which he ground into powder and made into pills with honey:

Zi He Che (Hominis Placenta), 30g

Lu Jiao Jiao (Cervi Cornus Gelatinum), 30g

Shan Zhu Yu (Corni Fructus), 30g

Fu Pen Zi (Rubi Fructus), 30g

Bu Gu Zhi (Psoraleae Fructus), 30g

Chao Gou Qi Zi (Lycii Fructus Fricta), 15g

Yi Zhi Ren (Alpiniae Oxyphyllae Fructus), 15g

Sha Ren (Amomi Fructus), 15g

Gou Ji (Cibotii Rhizoma), 60g

Du Zhong (Eucommiae Cortex), 30g

Wu Wei Zi (Schisandrae Fructus), 15g

Wu Bei Zi (Galla Chinensis), 15g

Ju Hua (Chrysanthemi Flos), 60g

Gui Zhi (Cinnamomi Ramulus), 30g

Zi Su Ye (Perillae Folium), 30g

Sang Piao Xiao (Mantidis Ootheca), 30g

She Chuang Zi (Cnidii Fructus), 15g

Shu Di Huang (Rehmanniae Radix Praeparata), 30g

Chao Yuan Zhi (Polygalae Radix Fricta), 30g

Shi Chang Pu (Acori Tatarinowii Rhizoma), 15g

Hu Tao Rou (Juglandis Semen), 60g

Sang Shen Zi (Mori Fructus), 30g

The method of preparation for the formula was to grind all the medicinals into a fine powder, combine with 180g of *Jin Ying Zi* (Rosae Laevigatae Fructus) paste[10] and 300g of honey, and form into pills. One pill was prescribed to be taken each morning with boiled water.

In his commentary on the case, Dr. Shi pointed out that in cases of dual vacuity of yin and yang, it is important to strike a balance between yang-warming and yin-enriching medicinals. Further, he described his use of medicinals with an affinity to flesh and blood in order to enrich essence and replenish marrow.

Gallbladder damp-heat

Long (1998) reported a case of liver-gallbladder damp-heat premature ejaculation in a 32 year-old male treated by Zhang Shou-Rui. The patient had reported premature ejaculation for two months after returning home from a business trip abroad. A doctor at a local clinic had prescribed him an unspecified kidney-supplementing formula, which he took for over a month with no improvement in his condition. The patient reported that when he felt a desire for sex, he readily developed an erection, but ejaculated very quickly after intromission. Further, he reported bitter fullness of the chest and rib-side, heart

---

[10] *Jin Ying Zi* paste is created by boiling it in water and reducing the solution until it thickens.

vexation and irascibility, and a tendency to sigh. His tongue was red with a
yellow slimy fur. He also had a long history of overindulgence in alcohol.

The diagnosis was liver-gallbladder damp-heat and the treatment principle was
to clear the liver and gallbladder and to disinhibit dampness and heat. The
prescription was based on *Long Dan Xie Gan Tang* (Gentian Liver-Draining
Decoction) and contained the following medicinals:
>   *Long Dan Cao* (Gentianae Radix), 12g
>   *Huang Qin* (Scutellariae Radix), 12g
>   *Shan Zhi Zi* (Gardenia Fructus), 9g
>   *Mu Tong* (Akebiae Trifoliatae Caulis), 9g
>   *Ze Xie* (Alsimatis Rhizoma), 12g
>   *Chai Hu* (Bupleuri Radix), 12g
>   *Sheng Di Huang* (Rehmanniae Radix Exsiccata seu Recens), 9g
>   *Che Qian Zi* (Plantaginis Semen), 12g
>   *Sheng Gan Cao* (Glycyrrhizae Radix Cruda), 9g
>   *Hua Shi* (Talcum), 15g

After taking 7 packets of the prescription, the patient had reduced libido and
other overall improvements. Dr. Zhang prescribed another 7 packets of the
same formula and also prescribed the following medicinals for external use as
a steam wash on the penis before having intercourse:
>   *Wu Bei Zi* (Galla Chinensis), 30g
>   *Di Gu Pi* (Lycii Cortex), 30g
>   *She Chuang Zi* (Cnidii Fructus), 30g
>   *Xi Xin* (Asari Herba), 30g
>   *Fang Feng* (Saposhnikoviae Radix), 30g
>   *Hua Jiao* (Zanthoxyli Pericarpium), 30g

After taking the formula and using the external steam wash for one week, the
patient returned reporting that he was able to have intercourse for a much
longer time before ejaculating. However, he also said that the firmness of his
erections had decreased. Dr. Zhang then discontinued the original prescription
and instead had the patient take 6 grams, three times per day of *Jin Suo Gu Jing
Wan* (Golden Lock Essence-Securing Pill) for one month. At the next visit one
month later, the patient stated that his sexual life had completely normalized.

Kidney yang vacuity and detriment and damage to kidney essence

Xie (1982) reports a case of premature ejaculation in a 34 year-old male who
also had infertility and yang wilt. He had been married for 10 years and was
still childless, had yang wilt and premature ejaculation, soreness and pain of
the lumbus, and exhaustion of essence-spirit. His tongue was pale tender and
enlarged with tooth marks, and his pulse was vacuous and lacked strength, especially in the cubit (*chi*) position.

The diagnosis was kidney yang vacuity and detriment and damage of kidney
essence. Dr. Xie prescribed a modification of *Jiu Zi Wan* (Chinese Leek Seed

Pill) and *Wu Zi Yan Zong Wan* (Five-Seed Progeny Pill). The ingredients were as follows:

Gou Shen (Dog Kidney), 1 kidney[11]
Jiu Cai Zi (Allii Tuberosi Semen), 15g
She Chuang Zi (Cnidii Fructus), 10g
Wu Wei Zi (Schisandrae Fructus), 10g
Tu Si Zi (Cuscutae Semen), 30g
Bu Gu Zhi (Psoraleae Fructus), 12g
Sang Piao Xiao (Mantidis Ootheca), 30g
Fu Pen Zi (Rubi Fructus), 15g
Shan Yao (Dioscoreae Rhizoma), 15g
Che Qian Zi (Plantaginis Semen), 9g
Yan Zhi Mu (Anemarrhenae Rhizoma Salsa), 9g
Yan Huang Bai (Phellodendri Cortex Salsa), 9g
Dang Gui (Angelicae Sinensis Radix), 12g

After taking over 60 packets of this prescription, the patient reported complete resolution of the yang wilt and premature ejaculation. Further, his essence-spirit had improved, and his pulse was stronger. Dr. Xie then added *Shu Di Huang* (Rehmanniae Radix Praeparata), *Bai Shao* (Paeoniae Radix Alba), and *Shan Zhu Yu* (Corni Fructus)—to strengthen the yin-nourishing and essence-enriching action of the formula—and prescribed another 20 packets. After 20 packets of this formula, he removed *Zhi Mu*, and added *Qiang Huo* (No-topterygii Rhizoma et Radix), *Yi Mu Cao* (Leonuri Herba), *Mu Dan Pi* (Moutan Cortex), and *Chuan Xiong* (Chuanxiong Rhizoma), and prescribed another 30 packets.

In all, this patient took 110 packets of Dr. Xie's prescriptions and experienced complete resolution of both yang wilt and premature ejaculation. As an aside, his semen analysis also showed marked improvement in that the percentage of motile sperm increased from 10–20% at the initiation of treatment to 80–90% at discharge, and this resulted in him fathering a son with his wife. In his commentary on the case, Dr. Xie stressed the importance of using channel-freeing, blood-quickening medicinals (especially *Qiang Huo*) along with supplementing medicinals when treating dual vacuity of yin and yang. In this way, treatment facilitates the mutual engendering of yin and yang.

Yin vacuity with hyperactive yang

Shi (1992), reports a case of yin vacuity with hyperactive yang type premature ejaculation in a 37 year-old man that was successfully treated by Chen Pei-Jia. The patient had been married since he was 28 years old and had been quite healthy. However, about seven months prior to the initial visit, he underwent surgery for kidney stones, and ever since then had suffered from seminal emission, premature ejaculation, and reduced libido. Additional symptoms included weight loss, vertigo, palpitations, low-level heat effusion and tidal

---

[11] Lamb kidneys can be used as a substitute.

redness, night sweats, dry throat, copious dreaming, seminal emission 3–4 times per week, bound stool and reddish urine. The tongue was red, dry, and peeled bare of fur, and the pulse was fine rapid.

The diagnosis was yin vacuity with hyperactive yang and the treatment principle was to enrich yin and drain fire. Dr. Chen prescribed 7 packets of the following formula:

Huang Qin (Scutellariae Radix), 3g
Tian Men Dong (Asparagi Radix), 9g
Di Gu Pi (Lycii Cortex), 9g
Sheng Di Huang (Rehmanniae Radix Exsiccata seu Recens), 15g
Shan Zhi Zi (Gardeniae Fructus), 9g
Chi Shao (Paeoniae Radix Rubra), 9g
Chi Fu Ling (Poria Rubra), 9g
Lian Zi (Nelumbinis Fructus), 20g
Wu Wei Zi (Schisandrae Fructus), 9g
Mu Tong (Akebiae Trifoliatae Caulis), 3g
Huang Bai (Phellodendri Cortex), 3g
Xian Zhu Ye (Lophatheri Folium Recens), 15 pieces

At the second visit, after taking 7 packets of the formula, the patient reported fewer incidents of seminal emission, and only one incident of dream emission. His tongue was red and his pulse was fine rapid. Dr. Chen continued with the method of enriching yin and supplementing the kidneys by prescribing 20 packets of the following formula:

Huang Bai (Phellodendri Cortex), 6g
Zhi Mu (Anemarrhenae Rhizoma), 9g
Sheng Di Huang (Rehmanniae Radix Exsiccata seu Recens), 12g
Shu Di Huang (Rehmanniae Radix Praeparata), 12g
Gui Ban (Testudinis Carapax et Plastrum), 12g
Bie Jia (Trionycis Carapax), 12g
Nu Zhen Zi (Ligustri Lucidi Fructus), 15g
Chi Shao (Paeoniae Radix Rubra), 10g
Shan Yao (Dioscoreae Rhizoma), 18g
Mu Dan Pi (Moutan Cortex), 9g
Lian Zi (Nelumbinis Semen), 15g
Yu Zhu (Polygonati Odorati Rhizoma), 15g
Rou Gui (Cinnamomi Cortex), 3g

At follow-up one year later, the patient stated that the seminal emission and premature ejaculation was completely resolved and had not returned. Further, he felt that he had recovered his general health.

Priapism

Western Medicine

Priapism[1] is characterized by persistent, abnormal, and painful erections without detumescence and is often unrelated to any sexual excitation or activity. It occurs not only in adult men but in young boys as well. Priapism can be distinguished from a normal erection in that the priapic erection lasts for much longer than usual, is painful, and the glans penis is not tumescent. Although the exact pathological mechanisms of priapism are not clearly understood, it often occurs in association with diseases such as sickle cell anemia, chronic granulocytic anemia, and spinal cord injury. However, nowadays it occurs most frequently as a side effect of (ED) treatments including oral PDE-5 inhibitors (such as sildenafil) and intraurethral alprostadil injection therapy. If left untreated for four or more hours, priapism can lead to fibrotic deposition in the corpus cavernosum which results in subsequent ED. In serious cases, penile necrosis and gangrene results; hence, true priapism is a urological emergency.

The dominant theory about the etiology of priapism involves complex vascular and neurologic mechanisms and according to Fauci *et al.* (1998), includes blood clots within the sinusoidal spaces of the corpora and abnormal adrenergic-mediated mechanisms for detumescence. Further, as is the case with researchers of ED, the role of nitric oxide in penile tumescence and detumescence is increasingly attracting the attention of priapism researchers (Burnett, 2006).

Diagnosis

According to Pryor *et al.* (2004), priapism should be differentiated into three types—ischemic (low-flow), nonischemic (high-flow), and recurrent (stuttering).

---

[1] Priapism is named for Priapus—the Greek god of fertility, horticulture, and viticulture. In Greco-Roman artwork, he is always depicted with a huge and perpetually erect penis.

• Ischemic (low-flow; venoocclusive) priapism

The most common cause of priapism is ischemic priapism, which is characterized by decrease or absence of penile blood flow. In these cases, the blood within the corpus cavernosa takes on a highly viscous quality and dark color that is sometimes likened to motor oil. Severe pain occurs, especially when ischemia has persisted for four or more hours. According to Beers *et al.* (2006), whereas in the past most cases were caused by pelvic vascular thrombosis, the most common cause in current clinical practice is ED therapy (including both oral PDE-5 inhibitors and intraurethral alprostadil injection). Other medications that sometimes cause ischemic priapism include cocaine, amphetamines, antihypertensive agents, anticoagulants, corticosteroids, antipsychotics, and rarely alpha-blockers that are prescribed for lower urinary tract symptoms associated with benign prostatic hyperplasia (BPH).[2] Finally, some cases of ischemic priapism are caused by pelvic tumors, prostatitis, cystitis, and urethritis. ED ensues in 90% of men in whom ischemic priapism has persisted for longer than 24 hours (Pryor *et al.*, 2004). The mechanism of causation for ED in such cases is the formation of fibrotic tissue (or possibly even necrosis or gangrene in severe cases) within the corpus cavernosum which interferes with penile tumescence.

• Nonischemic (high-flow) priapism

Some cases of priapism are nonischemic and occur in patients who have suffered penile trauma with significant vascular damage that results in a loss of regulation of arterial blood flow. This clinical type of priapism is not painful and does not usually lead to necrosis. However, nonischemic priapism is still a serious condition and is also often followed by ED (Beers *et al.*, 2006).

• Recurrent (stuttering) priapism

This type of priapism is characterized by repeated priapic events. The pathological mechanism may be either central (neurogenic) or local (as in sickle cell disease).

Treatment

The treatment of priapism depends on identifying which type of the disease the patient has and how long the condition has persisted. According to Beers *et al.* (2006), however, treatment is often unsuccessful, even when the cause has been identified.

Generally, treatment is initiated with ice packs applied directly to the penis, and the patient is advised to walk up stairs in an attempt to induce an "arterial steal" that could lead to detumescence. For patients with ischemic priapism, physicians additionally try a number of different medications to induce detumescence, but ultimately if these medications fail or if the condition persists for more than four hours, they must resort to inserting a large-bore needle

[2] See Sadeghi-Negad, H. and Jackson, I. (2007).

(12–16 gauge) directly into the corpora with the goal of draining the venous blood that has accumulated within the corpora. This is usually followed by irrigation to remove any possible clots that have formed.

More invasive surgical techniques are sometimes necessary including the creation of a fistula between the glans penis and the corpora cavernosa, saphenous vein shunt, or corpora or cavernosa-spongiosum shunt. The large-bore needle method is sometimes associated with complications including penile hematoma, penile infection and abscess, urethral stricture, and penile gangrene. Shunts are often associated with either temporary or permanent ED. For nonischemic priapism, the underlying cause must be determined. For sickle cell disease, transfusion may be necessary; for leukemia, chemotherapy may be required. Neurogenic causes are sometimes treated by continuous spinal or caudal anaesthesia (Beers *et al.*, 2006).

Western Complementary Medicine

Bansal, Godara, and Garg (2004) report that an ice-cold saline enema (after sedation) represents a useful low-cost treatment for initial and conservative management of priapism in underprivileged patients.

Chinese Medicine

Disease discrimination

There are three main Chinese andrological disease categories that are the closest correlates with priapism. They are rigid yang (*yang jiang* or *qiang yang*), rigid center (*qiang zhong*) and yin protraction (*yin zong*). These three disease categories are used synonymously in the Chinese literature and are characterized by persistent erection with either inability to ejaculate or with spontaneous seminal efflux. For purposes of simplicity and clarity, I will use the term rigid yang by default, unless a specific source I am translating from does otherwise.

In *Zhu Bing Yuan Hou Lun* (*On the Origin and Indicators of Disease*)[3]—one of the earliest texts to mention rigid center—we find the following quote: "[In] those with rigid center, the penis is elongated, raised, exuberant, and does not wilt, [and] semen is spontaneously discharged." In *Zheng Zhi Hui Bu* (*Supplemental Essays on Patterns and Treatments*),[4] it was reported that this condition can occur in men who ingest medicines made from gold and precious stones (called "*dan yao*" [elixir medicines]) as well as in men who consume excessive amounts of yang-supplementing medicinals. In both cases, ministerial fire becomes hyperactive and yin is debilitated; as a result, ministerial fire cannot be controlled and rigid yang results.

---

[3] *Zhu Bing Yuan Hou Lun* was written by Chao Yuan-Fang in 610 CE, during the Sui dynasty.
[4] *Zheng Zhi Hui Bu* was written by Li Yong-Cui in 1687, during the Qing dynasty.

It is important to note that the correlation between priapism and rigid yang, yin protraction, and rigid center is not exact. These disease categories are also used by Chinese andrologists to treat conditions such as hyperactive libido and sexual addiction. In such cases, the main pathological issue from a Chinese andrology perspective is that the penis is either erect to an uncomfortable degree, or too often, or at unusual times. At times, there is also hyperactive libido, seminal emission, and inability to ejaculate. Although the correlation between priapism and rigid yang is not exact, there are no other Chinese andrology disease categories that provide a better match with priapism. Hence, the disease causes, pathomechanisms, pattern discrimination, and treatments for rigid yang provide the best Chinese medical foundation for understanding and treating patients with the Western disease of priapism. Further, given the emergent nature of true priapismand the risk it carries for future morbidity, it should be managed carefully and usually together with Western urologists or emergency room physicians.

Disease causes and pathomechanisms

The disease causes and pathomechanisms for rigid yang are generally divided into repletion and vacuity. The primary vacuity cause is kidney yin-essence vacuity with hyperactivity of yang. Repletion causes include damp-heat pouring downward into the liver channel, traumatic injury, and static blood obstructing the anterior yin region. The main viscera involved in rigid yang are the kidneys, the liver, and the heart.

• Kidney essence debility and yin vacuity with hyperactivity of yang
Either due to insufficient natural endowment or constitutional vacuity of yin-essence, hyperactive libido and sexual intemperance, or excessive intake of yang-supplementing medicinals, ministerial fire within the kidneys is overstimulated and kidney yin-essence is debilitated. Because the liver is also ascribed to ministerial fire, when kidney yin-essence is depleted, and kidney ministerial fire moves frenetically, liver ministerial fire also stirs excessively. Since the ancestral sinew is closely linked with the liver, it becomes overly stimulated by yang qi, and rigid yang results.

• Affect-mind internal damage
When there is enduring anger, indignation, hatred, and unfulfilled desires, over time liver depression transforms fire. Likewise, when there is an isolated episode of fulminant anger, liver depression acutely transforms fire. In either case, depressed liver fire flames downward and harasses the anterior yin region, including the penis. Further, depressed liver fire transmits into the liver channel. Since the liver channel encircles the genitals, depressed liver channel fire harasses the ancestral sinew, overstimulates it and leads to rigid yang.

The kidney and the heart are intimately connected. They are physiologically related in several ways, including the fact that heart fire (sovereign fire) warms the kidney fire (ministerial fire). This important physiological connection plays out pathologically in rigid yang when sexual desire causes the sovereign fire to stir and ministerial fire stirs in turn. Ministerial fire then also conducts into the liver channel and the ancestral sinew and rigid yang results.

• Damp-heat pouring downward

Owing to dietary irregularities including excessive consumption of alcohol, greasy-fried and spicy-hot foods, and sweets and dairy products, damp-heat collects in the center burner. As dampness is a yin evil, it tends to pour downward along the course of the reverting yin liver channel and to collect in the anterior yin region. If it obstructs the free flow of qi and blood within the penis, rigid yang may result.

• Vanquished essence obstructing the orifice, static blood obstructing within the ancestral sinew

When there is sexual intemperance and ejaculation is withheld, there is stoppage and stagnation of vanquished essence. Or, if excessive masturbation leads to constant thoughts of sex, ministerial fire becomes hyperactive and scorches essence. As a result, essence is vanquished and then rots within the essence chamber and in the ancestral sinew and obstructs blood. Static blood in turn blocks the channels and network vessels within the ancestral sinew and causes rigid yang.

• Traumatic injury and static blood obstructing within the ancestral sinew

Either because of enduring erection or to traumatic injury to the anterior yin region, static blood can obstruct the channels and network vessels within the penis. If the blockage is severe enough, rigid yang results.

• Mutual binding of phlegm and blood stasis

Enduring kidney yang vacuity and debility of ministerial fire results in a lack of warmth and power for the anterior yin region. When there is lack of yang qi transformation, yin-fluid collects and blood congeals because without warmth, it cannot move. As a result, phlegm and blood stasis form and mutually bind in the anterior yin region. When they specifically collect in the ancestral sinew, rigid yang is the result.

Pattern discrimination

1.Yin vacuity with hyperactive yang

Signs: An erection that will not become soft, a swollen and painful penis, may occur after excessive sexual intercourse or along with seminal efflux, testicular distention, swelling, and pain, a history of spontaneous erections, easily getting an erection and premature ejaculation, tidal heat effusion and night sweats, dizzy head and eyes, heart vexation and insomnia, fatigued spirit and lack of strength, dry mouth and throat, red cheeks, soreness and limpness of the lumbus and knees, difficult micturition and short scanty urine, small red tender tongue with scanty fur, stringlike fine rapid pulse.

Treatment principles: Enrich yin and drain fire, quicken the blood and soften hardness

Guiding formula: Modified *Zhi Bai Di Huang Wan* (Anemarrhena, Phellodendron, and Rehmannia Pill)

Ingredients:
Yan Zhi Mu (Anemarrhenae Rhizoma Salsa), 10g
Yan Huang Bai (Phellodendri Cortex Salsa), 10g
Sheng Di Huang (Rehmanniae Radix Exsiccata seu Recens), 15g
Shan Zhu Yu (Corni Fructus), 10g
Shan Yao (Dioscoreae Rhizoma), 12g
Fu Ling (Poria), 12g
Ze Xie (Alismatis Rhizoma), 25g
Mu Dan Pi (Moutan Cortex), 12g
Chi Shao (Paeoniae Radix Rubra), 20g
Ze Lan (Lycopi Herba), 10g
Dang Gui (Angelicae Sinensis Radix), 10g
Niu Xi (Achyranthis Bidentatae Radix), 15g
Gui Ban (Testudinis Carapax et Plastrum), 15g
Bie Jia (Trionycis Carapax), 30g

Modifications: For patients with additional signs of qi and yin vacuity including a nonluxuriant facial complexion, more prominent fatigue and lack of strength, and more prominent dry mouth and throat, add *Tai Zi Shen* (Pseudostellariae Radix), 15g, *Xi Yang Shen* (Panacis Quinquefolii Radix), 15g, *Huang Qi* (Astragali Radix), 15g, *Mai Men Dong* (Ophiopogonis Radix), 10g, and *Wu Wei Zi* (Schisandrae Fructus), 10g, to boost qi and nourish yin.

2. Binding depression of liver qi with depressed heat

Signs: An erection that will not become soft, swelling and distention of the penis, a somber-colored penis, irascibility, a history of repressed anger, resentment, hatred, and indignation, fullness, distention, and pain of the rib-side, bitter oral taste and dry mouth, bound hard stool, reddish urine, a red tongue with redder sides or red spots on the sides, yellow tongue fur, stringlike rapid forceful pulse.

Treatment principles: Course the liver and rectify the qi, clear heat and resolve depression

Guiding formula: Modified *Chai Hu Qing Gan Tang* (Bupleurum Liver-Clearing Decoction)

Ingredients:
Chai Hu (Bupleuri Radix), 12g
Qing Pi (Citri Reticulatae Pericarpium Viride), 10g
Chuan Lian Zi (Toosendan Fructus), 10g

Huang Qin (Scutellariae Radix), 15g
Shan Zhi Zi (Gardeniae Fructus), 12g
Lian Qiao (Forsythiae Fructus), 12g
Shi Gao (Gypsum Fibrosum), 15g
Zhi Mu (Anemarrhenae Rhizoma), 12g
Sheng Gan Cao (Glycyrrhizae Radix Cruda), 6g

Modifications: For heart vexation, insomnia, and tongue sores, add *Lian Zi Xin* (Nelumbinis Plumula), 6g, *Huang Lian* (Coptidis Rhizoma), 6g, *Suan Zao Ren* (Ziziphi Spinosi Semen), 20g, and *Long Chi* (Mastodi Dentis Fossilia), 15g, to clear the heart and to anchor, settle and calm the spirit. For enduring anger and resentment, add *Mei Gui Hua* (Rosae Rugosae Flos), 10g, *Su Xin Hua* (Jasmini Officinalis Flos), 10g, and *Fo Shou* (Citri Sacrodactylis Fructus), 10g, to strengthen the liver-coursing and depression-resolving action of the formula.

3. Damp-heat pouring downward into the liver channel

Signs: An erection that will not become soft, a swollen, hot, and painful penis, a somber-colored penis, genital sweating and malodor, heavy cumbersome limbs, dizzy head accompanied by a distending sensation, soreness and distention of the abdomen and lumbus, bitter oral taste, dry mouth with no desire to drink, short reddish urine or yellow turbid urine, inhibited urination, bound stool or loose stools with ungratifying defecation, red tongue with yellow or slimy yellow fur, stringlike rapid or stringlike slippery pulse.

Treatment principles: Clear and drain damp-heat from the liver and gallbladder, cool the blood, and transform stasis and free the network vessels

Guiding formula: Modified *Long Dan Xie Gan Tang* (Gentian Liver-Draining Decoction)

Ingredients:
Long Dan Cao (Gentianae Radix), 15g
Shan Zhi Zi (Gardeniae Fructus), 10g
Huang Qin (Scutellariae Radix), 10g
Che Qian Zi (Plantaginis Semen), 30g
Ze Xie (Alismatis Rhizoma), 20g
Mu Tong (Akebiae Trifoliatae Caulis), 10g
Chi Shao (Paeoniae Radix Rubra), 15g
Dang Gui (Angelicae Sinensis Radix), 10g
Chuan Xiong (Chuanxiong Rhizoma), 10g
Sheng Di Huang (Rehmanniae Radix Exsiccata seu Recens), 12g
Mu Dan Pi (Moutan Cortex), 10g
Tao Ren (Persicae Semen), 15g
Sheng Gan Cao (Glycyrrhizae Radix Cruda), 6g

Modifications: For cases with inhibited urination and turbid urine, add *Shi Chang Pu* (Acori Tatarinowii Rhizoma), 15g, *Bi Xie* (Dioscoreae Hypoglaucae seu Semptemlobae Rhizoma), 12g, and *Yu Jin* (Curcumae Radix), 10g, to eliminate dampness, sweep away phlegm, and free the network vessels. For more prominent swelling and distention of the penis, add *Ru Xiang* (Olibanum), 6g, *Mo Yao* (Myrrha), 6g, *Niu Xi* (Achyranthis Bidentatae Radix), 15g, and *Wang Bu Liu Xing Zi* (Vaccariae Semen), 12g, to quicken blood, soften hardness, and free the network vessels. For dry bound stool, add *Da Huang* (Rhei Radix et Rhizoma), 10g, add at end, and *Lu Hui* (Aloe), 10g, to clear heat, cool the blood, and free the stools. For loose stools with ungratifying defecation, add *Da Huang* (Rhei Radix et Rhizoma), 10g, add at end, *Zhi Shi* (Aurantii Fructus Immaturis), 10g, and *Mu Xiang* (Aucklandiae Radix), 6g, to clear heat and dry dampness, and to free the intestinal qi dynamic.

4. Static blood obstructing the network vessels

Signs: A very firm erection that will not recede, a somber-colored penis that may have stasis macules, stabbing pain in the penis that is difficult to bear, pulling pain and urgency in the lesser abdomen, difficult and painful voidings of urine, vexation and agitation, purple tongue with stasis macules or points, sinking rough pulse.

Treatment principles: Transform stasis and free the network vessels, disperse swelling and relieve pain

Guiding formula: Modified *Tao Hong Si Wu Tang* (Peach Kernel and Carthamus Four Agents Decoction)

Ingredients:
    Tao Ren (Persicae Semen), 15g
    Hong Hua (Carthami Flos), 12g
    Dang Gui Wei (Angelicae Sinensis Radicis Extremitas), 15g
    Chuan Xiong (Chuanxiong Rhizoma), 15g
    Chi Shao (Paeoniae Radix Rubra), 15g
    Sheng Di Huang (Rehmanniae Radix Exsiccata seu Recens), 15g
    Su Mu (Sappan Lignum), 10g
    Ze Lan (Lycopi Herba), 12g
    Niu Xi (Achyranthis Bidentatae Radix), 15g
    Ru Xiang (Olibanum), 6g
    Mo Yao (Myrrha), 6g
    Sheng Da Huang (Rhei Radix et Rhizoma Crudi), 10g
    Chuan Lian Zi (Toosendan Fructus), 15g
    Zhi Ke (Aurantii Fructus), 10g
    Sheng Shui Zhi Fen (Hirudo Recens Pulverata), 5g, mixed with the
        strained decoction

Modifications: For urinary retention, add *Shi Chang Pu* (Acori Tatarinowii Rhizoma), 15g, *Yu Jin* (Curcumae Radix), 15g, *Hu Po Fen* (Succinum Pulverata), 3g, taken mixed with the strained decoction, and *Wang Bu Liu Xing* (Vaccariae Semen), 15g, to eliminate dampness, free the network vessels, and to open the orifice and disinhibit urination. When the penis is especially purplish and distended, add *Bie Jia* (Trionycis Carapax), 15g, *Tu Bie Chong*

(Eupolyphaga seu Steleophaga), 6g, and *E Zhu* (Curcumae Rhizoma), 20g, to strengthen the blood-moving, stasis-transforming, and swelling-dispersing actions of the formula.

5. Mutual binding of phlegm and blood stasis

Signs: An erection that will not become soft, a dark purple penis that is distended and firm, a cold sensation in the genitals, white slimy tongue fur, slippery pulse.

Treatment principles: Warm the yang and transform stasis, transform phlegm and free the network vessels

Guiding formula: Modified *Yang He Tang* (Harmonious Yang Decoction)

Ingredients:
> *Ma Huang* (Ephedrae Herba), 10g
> *Bai Jie Zi* (Sinapis Albae Semen), 10g
> *Rou Gui* (Cinnamomi Cortex), 6g
> *Lu Jiao Jiao* (Cervi Cornus Gelatinum), 10g, dissolved into strained
>   decoction
> *Pao Jiang* (Zingiberis Rhizoma Praeparatum), 6g
> *Shu Di Huang* (Rehmanniae Radix Praeparata), 15g
> *Xia Ku Cao* (Prunellae Spica), 20g
> *Bai Jiang Can* (Bombyx Batryticatus), 10g
> *Jiang Huang* (Curcumae Longae Rhizoma), 10g
> *Zhe Bei Mu* (Fritillariae Thunbergii Bulbus), 10g
> *Hong Hua* (Carthami Flos), 6g
> *Dang Gui* (Angelicae Sinensis Radix), 10g
> *Su Mu* (Sappan Lignum), 10g
> *Gan Cao* (Glycyrrhizae Radix), 6g

Modifications: For prominence of cold sensation of the penis and the lesser abdomen, add *Xiao Hui Xiang* (Foeniculi Fructus), 10g, and *Wu Zhu Yu* (Evodiae Fructus), 6g, to warm the liver channel and dissipate cold. If the erection is especially swollen and hard, add *Bie Jia* (Trionycis Carapax), 15g, *Sheng Mu Li* (Ostreae Concha Cruda), 30g, *Quan Xie* (Scorpio), 6g, and *Tu Bie Chong* (Eupolyphaga seu Steleophaga), 10g, to increase the blood-quickening and hardness-dispersing action of the formula.

Acumoxa therapy

Main points: *Guan Yuan* (CV-4), *Xing Jian* (LV-2), *Li Gou* (LV-5), *Zhao Hai* (KI-6), *San Yin Jiao* (SP-6), *Da Dun* (LV-1), *Tai Xi* (KI-3)

For yin vacuity with hyperactive yang, add *Shui Quan* (KI-5), *Zhong Ji* (CV-3), and *Qu Gu* (CV-2)

For binding depression of liver qi with depressed heat, add *Gan Shu* (BL-18), *Dan Shu* (BL-19), and *Tai Chong* (LV-3)

For damp-heat pouring downward into the liver channel, add *Tai Chong* (LV-3), *Yang Ling Quan* (GB-34), and *Pang Guang Shu* (BL-28)

For static blood obstructing the network vessels, add *Zhi Bian* (BL-54), *Ge Shu* (BL-17), *Shang Ju Xu* (ST-37), *Xia Ju Xu* (ST-39), *Da Zhu* (BL-11)

For mutual binding of phlegm and blood stasis, add *Feng Long* (ST-40), *Dan Shu* (BL-19), *Yin Ling Quan* (SP-9), *Shen Shu* (BL-23)

Experiential formulas

Clearing heat and transforming phlegm

He and Zhou (1997) provide Dr. Jin Shi-Hua's formula for treating rigid yang due to yin vacuity with vacuity heat, and phlegm-heat invading the liver channel and veiling the spirit-brightness. The formula is called *Qing Re Hua Tan Fang* (Heat-Clearing Phlegm-Transforming Formula) and contains the following medicinals:

Sheng Di Huang (Rehmanniae Radix Exsiccata seu Recens), 12g
Zhi Bai He (Lilii Bulbus cum Liquido Fricta), 12g
Zhi Mu (Anemarrhenae Rhizoma), 9g
Huang Bai (Phellodendri Cortex), 9g
Ju Hong (Citri Reticulatae Exocarpium Rubrum), 9g
Fu Ling (Poria), 9g
Dan Nan Xing (Arisaematis Rhizoma cum Bile), 9g
Zhu Ru (Bumbusae Caulis in Taenia), 9g
Gou Teng (Uncariae Ramulus cum Uncis), 12g
Yuan Zhi (Polygalae Radix), 9g
Gan Cao (Glycyrrhizae Radix), 3g

Clearing heat and cooling the blood

He and Zhou (1997) report on Dr. He Chuan-Yi's formula for treating a complex pattern of rigid yang due to heat toxin in the blood and phlegm-stasis obstructing the ancestral sinew. The formula is called *Qing Re Liang Xue Fang* (Heat-Clearing Blood-Cooling Formula) and contains the following medicinals:

Hu Zhang (Polygoni Cuspidati Rhizoma), 15g
Bing Pian (Borneolum), 3g
Xue Yu Tan (Crinis Carbonisatus), 10g
Jin Qian Cao (Lysimachiae Herba), 30g
Bai Shao (Paeoniae Radix Alba), 12g
Che Qian Zi (Plantaginis Semen), 10g
Tu Niu Xi (Achyranthis Radix), 15g
Zao Jiao Ci (Gleditsiae Spina), 12g
Wu Ling Zhi (Trogopteri Faeces), 10g
Bai Wei (Cynanchi Atrati Radix), 12g
Di Gu Pi (Lycii Cortex), 15g
Mu Dan Pi (Moutan Cortex), 12g

Clearing heat and drying dampness, and quickening the blood and transforming stasis

Zhang (1994) reported on a formula from Yu Zhi-Wei for treating rigid yang due to internal obstruction of damp-heat and blood stasis in the ancestral sinew. It is called *Dao Zhong Tang* (Inverted Center Decoction) and contains the following medicinals:

Long Dan Cao (Gentianae Radix), 12g
Sheng Di Huang (Rehmanniae Radix Exsiccata seu Recens), 18g
Dang Gui (Angelicae Sinensis Radix), 9g
Che Qian Zi (Plantaginis Semen), 15g
Shan Zhi Zi (Gardeniae Fructus), 12g
Hong Hua (Carthami Flos), 6g
Chai Hu (Bupleuri Radix), 12g
Huang Bai (Phellodendri Cortex), 12g
Ze Xie (Alismatis Rhizoma), 8g
Tao Ren (Persicae Semen), 15g
Gan Cao (Glycyrrhizae Radix), 9g

Counterflow and chaotic flow of qi and blood

Dr. Mou Lin-Mao (1994) reports on the efficacy of *Jia Wei Shao Yao Gan Cao Tang* (Modified Peony and Licorice Decoction) in the treatment of rigid yang due to evils (presumably liver channel qi depression and blood stasis) harassing the ancestral sinew causing "counterflow and chaotic" (*ni luan*) flow of qi and blood. The formula consists of the following medicinals:

Bai Shao (Paeoniae Radix Alba), 30g
Zhi Gan Cao (Glycyrrhizae Radix cum Liquido Fricta), 10g
Mu Gua (Chaenomelis Fructus), 30g
Wu Yao (Linderae Radix), 10g
Yan Hu Suo (Corydalis Rhizoma), 10g
Dan Shen (Salviae Miltiorrhizae Radix), 40g
Yi Mu Cao (Leonuri Herba), 30g
Che Qian Zi (Plantaginis Semen), 10g

Clearing and disinhibiting dampness, and enriching kidney yin

Qiao (1986) recommends a formula called *Zhi Bai Long Dan Xie Gan Tang* (Anemarrhena, Phellodendron, and Gentian Liver-Draining Decoction) for the treatment of rigid center. The formula consists of:

Long Dan Cao (Gentianae Radix), 15g
Shan Zhi Zi (Gardeniae Fructus), 10g
Huang Qin (Scutellariae Radix), 10g
Chai Hu (Bupleuri Radix), 6g
Sheng Di Huang (Rehmanniae Radix Exsiccata seu Recens), 12g
Che Qian Zi (Plantaginis Semen), 10g
Mu Tong (Akebiae Trifoliatae Caulis), 10g
Dang Gui (Angelicae Sinensis Radix), 10g
Zhi Mu (Anemarrhenae Rhizoma), 12g
Huang Bai (Phellodendri Cortex), 10g

External treatments

1. Make a paste the consistency of rice gruel by mixing pig's bile with equal parts of *Xuan Ming Fen* (Natrii Sulfas Exsiccatus) and *Han Shui Shi* (Gypsum seu Calcitum). Refrigerate and apply directly to the penis as a cold damp compress (Guo *et al.*, 1999).

2. For pediatric cases, make a decoction with *Che Qian Zi* (Plantaginis Semen), 50g, and *Qing Xiang Zi* (Celosiae Semen), 50g. Apply to the penis with a soft cloth soaked in the decoction, or use as a warm sitz bath (Zhang, 1998).

Preventive measures and lifestyle modification

1. Avoid excessive sexual activity

Excessive sexual activity (either with a partner or through masturbation) damages kidney yin-essence and leads to hyperactivity of ministerial fire. If ministerial fire within the kidneys and liver become hyperactive, the ancestral sinew is overstimulated and rigid yang may result. Also, if one holds back ejaculation for too long or completely refrains from ejaculation, qi stagnation, blood stasis, and vanquished essence may ensue and may cause rigid yang. Therefore, it is wise to have moderate sexual activity, and to avoid excessive sexual stimulation from books, magazines, and films with strong sexual content.

2. Avoid sexually-oriented supplementing medicinals

Chinese medicine—mostly from its nourishing life tradition (*yang sheng*)—has a deep knowledge of medicinals for enhancing male sexual performance. Many of these formulas have yang-warming ingredients and when taken for too long, or by men for whom they are inappropriate, can cause rigid yang. The pathomechanism is damage to kidney yin-essence leading to hyperactive stirring of ministerial fire. The ancestral sinew becomes abnormally erect and rigid yang can result. Therefore, men with a history of rigid yang or who are at high risk for it due to their constitution, should avoid such formulas.

3. Maintain good perineal hygiene

When there is a lack of perineal hygiene, evils can enter the penis through the urethra and can result in damp-heat and heat toxin conditions of the male anterior yin region, including acute and chronic prostatitis, strangury, dribbling urinary block, etc. As we have seen, damp-heat and heat toxin can obstruct within the ancestral sinew and can cause rigid yang. Hence, good perineal hygiene is essential to preventing this condition.

4. Maintain a clear bland diet

In order to prevent the formation, collection, or downward pour of damp-heat or phlegm, it is advisable to maintain a clear bland diet, and to avoid excessive intake of greasy-fried foods, hot-spicy foods, and alcohol.

Men with rigid yang from hyperactive ministerial fire should take a heat-clearing, hardness-softening, and blood-moving tea on a regular basis. One such recipe is: *Xia Ku Cao* (Prunellae Spica), 15g, and *Hong Hua* (Carthami Flos), 5g. This tea can be boiled for 10–15 minutes, strained, and taken on a regular basis (Chen and Jiang, 2000).

5. Maintain psychological wellness

The ancestral sinew is very closely resonant with the liver because the liver governs the sinews and the liver channel skirts the genitals. Therefore, rigid yang is often a disease of binding depression and sometimes also heat of the liver viscus and channel. The best way for men to maintain liver coursing and discharge (*shu xie*) and liver orderly reaching (*tiao da*) is to express their emotions and to avoid repressing anger and harboring resentment for long periods of time. When anger, resentment, hatred, and indignation endure, liver qi becomes bound and depressed, and fire transforms. These affects set the stage for rigid yang and should be diligently avoided. Rather, men at risk should schedule regular relaxation periods and engage in stress-reducing activities such as meditation and physical exercise, especially *qi gong*, yoga, and *tai ji chuan*, which have the added benefit of integrating physical exercise with stress-reducing breathing techniques and meditative focus.

Representative Chinese Research

Draining fire, flushing phlegm, and expelling stasis

Liu (1992) treated 12 cases of abnormal erections and hyperactive libido with a formula called *Meng Shi Zhi Bai Huang Ze Tang* (Chlorite, Anemarrhena, Phellodendron, and Alisma Decoction) to drain fire and enrich yin, and to flush phlegm and expel stasis. The ingredients were:

> *Meng Shi* (Chloriti seu Micae Lapis), 24g
> *Yan Chao Zhi Mu* (Anemarrhenae Rhizoma cum Salsa Fricta), 12g
> *Yan Chao Huang Bai* (Phellodendri Cortex cum Salsa Fricta), 9g
> *Sheng Da Huang* (Rhei Radix et Rhizoma Crudi), 9g, add at end
> *Ze Xie* (Alismatis Rhizoma), 15g

Modifications: For cases with effulgent liver fire, add *Long Dan Cao* (Gentianae Radix), 6g. For damp-heat pouring downward into the liver channel, add *Long Dan Xie Gan Wan* (Gentian Liver-Draining Pill), 6g, two times per day. For hyperactive heart fire and symptoms such as heart vexation, add *Huang Lian* (Coptidis Rhizoma), 6g, and *Shan Zhi Zi* (Gardeniae Fructus), 6g. For inability to house the spirit and symptoms such as insomnia, add *Fu Shen* (Poria cum Pini Radice), 24g, and *Zhu Sha* (Cinnabaris),[5] 1g, taken mixed with the strained decoction. For yin vacuity, add *Tian Men Dong* (Asparagi Radix), 15g, and *Xuan*

---

[5] *Zhu Sha* is toxic. Consider substituting *Long Chi* (Mastodi Dentis Fossilia), 15g, predecocted.

Shen (Scrophulariae Radix), 15g. For persistent rigid yang with penile swelling, distention, pain, and heat sensation, add *Ze Lan* (Lycopi Herba), 12g, and *Chuan Shan Jia* (Manitis Squama),[6] 18g. For persistent rigid yang and inability to ejaculate, add *Wang Bu Liu Xing* (Vaccariae Semen), 30g, *Lu Lu Tong* (Liquidambaris Fructus), 24g, and *Shi Chang Pu* (Acori Tatarinowii Rhizoma), 15g.

Results: The investigator reported that 10 cases were cured and that 2 cases had some results, though specific criteria for determining effectiveness were not provided.

Quickening the blood and transforming stasis

Li (1990) investigated the use of a formula called *Hua Yu Xiao Qiang Tang* (Stasis-Transforming Rigidity-Dispersing Decoction) for the treatment of 5 cases of abnormal erections by quickening the blood and transforming stasis, and by freeing the network vessels. The ingredients were:

Hu Zhang (Polygoni Cuspidati Rhizoma), 30g
Liu Ji Niu (Artemisiae Anomalae Herba), 30g
Ze Lan (Lycopi Herba), 24g
Tao Ren (Persicae Semen), 12g
Chi Shao (Paeoniae Radix Rubra), 12g
Dan Shen (Salviae Miltiorrhizae Radix), 15g
Su Mu (Sappan Lignum), 15g
Ru Xiang (Olibanum), 9g
Da Huang (Rhei Radix et Rhizoma), 9g

Results: The researcher reported that among the 5 cases he treated, all had chronic prostatitis and low libido, and that 4 cases were cured and 1 case had no result.

Representative Case Studies

Effulgent liver fire

Qin (1989) reported on a case of rigid center in a 26 year-old male due to effulgent liver fire. The patient had been married one week and had an erection that would not recede. When he and his wife had intercourse, he was unable to ejaculate, but during the day, he had leakage of turbid semen from his penis. He also had distention and pain of the penis, and urinary frequency and urgency. He went to a hospital and was diagnosed with seminal vesiculitis, and took antibiotics without effect. Further, he had redness of the cheeks, face, and lips, heart vexation, bitter oral taste and dry mouth, yellowish urine, oozing of turbid white fluid from his penis, yellow slimy tongue fur, and a stringlike rapid pulse.

The diagnosis was effulgent liver fire conducting downward to the bladder, running rampant in the essence chamber, and causing essence to be forced outward. The representative formula was *Long Dan Xie Gan Tang* (Gentian Liver-Draining

---

[6] Wild *Chuan Shan Jia* is derived from a threatened species. Only farm-raised pangolins should be used as a source for this medicinal.

Decoction), which Dr. Qin modified according to the pattern. The prescription was as follows:

Long Dan Cao (Gentianae Radix), 10g
Dang Gui Wei (Angelicae Sinensis Radicis Extremitas), 10g
Chai Hu (Bupleuri Radix), 10g
Mu Tong (Akebiae Trifoliatae Caulis), 10g
Bi Xie (Dioscoreae Hypoglaucae seu Semptemlobae Rhizoma), 10g
Che Qian Zi (Plantaginis Semen), 10g
Shan Zhi Zi (Gardeniae Fructus), 10g
Huang Qin (Scutellariae Radix), 10g
Ze Xie (Alismatis Rhizoma), 10g
Dan Shen (Salviae Miltiorrhizae Radix), 15g
Mu Li (Ostreae Concha), 15g
Sheng Di Huang (Rehmanniae Radix Exsiccata seu Recens), 20g
Gan Cao (Glycyrrhizae Radix), 5g

After taking 4 packets of the prescription, the patient reported that the erection had receded, the white turbid ooze had virtually disappeared, and the urine was clear and bright. After an additional 5 packets, all the symptoms completely disappeared, and his sexual function returned to normal. Dr. Qin then advised him to take *Zhi Bai Di Huang Wan* (Anemarrhena, Phellodendron, and Rehmannia Pill) to consolidate the effects.

In his commentary for this case, Dr. Qin pointed out that very often rigid yang is due to liver repletion heat and therefore *Long Dan Xie Gan Tang* is a good representative formula. Moreover, he stated that one should always add blood-quickening medicinals to the formula to free the network vessels so that the erection can recede.

Rampant phlegm-fire

Wang (1997) reported on a case study of Xu Fu-Song, who treated a case of rigid center due to rampant phlegm fire. The patient reported that for about the past year, he had an erection for about 6–7 hours per night that disturbed his sleep. Generally speaking, he had a repressed and depressed demeanor, and was irascible. Further, he had dizzy head, headache, copious dreaming, occasional tinnitus, weakness and limpness of the lumbus and knees, fatigued limbs and lack of strength, dry mouth with a bitter sticky taste, short reddish urine, red tongue with dry thin yellow fur which was slimy at the root, and a stringlike fine slippery pulse.

The diagnosis was rampant phlegm fire in the liver channel and detriment to heart and kidney yin due to hyperactive yang. The treatment principle was to drain fire and flush phlegm, enrich yin and settle the yang, and to heavily settle and quiet the spirit. The prescription was as follows:

Dan Nan Xing (Arisaema cum Bile), 10g
Shan Zhi Zi (Gardeniae Fructus), 10g
Chuan Lian Zi (Toosendan Fructus), 10g
Yuan Zhi (Polygalae Radix), 10g

Zhe Bei Mu (Fritillariae Thunbergii Bulbus), 10g
Sheng Di Huang (Rehmanniae Radix Exsiccata seu Recens), 10g
Shu Di Huang (Rehmanniae Radix Praeparata), 10g
Mai Men Dong (Ophiopogonis Radix), 10g
Huang Bai (Phellodendri Cortex), 10g
Sheng Long Chi (Mastodi Dentis Fossilia Cruda), 30g
Sheng Mu Li (Ostreae Concha Cruda), 30g
Shi Hu (Dendrobii Herba), 15g
Shi Chang Pu (Acori Tatarinowii Rhizoma), 6g
Wu Wei Zi (Schisandrae Fructus), 6g
Huang Lian (Coptidis Rhizoma), 4g

After taking 30 packets of the prescription, modified occasionally according to changes in the pattern, the patient was completely cured.

In the commentary for the case, Dr. Xu pointed out that rigid yang is mainly a disease of the liver and kidney. He backed up his position by quoting two dictums in Chinese medicine: "the liver governs the sinews" and the "kidney governs the two yin."

Kidney yin vacuity with hyperactive stirring of ministerial fire

Liu (1994) reported on the treatment of one case of rigid yang occurring in a 72-year-old male. One day prior to visiting Dr. Liu, the patient developed a very painful erection. Additional symptoms included dizzy eyes and head, tinnitus, soreness and limpness of the lumbus and knees, and heat effusion in the heart of the palms and soles. Further, it was noteworthy that although the patient was over 70 years old, his libido was still quite strong. His tongue was red with scanty fur and dry, and the pulse was stringlike fine.

The diagnosis was insufficiency of kidney yin with hyperactive stirring of ministerial fire and the treatment principle was to enrich yin and downbear fire. The prescription was based on *Zhi Bai Di Huang Wan* (Anemarrhena, Phellodendron, and Rehmannia Pill) and contained the following medicinals:

Zhi Mu (Anemarrhenae Rhizoma), 15g
Huang Bai (Phellodendri Cortex), 15g
Shu Di Huang (Rehmanniae Radix Praeparata), 20g
Sheng Di Huang (Rehmanniae Radix Exsiccata seu Recens), 20g
Shan Zhu Yu (Corni Fructus), 15g
Shan Yao (Dioscoreae Rhizoma), 30g
Mu Dan Pi (Moutan Cortex), 10g
Fu Ling (Poria), 15g
Ze Xie (Alismatis Rhizoma), 10g
Sha Shen (Adenophorae seu Glehniae Radix), 20g
Mai Men Dong (Ophiopogonis Radix), 20g
Gan Cao (Glycyrrhizae Radix), 5g

After taking 3 packets of the prescription, the erection receded and the patient was cured.

Treating penile swelling and pain with an external plaster

Shi (2002) used an external plaster to treat one case of penile swelling and pain. The patient was a 40 year-old male who had been having lesser abdominal distention and sagging for three days. At times, there was also pain and a scorching heat sensation in the same area. Subsequently, his penis became swollen and painful, and subjectively felt scorching hot. He took antibiotics for three days without effect. Upon examination, he had a fever of 39°C and had elevated white blood cells. His tongue was red with a yellow slimy fur, and his pulse was slippery rapid. The diagnosis was damp-heat pouring downward and the treatment principle was to clear heat and disinhibit dampness and to resolve toxicity. The ingredients of the external plaster were:

> *Che Qian Zi* (Plantaginis Semen), 50g
> *Tu Fu Ling* (Smilacis Glabrae Rhizoma), 50g
> *Qing Xiang Zi* (Celosiae Semen), 50g
> *Long Dan Cao* (Gentianae Radix), 20g

The medicinals were ground into powder and mixed with a small amount of egg white to reach the consistency of rice gruel, and then applied directly to the penis once per day. After using the paste for two days, the penile swelling and pain had greatly reduced, the redness and swelling disappeared, and the fever was gone. After five more days of use, the symptoms all completely disappeared. Follow-up one month later indicated no recurrence.

Acumoxa treatment

Using *Tai Chong* (LV-3) and *San Yin Jiao* (SP-6)

Wang, Wang, and Miao (1997) reported on the successful treatment of a case of rigid center with the use of *Tai Chong* (LV-3) and *San Yin Jiao* (SP-6). Both points were needled with the draining method.

Treating the kidney, bladder, and heart channels, as well as the conception vessel

Xu (1995) reported on Yang Jie-Bin's experience treating a case of rigid center with two different groups of acumoxa points which were alternated on different days. The first group consisted of *Tai Chong* (LV-3) needled through to *Yong Quan* (KI-1), *Tai Xi* (KI-3), and *Ci Liao* (BL-32). The second group comprised *San Yin Jiao* (SP-6), *Shen Men* (HT-7), *Zhao Hai* (KI-6), and *Hui Yin* (CV-1). Treatment was given every day with strong draining technique. The patient was reportedly cured after 12 treatments. Follow-up in 6 months indicated no recurrence of the condition.

Using *Zhong Ji* (CV-3) and *Li Gou* (LV-5)

Yuan (1988) reported on the successful treatment of one case of penile distention and pain induced by injected papaverine. The points were *Zhong Ji* (CV-3) and *Li Gou* (LV-5) and were needled with cooling and draining technique.

Hematospermia

Western Medicine

Hematospermia (hemospermia) is characterized by the presence of blood in the ejaculate, and usually manifests as pinkish-red semen. It can occur in men in any age group and can be due to a variety of causes including prostatic, epididymal, or urethral inflammation or infections, traumatic injury (including from surgery or urological instrumentation such as transrectal ultrasound [TRUS]-guided prostatic biopsy or transurethral resection of the prostate [TURP], and from sexual activity), benign or malignant tumors of the male genitourinary tract, renal malformations and cysts, bleeding disorders, radioactive seed therapy for prostate cancer, prostate stones, and systemic diseases such as hypertension, chronic liver disease, amyloidosis, lymphoma, and bleeding diatheses (von Willebrand disease).

In the majority of cases, hematospermia is idiopathic, benign, and requires no specific treatment other than reassuring the patient that it is not usually a sign of prostate cancer and it is not associated with sexual dysfunction (Beers *et al.*, 2006). This is especially true for men under 40 years of age, but even in older men it is very rarely thought to be associated with malignancy. However, some studies suggest that the perception among physicians that hematospermia is usually benign may be blinding them to existing associations with more severe diseases such as prostate cancer (Schiff and Mulhall, 2006). Hence, physicians should remain alert to the fact that sometimes hematospermia is a symptom of a more serious urologic or systemic disease process that requires careful diagnosis and treatment.

History

According to Schiff and Mulhall (2006), the main points requiring attention in the history of patients with hematospermia include trauma, prostatitis or seminal vesiculitis, and bleeding disorders. The duration of the condition typically is from 1–24 months, and most men presenting with hematospermia are under 40 years of age. Although some controversy exists, as a general rule hematospermia that persists for more than two months or that has occurred in more than ten ejaculations requires urological workup (Schiff and Mulhall, 2006).

Physical examination

Physical examination should include close inspection of the penis so as to rule out any lesions that could possibly be bleeding and therefore contributing to the ejaculate. This is especially important when the history reveals recent penile trauma. Further, physicians should palpate the vas deferens along its entire course with an eye towards detecting any nodules or induration. Nodules along the vas are expected in men with a history of vasectomy, but in men with an intact vas they can be a sign of primary or extended malignancy, or even tuberculous (TB) infection. The digital rectal examination (DRE) is used to detect abnormalities of the prostate and seminal vesicles, including prostate cancer and seminal vesiculitis.

Laboratory examination

• Urinalysis and culture

In men with hematospermia, urinalysis and culture can establish an infectious etiology. For men with a history of exposure to TB, specific culture for acid-fast bacilli should be ordered to detect their presence. Men who have multiple sexual partners sometimes present with hematospermia as a result of nonspecific or gonococcal urethritis; therefore, for these men, physicians use a urethral swab to collect a sample for culture.

• Semen analysis and culture

Physicians may use semen analysis and culture to help make an accurate diagnosis of hematospermia. For example, semen analysis can help to discriminate hematospermia from melanospermia, which can occur in malignant melanoma (Schiff and Mulhall, 2006). If the semen culture is positive, prostatic infection is indicated, though the possibility that the culture has been contaminated with urethral organisms must be considered. Further, in men who have traveled to endemic areas, schistosomiasis has been reported as an etiology (Corachan et al., 1994).

• Blood work

Whenever there is chronic unexplained hematospermia or when the patient is over 40 years of age and especially if he has a family history of prostate cancer, physicians should order a prostate specific antigen (PSA) test. Although PSA is certainly not a fool-proof test for prostate cancer, it is one helpful tool in the diagnostic process. Further, for men with chronic unexplained hematospermia, coagulation studies can be helpful in diagnosing coagulation disorders.

Imaging

• Transrectal ultrasound (TRUS) of the prostate

TRUS is an extremely valuable tool for the differential diagnosis of hematospermia. It allows the physician to view the morphology of the prostate, seminal vesicles, and portions of the vas. Hence, it can establish the diagnosis of prostatic, epididymal, or ejaculatory duct calculi, as well as other structural abnormalities of these tissues.

• MRI

Similar to TRUS, MRI can be used to study the morphology of the prostate, seminal vesicles, and the vas. According to Schiff and Mulhall (2006), the main advantage of MRI over TRUS is that it can detect bleeding within the prostate and vas.

• Cystourethroscopy

Usually reserved for chronic unexplained cases without known infection, and for all cases with hematuria, cystourethroscopy can provide direct visualization of prostatic and urethral causes of hematospermia.

Treatment

Because hematospermia—especially the first occurrence—is associated with significant patient anxiety, the first therapeutic goal is to allay the patient's fear that he has prostate cancer or is destined for sexual dysfunction. As we have seen, this condition is more often than not benign, especially in younger men; in such cases, watchful waiting is the main treatment (Ahmad and Kirshna, 2007). Generally speaking, the three main factors in determining the appropriate therapeutic intervention for hematospermia are: 1) the patient's age; 2) its duration and frequency and; 3) the presence or absence of hematuria (Schiff and Mulhall, 2006). When hematuria is present, a more detailed analysis is warranted with an eye towards detecting renal or coagulation disorders. Treatment then follows logically from the conclusions drawn from the workup.

When infection is detected and the offending organism is identified, appropriate antibiotic therapy should be used. When no infection can be detected and prostatic or epididymal inflammation is discovered or suspected, nonsteroidal antiinflammatory agents such as ibuprofen are recommended. When prostatic hyperplasia or inflammation results in significant bladder outlet obstruction, a 5 alpha-reductase inhibitor is often prescribed. For men with cysts in the prostatic urethra or seminal vesicles, transrectal aspiration is sometimes used. For men with bleeding varices in the prostate, surgical fulguration is used, which consists of using an electrode to destroy the affected tissue.

Western Complementary Medicine[1]

• Yoga therapy

Ripoll, and Mahowald (2002), suggest that yoga therapy can be effective in managing chronic and difficult to diagnose male urological conditions such as

[1] Also see Book 2, Chapter 1 on prostatitis for additional recommendations.

epididymitis and chronic prostatitis. These conditions are among the most common causes of hematospermia, so it is logical to conclude that yoga may have some value for hematospermia.

Chinese Medicine

Disease discrimination

The Chinese medical disease category that directly correlates with hematospermia is hematospermia (*xue jing*), which is characterized by the ejaculation of semen containing blood. One of the earliest mentions of hematospermia occurs in *Zhu Bing Yuan Hou Lun* (*On the Origin and Indicators of Disease*),[2] where we find the following discussion: "This [condition] is caused by taxation damage to the kidney qi. The kidney stores essence, and essence is formed from blood. Vacuity taxation engenders the seven damages and six extremes.[3] Those with kidney [disease] are relatively vacuous and are unable to store essence; hence essence and blood are discharged together."

In clinical practice, it is important to distinguish hematospermia from bloody strangury and hematuria. In bloody strangury, there is rough painful voiding of urine containing blood, and in hematuria there is painless voiding of urine containing blood.

Disease causes and pathomechanisms

• Kidney yin vacuity with hyperactive ministerial fire

Either due to natural endowment insufficiency, constitutional vacuity, excessive sexual activity, or excessive intake of warm dry yang-supplementing medicinals, kidney yin-essence may become vacuous. As a result, ministerial fire becomes hyperactive and yin vacuity fire stirs in the interior and scorches the network vessels within the essence chamber. Blood moves frenetically from within these network vessels and mixes with semen in the essence chamber. When the semen is discharged, blood is discharged along with it and the disease of hematospermia results.

• Spleen-kidney dual vacuity

When there is overwork, dietary irregularities, or excessive thought and preoccupation, spleen qi—the later heaven source for the engenderment and transformation of qi and blood—becomes vacuous. When qi and blood become

---

[2] *Zhu Bing Yuan Hou Lun* was written by Chao Yuan-Fang and published in 610 CE, during the Sui dynasty.

[3] In *Zhu Bing Yuan Hou Lun* the seven damages (*liu shang*) refers to seven disease patterns of vacuity taxation: 1) cold genitals; 2) yin wilt; 3) abdominal urgency; 4) continuous [loss of] essence; 5) scanty essence and dampness in the genitals; 6) cold semen and; 7) painful frequent micturition. In the same text, the six extremes (*liu ji*) refers to six possible disease patterns of vacuity taxation: 1) qi extreme; 2) vessel extreme; 3) sinew extreme; 4) flesh extreme; 5) bone extreme and; 6) essence extreme. The term "extreme" in this context essentially means "vacuity"; hence, each of the six extremes has its own specific signs. (See Wiseman and Feng, 1998, p. 535.)

vacuous, essence eventually becomes vacuous. This is because qi engenders blood, and essence and blood share the same source. Hence, when blood is vacuous, yin-essence becomes vacuous in turn, and the kidney loses its nourishment. As a result, spleen qi is unable to restrain blood and kidney qi becomes insecure and unable to seal and store essence. Hence, blood and semen are discharged together and the disease pattern of hematospermia results.

• **Enduring depression of liver qi transforming fire**
When anger, indignation, hatred, and resentment endure for long periods of time, depressed liver qi transforms fire. Liver fire may flame downward along the liver channel into the anterior yin region and the essence chamber. If it scorches and harasses the network vessels within the essence chamber, blood moves frenetically from within them and mixes with semen. Hence, the disease pattern of hematospermia results.

• **Damp-heat pouring downward to the lower burner**
Due to dietary irregularities such as excessive intake of greasy-fried, spicy-hot, and sweet foods, as well as alcohol, or from external contraction of damp-heat, damp-heat collects in the center burner and pours downward into the lower burner. Once there, it may harass and scorch the network vessels in the essence chamber. This results in frenetic movement of blood out from the network vessels into the semen, and the disease pattern of hematospermia results.

• **Internal obstruction of static blood**
Either due to traumatic injury to the anterior yin region, or to enduring affect-mind irregularities, qi stagnation and blood stasis may form within the essence chamber. During sexual activity, the activating function of qi aroused by sexual desire pushes against the static blood. This causes the network vessels within the essence chamber to become damaged, and blood to leak out from within them; when this blood mixes with semen, the disease pattern of hematospermia results.

Pattern discrimination

1. Kidney yin vacuity with hyperactive ministerial fire

Signs: Seminal efflux with reddish semen or ejaculation of reddish semen during sexual activity, a sensation of sagging and distention in the genital region, soreness and limpness of the lumbus and knees, dizzy head and flowery vision, night sweats, heart vexation and dry mouth, short reddish urine, tender red tongue with either scanty dry or thin yellow tongue fur, stringlike fine rapid pulse.

Treatment principles: Enrich yin and downbear fire, cool the blood and stanch bleeding

Guiding formulas: Modified *Zhi Bai Di Huang Wan* (Anemarrhena, Phellodendron, and Rehmannia Pill) plus *Er Zhi Wan* (Double Supreme Pill)

Ingredients:
> *Sheng Di Huang* (Rehmanniae Radix Exsiccata seu Recens), 15g
> *Zhi Mu* (Anemarrhenae Rhizoma), 10g
> *Huang Bai* (Phellodendri Cortex), 10g
> *Mu Dan Pi* (Moutan Cortex), 10g
> *Gui Ban Jiao* (Testudinis Carapax et Plastrum), 10g, dissolved into the strained decoction
> *Ze Xie* (Alismatis Rhizoma), 10g
> *Fu Ling* (Poria), 10g
> *Huai Hua* (Sophorae Flos), 12g
> *Bai Mao Gen* (Imperatae Rhizoma), 30g
> *Nu Zhen Zi* (Ligustri Lucidi Fructus), 12g
> *Han Lian Cao* (Ecliptae Herba), 12g
> *Xiao Ji* (Cirsii Herba), 12g

Modifications: With pronounced pain during ejaculation, add *Chuan Lian Zi* (Toosendan Fructus), 12g, and *Fo Shou* (Citri Sacrodactylis Fructus), 12g, to rectify qi and stop pain. For more pronounced signs of fluid damage from yin vacuity fire, including dry mouth and throat and scanty semen, remove *Ze Xie*, *Xiao Ji*, and *Fu Ling*, and add *Tian Hua Fen* (Trichosanthis Radix), 12g, and *Mai Men Dong* (Ophiopogonis Radix), 10g.

2. Spleen-kidney dual vacuity

Signs: Ejaculation of semen mixed with pale red blood, low libido, soreness and encumbrance of the lumbus, shortness of breath, low appetite and torpid intake, dizziness of the head and eyes, lack of strength and lassitude, cold limbs, palpitations and insomnia, susceptibility to fright and fear, pale tongue with white fur, deep fine forceless pulse.

Treatment principles: Supplement the spleen and kidneys, nourish essence-blood, boost qi to contain blood

Guiding formulas: Modified *Gui Pi Tang* (Spleen-Returning Decoction) plus *You Gui Wan* (Right-Restoring [Life Gate] Pill)

Ingredients:
> *Dang Shen* (Codonopsis Radix), 15g
> *Bai Zhu* (Atractylodis Macrocephalae Rhizoma), 12g
> *Zhi Huang Qi* (Astragali Radix cum Liquido Fricta), 15g
> *Dang Gui* (Angelicae Sinensis Radix), 12g
> *Gou Qi Zi* (Lycii Fructus), 15g
> *Shu Di Huang* (Rehmanniae Radix Praeparata), 12g
> *Shan Yao* (Dioscoreae Rhizoma), 15g
> *Shan Zhu Yu* (Corni Fructus), 12g
> *Lu Jiao Jiao* (Cervi Cornus Gelatinum), 10g
> *Du Zhong* (Eucommiae Cortex), 15g
> *Tu Si Zi* (Cuscutae Semen), 15g

Suan Zao Ren (Ziziphi Spinosi Semen), 12g
Yuan Zhi (Polygalae Radix), 10g
Ce Bai Ye (Platycladi Cacumen), 12g
Xue Yu Tan (Crinis Carbonisatus), 12g
Zhi Gan Cao (Glycyrrhizae Radix cum Liquido Fricta), 6g

Modifications: For center qi fall, remove *Dang Gui* and *Suan Zao Ren* and add *Sheng Ma* (Cimicifugae Rhizoma), 6g, and *Chai Hu* (Bupleuri Radix), 6g, to raise the spleen yang. For more pronounced insufficiency of essence, add *Zi He Che* (Hominis Placenta), 6g, to further replenish and enrich essence. For seminal efflux or premature ejaculation, add *Qian Shi* (Euryales Semen), 10g, *Jin Ying Zi* (Rosae Laevigatae Fructus), 15g, *Duan Long Gu* (Mastodi Ossis Fossilia Calcinata), 15g, and *Duan Mu Li* (Ostreae Concha Calcinata), 15g, to secure essence.

3. Depression of liver qi transforming fire

Signs: Semen containing fresh red blood or semen with fresh red threads of blood, red face and distended eyes, irascibility, chest oppression, headache, vague discomfort or sagging distention in the lesser abdomen, perineum, or testes, dry mouth and bitter taste, yellowish-red and hot urine, stabbing pain in the penis, red tongue with redder margins and yellow fur, stringlike rapid pulse.

Treatment principles: Clear and drain liver fire, cool the blood and stanch bleeding

Guiding formula: Modified *Long Dan Xie Gan Tang* (Gentian Liver-Draining Decoction)

Ingredients:
Long Dan Cao (Gentianae Radix), 12g
Huang Qin Tan (Scutellariae Radix Carbonisata), 12g
Zhi Zi Tan (Gardeniae Fructus Carbonisatus), 12g
Chai Hu (Bupleuri Radix), 10g
Ze Xie (Alismatis Rhizoma), 12g
Mu Tong (Akebiae Trifoliatae Caulis), 10g
Che Qian Zi (Plantaginis Semen), 15g
Sheng Di Huang (Rehmanniae Radix Exsiccata seu Recens), 15g
Dang Gui (Angelicae Sinensis Radix), 10g
Xiao Ji (Cirsii Herba), 12g
Sheng Gan Cao (Glycyrrhizae Radix Cruda), 6g

Modifications: For more pronounced dry mouth and throat from liver fire scorching stomach fluids, add *Mai Men Dong* (Ophiopogonis Radix), 10g, *Tian Hua Fen* (Trichosanthis Radix), 12g, and *Bai Mao Gen* (Imperatae Rhizoma), 12g, to nourish yin and engender fluids. When depressed liver fire engenders heat toxin causing redness, swelling, and pain in the anterior yin region, add *Pu Gong Ying* (Taraxaci Herba), 15g, *Jin Yin Hua* (Lonicerae Flos), 15g, and *Chi Shao* (Paeoniae Radix Rubra), 12g, to clear heat and resolve toxicity and to reduce swelling.

4. Damp-heat pouring downward to the lower burner

Signs: Reddish-yellow semen that is scanty and viscous, heavy encumbered lumbus and knees, frequent urgent and yellowish-red and turbid urine, possible urinary dribbling and inhibited urination, red tongue with yellow slimy fur, soft rapid or stringlike slippery pulse.

Treatment principles: Clear and disinhibit damp-heat, cool the blood and stanch bleeding

Guiding formula: Modified *Ba Zheng San* (Eight Corrections Powder)

Ingredients:
    Bian Xu (Polygoni Avicularis Herba), 15g
    Qu Mai (Dianthi Herba), 15g
    Mu Tong (Akebiae Trifoliatae Caulis), 12g
    Zhi Zi Tan (Gardeniae Fructus Carbonisatus), 12g
    Huang Bai Tan (Phellodendri Cortex Carbonisatus), 12g
    Da Huang (Rhei Radix et Rhizoma), 6g
    Hua Shi (Talcum), 15g
    Che Qian Zi (Plantaginis Semen), 15g
    Deng Xin Cao (Junci Medulla), 10g
    Xiao Ji (Cirsii Herba), 12g
    Sheng Gan Cao (Glycyrrhizae Radix Cruda), 6g

Modifications: With pronounced signs of spleen-stomach damp-heat, add *Huang Lian* (Coptidis Rhizoma), 6g, *Cang Zhu* (Atractylodis Rhizoma), 12g, *Hou Po* (Magnoliae Officinalis Cortex), 10g, and *Shen Qu* (Massa Medicata Fermentata), 10g.

5. Internal obstruction of static blood

Signs: Semen containing dark purplish blood and/or blood clots, stabbing pain in the perineum and anterior yin region, an abundance of reddish or purplish threads visible on the penis or scrotum, palpable nodules in the scrotum, dark purple tongue with purplish points or macules, rough pulse.

Treatment principles: Quicken the blood and transform stasis

Guiding formula: Modified *Tao Hong Si Wu Tang* (Peach Kernel and Carthamus Four Agents Decoction)

Ingredients:
    Tao Ren (Persicae Semen), 10g
    Hong Hua (Carthami Flos), 10g
    Dang Gui Wei (Angelicae Sinensis Radicis Extremitas), 12g
    Chuan Xiong (Chuanxiong Rhizoma), 12g
    Chi Shao (Paeoniae Radix Rubra), 10g
    Sheng Di Huang (Rehmanniae Radix Exsiccata seu Recens), 12g

San Qi (Notoginseng Radix), 10g
Ou Jie (Nelumbinis Rhizomatis Nodus), 10g

Modifications: When there is swelling and pain of the perineum or anterior yin region, add *Ru Xiang* (Olibanum), 6g, *Mo Yao* (Myrrha), 6g, *Pu Huang* (Typhae Pollen), 10g, and *Wu Ling Zhi* (Trogopteri Faeces), 10g, to further quicken the blood and transform stasis and to disperse swelling and relieve pain. When blood stasis has formed as result of enduring liver depression, add *Chai Hu* (Bupleuri Radix), 6g, *Fo Shou* (Citri Sacrodactylis Fructus), 10g, *Chuan Lian Zi* (Toosendan Fructus), 10g, and *Yu Jin* (Curcumae Radix), 10g, to course the liver and rectify qi and to resolve depression.

Acumoxa therapy

Main points: *Hui Yin* (CV-1), *Shen Shu* (BL-23), *San Yin Jiao* (SP-6)

Vacuity patterns

For yin vacuity with hyperactive ministerial fire, add *Tai Chong* (LV-3), *Zhao Hai* (KI-6), *Ran Gu* (KI-2), and *Qu Gu* (CV-2)

For spleen-kidney dual vacuity, add *Zu San Li* (ST-36), *Pi Shu* (BL-20), *Wei Shu* (BL-21), *Qi Hai* (CV-6), *Zhong Wan* (CV-12), *Shan Zhong* (CV-17), *Tai Xi* (KI-3), *Fu Liu* (KI-7), and *Ming Men* (GV-4)

Repletion patterns

For enduring liver depression with depressed fire, add *Xing Jian* (LV-2), *Li Gou* (LV-5), *Yang Ling Quan* (GB-34), *Gan Shu* (BL-18), and *Dan Shu* (BL-19)

For damp-heat pouring downward, add *Yin Ling Quan* (SP-9), *Li Gou* (LV-5), *Tai Chong* (LV-3), *Xing Jian* (LV-2), and *Zhong Ji* (CV-3)

For blood stasis obstructing the network vessels, add *San Yin Jiao* (SP-6), *Ge Shu* (BL-17), *Xue Hai* (SP-10), *Shang Ju Xu* (ST-37), *Xia Ju Xu* (ST-39), *Da Zhu* (BL-11),[4] *Wei Zhong* (BL-40), and *Ci Liao* (BL-32)

Experiential formulas

Treating complex patterns

Liu and Liu (2001) report on a formula created by Dr. Wang Zheng-Yu called *Li Shui Tong Lin Tang* (Water-Disinhibiting Strangury-Freeing Decoction) for treating hematospermia associated with epididymitis and prostatitis. It has complex functions including clearing heat and expelling dampness, dispersing inflammation and relieving pain, disinhibiting urination and freeing strangury, nourishing yin, and fortifying the spleen. The ingredients are as follows:

---

[4] ST-37, ST-39, and BL-11 are points corresponding to the sea of blood and can be used for all blood disorders.

Hua Shi (Talcum), 20g
Che Qian Zi (Plantaginis Semen), 20g
Niu Xi (Achyranthis Bidentatae Radix), 20g
Jin Yin Hua (Lonicerae Flos), 20g
Shan Zhi Zi (Gardeniae Fructus), 12g
Bai Shao (Paeoniae Radix Alba), 12g
Ze Xie (Alismatis Rhizoma), 12g
Fu Ling (Poria), 12g
Huang Bai (Phellodendri Cortex), 12g
Sheng Di Huang (Rehmanniae Radix Exsiccata seu Recens), 12g
Huang Qin (Scutellariae Radix), 12g
Dang Gui (Angelicae Sinensis Radix), 10g
Mu Tong (Akebiae Trifoliatae Caulis), 10g
Gan Cao (Glycyrrhizae Radix), 6g

Modifications: For patients with yang vacuity, add a small amount of *Fu Zi* (Aconiti Radix Lateralis Praeparata) and *Rou Gui* (Cinnamomi Cortex). For vomiting, add *Gan Jiang* (Zingiberis Rhizoma). For qi vacuity, add *Huang Qi* (Astragali Radix) and *Dang Shen* (Codonopsis Radix). For kidney vacuity, add *Tu Si Zi* (Cuscutae Semen) and *Yin Yang Huo* (Epimedii Herba).

Transforming turbidity, eliminating stasis, and stanching bleeding

Wang *et al.* (1990) reported on an experiential formula called *Cheng Jing Tang* (Clear Essence Decoction) for treating hematospermia associated with epididymitis with turbidity and stasis. The ingredients are as follows:
Chi Xiao Dou (Phaseoli Semen), 30g
Bai Mao Gen (Imperatae Rhizoma), 30g
Dan Shen (Salviae Miltiorrhizae Radix), 15g
Wang Bu Liu Xing (Vaccariae Semen), 15g
Tao Ren (Persicae Semen), 15g
Da Huang (Rhei Radix et Rhizoma), 10g, add at end
Hong Hua (Carthami Flos), 10g
Dang Gui (Angelicae Sinensis Radix), 10g
Bi Xie (Dioscoreae Hypoglaucae seu Semptemlobae Rhizoma), 10g
Fu Ling (Poria), 10g
Ze Xie (Alismatis Rhizoma), 10g
Niu Xi (Achyranthis Bidentatae Radix), 10g
Gan Cao (Glycyrrhizae Radix), 6g
San Qi (Notoginseng Radix), 6g, taken mixed with the strained decoction
Mang Xiao (Natrii Sulfas), 6g, dissolved into the strained decoction
Wu Gong (Scolopendra), 1 piece

Modifications: For pain during ejaculation add *Shi Xiao San* (Sudden Smile Powder). For pain in the lumbus, add *Xu Duan* (Dipsaci Radix) and *Gou Ji* (Cibotii Rhizoma). For damp-heat pouring downward, add *Che Qian Zi* (Plantaginis Semen), *Mu Tong* (Akebiae Trifoliatae Caulis), and *Bai Jiang Cao* (Patriniae Herba). For yang wilt, add *Yin Yang Huo* (Epimedii Herba), *Yang*

Qi Shi (Actinolitum), and *Gou Qi Zi* (Lycii Fructus). For seminal efflux or premature ejaculation, add *Bai Ji Li* (Tribuli Fructus), *Jin Ying Zi* (Rosae Laevigatae Fructus), and *Suo Yang* (Cynomorii Herba). For low libido, add *She Chuang Zi* (Cnidii Fructus) and *Yin Yang Huo* (Epimedii Herba). For insomnia and poor memory, add *Long Gu* (Mastodi Ossis Fossilia), *Mu Li* (Ostreae Concha), *Yuan Zhi* (Polygalae Radix), and *Shi Chang Pu* (Acori Tatarinowii Rhizoma). For heat effusion and aversion to cold, add *Chai Hu* (Bupleuri Radix), *Lian Qiao* (Forsythiae Fructus), and *Huang Qin* (Scutellariae Radix). For low-grade fever, add *E Jiao* (Asini Corii Colla), *Zhi Mu* (Anemarrhenae Rhizoma), *Huang Bai* (Phellodendri Cortex), and *Sheng Di Huang* (Rehmanniae Radix Exsiccata seu Recens).

Resolving toxicity, disinhibiting dampness, freeing strangury and stanching bleeding

Liu and Liu (2001) provide a formula from Dr. Wei Hong-Yun called *Bi Xie Jie Du Li Shi Tang* (Fish Poison Yam Toxin-Resolving Dampness-Disinhibiting Decoction) which treats hematospermia by resolving toxicity, disinhibiting dampness, freeing strangury, and stanching bleeding. The ingredients are:

> *Bi Xie* (Dioscoreae Hypoglaucae seu Semptemlobae Rhizoma), 20g
> *Tu Fu Ling* (Smilacis Glabrae Rhizoma), 15g
> *Bai Zhu* (Atractylodis Macrocephalae Rhizoma), 15g
> *Shi Chang Pu* (Acori Tatarinowii Rhizoma), 15g
> *Shi Wei* (Pyrrosiae Folium), 15g
> *Bai Jiang Cao* (Patriniae Herba), 15g
> *Dong Kui Zi* (Malvae Semen), 15g
> *Che Qian Zi* (Plantaginis Semen), 15g
> *Lian Zi Xin* (Nelumbinis Plumula), 12g
> *Huang Bai* (Phellodendri Cortex), 12g

In addition to the decoction, Dr. Wei had patients take 10 grams per day, in 2 divided doses, a finely-ground powder consisting of *Da Huang Tan* (Rhei Radix et Rhizoma Carbonisatus), 4g, *Hu Po* (Succinum), 4g, and *E Jiao* (Asini Corii Colla), 2g.

Modifications: For pain in the lumbus, add *Xu Duan* (Dipsaci Radix), 15g, *Gou Ji* (Cibotii Rhizoma), 15g, and *Du Zhong* (Eucommiae Cortex), 15g. For sagging distention in the testes, add *Li Zhi He* (Litchi Semen), 12g, and *Wu Yao* (Linderae Radix), 12g. For insomnia, add *Bai Zi Ren* (Platycladi Semen), 15g, and *Suan Zao Ren* (Ziziphi Spinosi Semen), 15g. For yang wilt, add *Wu Gong* (Scolopendra), 2 pieces. For seminal efflux, add *Suo Yang* (Cynomorii Herba), 15g, and *Qian Shi* (Euryales Semen), 15g. For a prostate that is hard to palpation, add *San Leng* (Sparganii Rhizoma), 12g, and *E Zhu* (Curcumae Rhizoma), 12g.

External treatments

1. For a combination damp-heat and blood stasis pattern, boil 250 grams

of fresh *Lu Cao* (Humuli Scandentis Herba)[5] in 2500 ml of water until 200 ml remains. Cool to a comfortably warm temperature, and use as a foot soak for 30 minutes, 1–2 times per day, for at least 10 days. Repeat as necessary. Maintain the warmth of the foot soak solution by re-warming as needed (Liu and Liu, 2001).

2. Bathe in hot water 1–2 times per day for 20–30 minutes at a time. Thirty days comprises one treatment course. After 30 days, rest for 10 days and repeat the treatment. According to Ma and An (2001), this procedure can relieve chronic inflammation in the male genitourinary tract and reduce hematospermia.

3. For hematospermia associated with chronic prostatitis and/or epididymitis, perform epididymal and prostatic massage 1–2 times per week for 4 weeks.

4. For heat and damp-heat patterns, make a decoction using 15–30 grams of *Jin Huang San* (Golden Yellow Powder),[6] boiled in enough water to yield a 1500–200 ml of medicinal solution. Use as a sitz bath twice per day for 2–3 weeks.

Preventive measures and lifestyle modification

1. Temporarily refrain from sexual activity

During treatment, patients should refrain from sexual activity of any kind for at least 1–2 weeks. They may slowly resume gentle sexual activity after this rest period, but remain alert for recurrence. For men who are not seeking to impregnate their female partner, temporarily wearing a condom is a useful way to capture ejaculated semen for easier tracking of recurrences.

2. Dietary modifications

To avoid the formation of depressed heat and dampness in the essence chamber, patients with hematospermia should avoid all spicy-hot, greasy-fried, sweet, and otherwise thick-flavored foods. Further, they should avoid drinking alcohol and smoking cigarettes.

3. Avoid long bicycle and horse rides

Prolonged or rough bicycle or horse riding subjects the anterior yin region to trauma and hence to qi stagnation and blood stasis. This can directly injure the network vessels and cause hematospermia, and can lead to depressed heat

---

[5] *Lu Cao* is sweet, bitter, and cold. It is being used in this instance to clear heat and free stran-gury.

[6] *Jin Huang San* consists of *Da Huang* (Rhei Radix et Rhizoma), *Huang Bai* (Phellodendri Cortex), *Jiang Huang* (Curcumae Longae Rhizoma), *Bai Zhi* (Angelicae Dahuricae Radix), *Tian Nan Xing* (Arisaematis Rhizoma), *Chen Pi* (Citri Reticulatae Pericarpium), *Hou Po* (Magnoliae Officinalis Cortex), *Gan Cao* (Glycyrrhizae Radix), and *Tian Hua Fen* (Trichosanthis Radix).

from stasis and stagnation. One can offset some of the trauma suffered during bike rides by using a softer bike seat with a "prostate-relief zone."

Representative Chinese Research

Supplementing the kidneys and eliminating dampness and clearing heat

Zhang et al. (1996) report on the treatment of 16 cases of hematospermia due to kidney vacuity and damp-heat. The formula is called Xue Jing Jie Du Yin (Bloody Essence Toxin-Resolving Beverage) and contains the following medicinals:

   Di Jin Cao (Euphorbiae Humifusae Herba), 30g
   Lu Xian Cao (Pyrolae Herba),[7] 30g
   Shi Wei (Pyrrosiae Folium), 40g
   Ma Bian Cao (Verbenae Herba), 40g
   Tu Fu Ling (Smilacis Glabrae Rhizoma), 20g

Results: Among the 16 cases treated, 15 were cured and 1 had no result, for a 93.7% total amelioration rate. The treatment period lasted from 1–2 weeks.

Enriching and boosting kidney yin, clearing heat and cooling blood, and stanching bleeding

Yuan *et al.* (1995) treated 34 cases of hematospermia with a formula called *Qing Shen Tang* (Kidney-Clearing Decoction). The ingredients were:

   Zhi Mu (Anemarrhenae Rhizoma), 15g
   Huang Bai (Phellodendri Cortex), 15g
   Bai Shao (Paeoniae Radix Alba), 12g
   Qian Cao Gen (Rubiae Radix), 12g
   Sheng Long Gu (Mastodi Ossis Fossilia Cruda), 30g
   Ze Xie (Alismatis Rhizoma), 30g
   Shan Yao (Dioscoreae Rhizoma), 30g
   Nu Zhen Zi (Ligustri Lucidi Fructus), 30g
   Han Lian Cao (Ecliptae Herba), 30g
   Tu Fu Ling (Smilacis Glabrae Rhizoma), 30g

During the study period, all patients were asked to refrain from indulging in sexual activity and spicy-hot foods and alcohol.

Modifications: For patients with prevalence of damp-heat, add *Long Dan Cao* (Gentianae Radix), 15g, and *Da Huang* (Rhei Radix et Rhizoma), 12g. For concurrent heart-spleen dual vacuity, add *Huang Qi* (Astragali Radix), 12g, and *Bai Zhu* (Atractylodis Macrocephalae Rhizoma), 12g, and have the patient take a 20-minute warm sitz bath 1–2 times per day.

---

[7] According to the *Zhang et al.* (1996), *Lu Xian Cao* boosts the kidneys, eliminates dampness, and stops bleeding.

Results: From among the 34 cases treated, 30 cases were completely cured (as established by normal-looking ejaculate, complete disappearance of clinical symptoms, and no red blood cells in the semen upon semen analysis), 4 cases had good results (as measured by disappearance of overt visible signs of blood in the ejaculate and fewer than 5/HP red blood cells in the ejaculate upon laboratory examination). Most patients noticed results within 3–10 days of initiating treatment.

Clearing heat and resolving toxicity, cooling and quickening blood, disinhibiting dampness and enriching yin

Zheng (1991) treated 26 cases of hematospermia with a formula called *Qing Jing Li Xue Tang* (Essence-Clearing Blood-Regulating Decoction), which was designed to clear heat and resolve toxicity, cool and quicken blood, and disinhibit dampness and enrich yin. The ingredients were as follows:

Bai Hua She She Cao (Oldenlandiae Diffusae Herba), 30g

Jin Yin Hua (Lonicerae Flos), 15g

Bi Xie (Dioscoreae Hypoglaucae seu Semptemlobae Rhizoma), 15g

Lian Qiao (Forsythiae Fructus), 15g

Sheng Di Yu (Sanguisorbae Radix Cruda), 15g

Qian Cao Gen (Rubiae Radix), 15g

Hu Zhang (Polygoni Cuspidati Rhizoma), 20g

Jin Qian Cao (Lysimachiae Herba), 20g

Bai Mao Gen (Imperatae Rhizoma), 20g

Che Qian Zi (Plantaginis Semen), 12g

Chi Shao (Paeoniae Radix Rubra), 12g

Mu Dan Pi (Moutan Cortex), 12g

Zhi Mu (Anemarrhenae Rhizoma), 12g

Huang Bai (Phellodendri Cortex), 12g

San Qi Fen (Notoginseng Radix Pulverata), 10g, stirred into the strained decoction

Shen Gan Cao Shao (Glycyrrhizae Radix Tenuis Cruda), 10g

Modifications: For pain in the lumbus referring to the perineum, add *Yan Hu Suo* (Corydalis Rhizoma), *Chuan Lian Zi* (Toosendan Fructus), *Wu Ling Zhi* (Trogopteri Faeces), and *Sheng Pu Huang* (Typhae Pollen Crudum). For enduring cases that are accompanied by blood stasis, add *Dan Shen* (Salviae Miltiorrhizae Radix), *Ji Xue Teng* (Spatholobi Caulis), *Tao Ren* (Persicae Semen), and *Hong Hua* (Carthami Flos). For kidney yin vacuity, add *Han Lian Cao* (Ecliptae Herba), *Nu Zhen Zi* (Ligustri Lucidi Fructus), *Gui Ban* (Testudinis Carapax et Plastrum), and *E Jiao* (Asini Corii Colla). For center burner qi vacuity, add *Sheng Huang Qi* (Astragali seu Hedysari Radix Cruda), *Sheng Bai Zhu* (Atractylodis Ovatae Rhizoma Crudum), *Huang Jing* (Polygonati Rhizoma), and *Shan Yao* (Dioscoreae Rhizoma).

Results: Among the 26 cases treated with variations of this formula for an average of 30 days, 20 were cured and 6 had good results.

Acumoxa therapy

Li *et al.* (1994) reported on 11 cases of hematospermia with acumoxa treatment based on pattern discrimination. For yin vacuity fire damaging the network vessels, they used *Shen Shu* (BL-23), *Xue Hai* (SP-10), *Tai Chong* (LV-3), *Yang Gu* (SI-5) and *San Yin Jiao* (SP-6). For qi and blood vacuity with insecurity of kidney qi, they used *Shen Shu* (BL-23), *Shen Que* (CV-8), *Qi Hai* (CV-6), *Zu San Li* (ST-36), and *Hui Yin* (CV-1). For damp-heat pouring downward, they used *Shen Shu* (BL-23), *Zhong Ji* (CV-3), and *Yin Ling Quan* (SP-9). In general, the investigators used supplementing and draining needle technique as appropriate to the condition, and added 3–5 minutes of moxa treatment as necessary.

Results: The researchers reported a 100% cure rate for the 11 cases they treated.

Representative Case Studies

Noninteraction of the heart and kidneys with hyperactive ministerial fire (Guo *et al.*, 1999)

A 28 year-old male was treated for hematospermia from noninteraction of the heart and kidneys and hyperactive ministerial fire with a variation of *Huang Lian E Jiao Tang* (Coptis and Ass Hide Glue Decoction). After returning home from a period of traveling abroad, he attended a banquet with friends and family at which he consumed a large quantity of alcohol. That night, he and his wife had sexual intercourse and they discovered blood in his semen. Also, he experienced a rough and obstructed sensation during ejaculation. At that time, he sought medical care at a hospital outpatient clinic and was diagnosed with epididymitis. He underwent a urinalysis at that time for acid-fast bacilli and the test was negative. He took many courses of antibiotics and hemostatic medicines (unspecified in the case report) for a period of three months and had no positive results. Hence, he came for Chinese medical treatment.

Upon examination he appeared emaciated, had soreness of the lumbus, dizzy head and copious dreaming, a red tongue with scanty fur, and a fine rapid pulse. The diagnosis was vacuity of kidney water below and hyperactive heart fire above, noninteraction of the heart and kidneys, and loss of benefit between water and fire leading to effulgent fire scorching the network vessels.

The physician prescribed a variation of *Huang Lian E Jiao Tang* which consisted of the following medicinals:
   Huang Lian (Coptidis Rhizoma), 5g
   Huang Qin (Scutellariae Radix), 10g
   E Jiao (Asini Corii Colla), 10g, dissolved into the strained decoction
   Bai Shao (Paeoniae Radix Alba), 30g
   Sheng Di Huang (Rehmanniae Radix Exsiccata seu Recens), 30g
   Nu Zhen Zi (Ligustri Lucidi Fructus), 30g
   Han Lian Cao (Ecliptae Herba), 30g
   Ji Zi Huang (Galli Vitellus), 1 yolk

Upon initiating treatment, the patient was advised to stop taking all Western medications. After taking 28 packets of the prescription, the symptoms completely disappeared.

Spleen and kidney qi vacuity with static blood and vanquished essence obstructing the network vessels

In Zhu (2001), a 63 year-old male with hematospermia was diagnosed with spleen and kidney qi vacuity with static blood and vanquished essence obstructing the network vessels. For the past two years, he had been experiencing hematospermia which was either brownish-red, dark purplish, or fresh red with bloody threads. Further, he had rough reddish urine, pain in the penis, a purple tongue with tooth marks on the margins and a slimy yellow fur, and a rough pulse.

The prescription was based on an experiential formula called *Xue Jing Fang* (Bloody Semen Formula) and *Xue Fu Zhu Yu Tang* (House of Blood Stasis-Expelling Decoction). The ingredients were as follows:

    Huang Qi (Astragali Radix), 30g
    Pao Jiang (Zingiberis Rhizoma Praeparatum), 3g
    Che Qian Zi (Plantaginis Semen), 12g
    Huang Bai (Phellodendri Cortex), 12g
    Shu Di Huang (Rehmanniae Radix Praeparata), 30g
    Pao Chuan Shan Jia (Manitis Squama Praeparatum), 10g
    Jing Jie Tan (Schizonepetae Herba et Flos Carbonisatae), 10g
    Pu Huang (Typhae Pollen), 9g
    Shan Zhu Yu (Corni Fructus), 15g
    Wang Bu Liu Xing (Vaccariae Semen), 15g
    Pu Gong Ying (Taraxaci Herba), 10g
    Gan Cao (Glycyrrhizae Radix), 5g

Note: Some medicinals from *Xue Fu Zhu Yu Tang* were also added, though the case report was less than clear which specific medicinals were chosen.

The patient took 14 packets of medicine and the hematospermia disappeared. Follow-up two years later indicated no recurrence of the problem.

Damp-heat pouring downward and mutual binding of heat and blood stasis

Chang and Sun (1997) provide a brief summary of a case reported in Fan (1989). The patient was diagnosed with damp-heat pouring downward and mutual binding of heat stasis in the network vessels of the essence chamber. The treatment principle was to clear and disinhibit damp-heat, to transform stasis and quicken the blood, and to cool the blood and stanch bleeding.

The prescription was based on an experiential formula called *Fan Shi Yi Pu Hui San* (Master Fan's Typha Pollen Cinders Powder) and contained the following medicinals:

Sheng Pu Huang (Typhae Pollen Crudum), 70g
Hua Shi (Talcum), 30g
Chao Shan Zhi Zi (Gardeniae Fructus Frictus), 30g
Chi Shao (Paeoniae Radix Rubra), 30g
Dang Gui (Angelicae Sinensis Radix), 30g
Sheng Di Huang (Rehmanniae Radix Exsiccata seu Recens), 30g
Mu Tong (Akebiae Trifoliatae Caulis), 30g
Chi Fu Ling (Poria Rubra), 30g
Sheng Gan Cao (Glycyrrhizae Radix Cruda), 30g

The medicinals were combined and ground into a fine powder and the patient was advised to boil 15 grams in water 3 times per day and to swallow the dregs along with the decoction. After 6 days, the condition was greatly improved. Doctor Fan then changed the prescription to:

Sheng Pu Huang (Typhae Pollen Crudum), 280g
Hua Shi (Talcum), 120g
Chao Shan Zhi Zi (Gardeniae Fructus Frictus), 120g

The patient took 10 grams of powder 3 times per day in the same manner as previously. After a little over two weeks, when the prescription was gone, the hematospermia completely disappeared.

Male Infertility

Western Medicine

When a man presents to his physician with at least a one-year history of unprotected intercourse without having impregnated his partner, and no determinable female factor has been found, male factor infertility is suspected. Estimates vary among different sources, but according to Greene, Johnston, and Lemcke (1998), male infertility may be a factor for 30–50% of the 5 million infertile couples in the United States, and the cause of male infertility is undetermined in 60–80% of all cases. According to Kasper, Braunwald, and Fauci *et al.*, (2005), the cause of infertility in about 17% of infertile couples in the United States is undetermined and the rate of infertility has remained stable over the past 30 years.

From among the known causes and manifestations of male infertility, 15–35% of cases are caused by varicocele, 8–10% of cases are caused by primary testicular failure, and the remaining 1–5% of cases are caused by one or more of the following factors: 1) chromosomal disorders (including Klinefelter's syndrome); 2) undescended testes; 3) radiation damage; 4) orchitis; 5) genital tract obstruction; 6) congenital absence of the vas deferens; 7) vasectomy; 8) epididymal obstruction; 9) hypogonadotropic hypogonadism; 10) pituitary adenomas; 11) panhypopituitarism; 12) hyperprolactinemia; 13) sperm autoimmunity; 14) drugs; 15) toxins; 16) subclinical *Chlamydia* infection and; 17) other systemic illnesses. Needless to say, the diagnosis in these cases can be quite complicated and usually requires more than one specialist for complete evaluation. Even then, exact diagnosis is often evasive.

The role of sexually-transmitted pathogens

According to Boggs (2007), as many as 18% of men with idiopathic infertility may have a subclinical sexually-transmitted disease (STD). This conclusion is based on finding the DNA of various sexually-transmitted pathogens including human papilloma virus (HPV), cytomegalovirus (CMV), herpes simplex virus (HSV), human herpes virus type 6 (HHV-6), Epstein-Barr virus (EBV), hepatitis

B virus (HBV) and *Chlamydia trachomatis* in the semen of men with idiopathic infertility.

The role of environmental estrogens

Some researchers have suggested that the increased entrance into the environment of plastics and other household and industrial chemicals and pesticides which contain xenoestrogens[1] such as polychlorinated biphenyls (PCBs) and phthalate esters (PEs) is having a detrimental effect on male fertility. Rozzati, Reddy, Reddanna, and Mujtaba (2002) found that infertile men had higher proportions of xenoestrogens in their semen than fertile men did. More than one study has shown that the main route of entry appears to be through intake of contaminated fish in the diet, though other sources suggest that overused plastic water bottles, and plastic food wrappings and containers (especially when washed with harsh detergents and reused) are also at fault. The leeching of these materials into food may be enhanced in the presence of heat, including when hot foods are placed in plastic immediately after cooking, or have contact with plastic during cooking as occurs when using microwave ovens.

History

Many factors and conditions can affect male fertility. Hence, when taking a thorough history, the physician will note factors such as history of paternity, frequency, timing, and technique of sexual intercourse, and use of contraceptives and spermicidal lubricants, chemotherapy, radiation exposure, medications (including over-the-counter medications), exposure to occupational and environmental toxins, recent infections and febrile illnesses, surgeries, and use of anabolic steroids or recreational drugs such as cocaine and cannabis.

Physical examination

The main goal of a physical examination in the evaluation of an infertile male is to detect any evidence of androgen deficiency or anatomical abnormality that would cause infertility. Findings that would raise the physician's suspicion include: 1) eunuchoidal features including underdeveloped testes, and decrease or absence of secondary sexual characteristics including pubic, axillary, and chest hair; 2) increased body fat and decreased muscle mass; 3) gynecomastia; 4) abnormal exam of the epididymis or vas deferens; 5) palpation of a varicocele, which is classically described as feeling like a "bag of worms" and; 6) the detection of an abnormal prostate upon digital rectal examination (DRE). Any abnormal findings on physical examination are correlated with laboratory and other findings in order to support proper diagnosis. For example, physicians: 1) order testicular ultrasound to confirm the presence of a varicocele suggested by physical examination. And if confirmed they will usually refer the patient for a surgical consult; 2) order laboratory examination to assess the degree of androgen insufficiency when they observe eunuchoidal features during physical examination and; 3) order genetic testing when they suspect Klinefelter's syndrome or other genetic abnormalities.

---

[1] Xenoestrogens are estrogens that are present in the human body but should not be, and that originate from external sources.

Diagnosis

I. Laboratory examination

• Semen analysis (SA)

Although the diagnosis of male infertility is dependent on history and the correlation of physical and laboratory examination, the first step in making a diagnosis is to obtain a semen analysis (SA), because it gives an objective picture to the evaluating physician. When a couple states that they have already had a normal semen analysis, fertility specialists (and specialists of Chinese andrology) should insist on obtaining the records themselves and should carefully scrutinize the results. Sometimes a "normal" result in the past turns out on closer inspection to be subnormal, indicating subfertility that is amenable to treatment. Many men are embarrassed to admit that they might have a fertility challenge, and this sometimes leads to delay in diagnosis, and premature commencement of costly and potentially risky female infertility treatments. Further, most authorities recommend the collection of at least two samples, separated by at least one week, when the initial SA is abnormal.

To perform an SA, semen is collected by masturbation after at least a 48–hour period of abstinence and is evaluated for volume, sperm density, sperm motility, percentage of normal morphology, and the presence or absence of agglutination, pyospermia, or hyperviscosity. According to the World Health Organization (WHO), 1994, normal values for semen analysis are as follows:

Normal Values for Semen

- **Seminal volume:** 2.0–5ml
- **Seminal pH:** 7.2–8.0
- **Sperm density (sperm concentration; sperm count):** >20 million/ml or ≥ 40 million per ejaculate
- **Sperm motility:** ≥50% forward-moving sperm or ≥20% total motile sperm
- **Sperm morphology:** ≥30% normal
- **Sperm vitality:** >75% of sperm are alive
- **Semen liquefaction time:** <30 minutes
- **Seminal white blood cells:** <1 million/ml

• Blood work

Serum testosterone levels are evaluated, especially when a man has low sperm concentration on repeated semen analysis. When testosterone is low, luteinizing hormone (LH) and follicle stimulating hormone (FSH) are also checked; when elevated, this suggests primary gonadal deficiency. Prolactin levels should be considered, especially when gynecomastia is present; elevated serum prolactin suggests other conditions, most notably pituitary adenoma.

• Imaging studies

When varicocele is suspected, testicular ultrasound is used to ascertain its presence. If hypothalamic or pituitary disease is suggested by other findings, MRI is usually ordered.

• Testicular biopsy

When diagnosis is evasive and treatment has failed, and when other clinical suspicions exist, a specialist may order a testicular biopsy to evaluate otherwise unexplained spermatogenic malfunction. Testicular biopsy is also used as a means of harvesting sperm for intra-cytoplasmic sperm injection (ICSI).

Treatment

1. General approach to treatment

• Psychological treatment

Once a definitive diagnosis is established, treatment logically follows. As we have seen, however, the majority of cases of male infertility are idiopathic. This often makes for a stressful experience for the man and his partner. He is sometimes faced with feelings of inadequacy, anger and frustration, and at times these feelings can be present to the extent that they constitute formidable challenges to the ongoing health of a couple's relationship. Because of this, individual and/or couple's counseling is suggested early in the process of treatment of male infertility. The focus of treatment should be on stress management, the development and maintenance of communication skills, and acceptance of personal limitations when treatment is unsuccessful. Exploring the couple's openness and/or resistance to adoption as an alternative is also reasonable, especially when clinical success is delayed or absent.

• Timing and frequency of intercourse

Infertile couples should be counseled on the importance of having intercourse frequently (though not too frequently so as to insure adequate sperm concentration at the time of intercourse), and especially around ovulation. Using an ovulation detection kit and tracking the woman's basal body temperature (BBT) can be helpful, especially for women who have erratic menstrual cycles. In some cases, however, especially when a couple has been struggling with fertility issues for some time, intercourse may begin to take on the nature of a goal-oriented task rather than being a spontaneous and loving exchange. In such cases, simply having intercourse 2–3 times per week, every week, may be a more comfortable option than the potentially-stressful experience of closely tracking ovulation and BBT and matching intercourse with this data.

2. Specific treatments

• Mild male-factor infertility

According to Kasper, Braunwald, and Fauci et al. (2005), mild male factor infertility is characterized by a sperm count of 15–20 million/ml and normal sperm motility. No specific management is necessary other than expectant waiting.

• Moderate male factor infertility

Moderate male factor infertility is characterized by a sperm count of 10–15 million/ml and 20–40% sperm motility. The recommended treatment is intrauterine insemination (IUI), possibly combined with pharmaceutical treatment of the female partner with clomiphene citrate or gonadotropins to increase the chances of successful fertilization, or *in vitro* fertilization (IVF)[2] with or without intra-cytoplasmic sperm injection (ICSI)[3] (Kasper, Braunwald, and Fauci *et al.*, 2005).

• *Severe male-factor infertility*

Severe male factor infertility is defined by a sperm count of less than 10 million/ml and 10% sperm motility. The recommended management is *in vitro* fertilization (IVF) with intra-cytoplasmic sperm injection (ICSI) or donor sperm (Kasper, Braunwald, and Fauci *et al.*, 2005).

3. Surgery

Surgery is primarily used for disorders of sperm transport, namely, varicocele or vas deferens obstruction.

• *Varicocele*

Varicocele is a condition in which a varicosity forms within a vein in the pampinoform plexus in the spermatic cord. This results in a higher intra-testicular temperature and impaired spermatogenesis. Varicocele may be present in one or both testes. Interestingly, a varicocele in one testicle can also raise the temperature in the neighboring testicle due to proximity. Although varicocele without infertility does not require specific treatment unless it causes significant discomfort, when it is present in an infertile male, it is removed by surgery (varicocelectomy).

• *Vas deferens obstruction*

Vas deferens obstruction may be caused a number of factors including vasectomy, accidental ligation or injury of the vas during inguinal surgery, and congenital anomalies. A surgical procedure called vasovasostomy is sometimes helpful in correcting the obstruction by making the vas patent.

4. Gonadotropin-releasing hormone (GnRH) or gonadotropins

GnRH or gonadotropin treatment is used for the treatment of male infertility when testosterone levels are low due to primary or secondary hypogonadism. Primary hypogonadism means that there is congenital or acquired primary testicular failure with low testosterone levels and high levels of the pituitary hormones luteinizing hormone (LH) and follicle-stimulating hormone (FSH), which normally stimulate the Leydig cells within the testes to produce testosterone. It may be caused by genetic disorders (especially by Klinefelter's syndrome or Y

---

[2] In *in vitro* fertilization, the woman is usually hormonally stimulated with gonadotropins to stimulate multiple ovarian follicles, and some of the eggs are removed from her ovaries. They are then fertilized by sperm in a fluid medium outside the womb and implanted into the uterus.
[3] This procedure consists of injecting a single sperm into the cytoplasm of the egg using a tiny hollow needle.

chromosome microdeletions), by uncorrected cryptorchidism (undescended testes), testicular trauma or torsion, infectious orchitis, radiation damage, pharmaceutical damage, environmental hazards and chemical toxicity, and many other conditions. Secondary hypogonadism is characterized by low testosterone levels and low FH and FSH. It is usually caused by a hypothalamic-pituitary defect such as pituitary microadenoma or hypothalamic tumor.

GnRH or gonadotropin treatment is mostly used for male infertility due to secondary hypogonadism, and only occasionally for that due to primary hypogonadism. However, according to Attia *et al.* (2007), gonadotropin treatment for idiopathic subfertility has been associated with increased pregnancy rates during and within three months of beginning treatment.

Western Complementary Medicine

Because many cases of male infertility are from unknown causes and therefore mainstream medical treatment is often unsuccessful, many researchers are looking to alternative and complementary medicine for some new ideas about causation and for new treatments of male infertility.

• Folic acid and zinc sulfate

More than one study has found that folic acid and zinc sulfate supplementation can improve sperm counts in subfertile men. For example, Wong, Merkus, and Thomas, *et. al.* (2002) found that oral administration of 5mg of folic acid and 66mg of zinc sulfate significantly increased total sperm count (by 74%) in both the fertile and subfertile men in their study.

• L-carnitine (LC), acetyl-L-carnitine (ALC), or combined LC and ALC

According to Agarwal and Said (2005), "L-carnitine (LC) and acetyl-L-carnitine (ALC) are highly concentrated in the epididymis and play a crucial role in sperm metabolism and maturation. They are related to sperm motility and have antioxidant properties." There has been some conflicting evidence about the efficacy of these amino acids for male infertility, but recently a study by Balercia, Regoli, and Koverich *et al.* (2005) found that oral administration of LC and ALC—either alone or in combination—significantly improved sperm motility in men with asthenozoospermia. Among the studies that show positive outcome, at least 3g per day were used.

• Vitamin E and selenium

One area of research in unexplained male infertility is the causative role of oxidative stress on sperm. Kessoupoulu, Powers, and Sharma, *et al.* (1995) found that 600mg per day of vitamin E "significantly improves the *in vitro* function of human spermatozoa as assessed by the sperm–zona pellucida (ZP) binding assay."[4]

---

[4] The sperm–zona pellucida (ZP) binding assay is a means of measuring the ability of sperm to bind to the zona pellucida—the membrane that forms around the ovum as it develops in the ovary.

Kesskes-Ammar and Feki-Chakroun *et al.* (2003) found that three-month oral supplementation with 400mg per day of vitamin E and 225mcg per day of selenium significantly improved sperm motility.

• Vitamin C and beta-carotene

Eskenazi and Kidd *et al.* (2005) report that higher sperm quality and therefore improved fertility is associated with higher intake of antioxidants including zinc, folate, vitamins E and C, and beta-carotene.

Chinese Medicine

Disease discrimination

In Chinese andrology, male infertility is suspected when a couple has been having unprotected intercourse for two or more years, and there are no known female factors at play.[5] There are several traditional Chinese disease categories that apply to male infertility, including [male] infertility (*bu yu* and *jue yu*), childlessness (*wu zi*), and male difficulty in [producing] an heir (*nan zi nan ci*).

The earliest mention of infertility in Chinese literature is in the *Yi Jing* (*Canon of Change*),[6] which uses the term female infertility (*nu yun bu yu*), but more specific discussions of male infertility are found in the *Nei Jing* (*Inner Canon*).[7] For example, in chapter 1 of *Su Wen* (*Plain Questions*),[8] it states: "At seven times eight [*i.e.*, 56 years of age], a man's essence is scant. At eight times eight [*i.e.*, 64 years of age], heavenly tenth is expired and [he is] unable to have children." In Chao Yuan-Fang's Tang dynasty masterpiece—*Zhu Bing Yuan Hou Lun* (*On the Origin and Indicators of Disease*)[9]—we find additional discussions of the disease causes and pathomechanisms of male infertility. In the *Bei Ji Qian Jin Yao Fang* (*A Thousand Gold Pieces Emergency Formulary*),[10] we find discussions of male infertility due to insufficiency of essence under the heading of seeking children (*qiu zi*), and seed (*zi*) medicinals are recommended for its treatment.[11] Later in the Ming dynasty, Ye Tian-Shi, began using the term male difficulty in [producing] an heir (*nan zi nan ci*). Nowa-

---

[5] It is interesting to note that the Chinese definition of infertility requires two years of unprotected intercourse and the Western definition only requires one year.

[6] The *Yi Jing* was probably written some time during the early Zhou dynasty (around 1000 BCE), though the exact date of its publication is uncertain. Legend attributes authorship to Fu Xi, one of the three legendary emperors of China.

[7] The *Nei Jing* was written in the 1st century CE.

[8] *Su Wen* is the first section of the *Nei Jing*.

[9] *Zhu Bing Yuan Hou Lun* was published by Chao Yuan-Fang in 610 CE, during the Sui dynasty.

[10] *Bei Ji Qian Jin Yao Fang* was written by Sun Si-Miao, and published during the 7th century CE, during the Tang dynasty.

[11] Seed medicinals, along with medicinals with an affinity to flesh and blood (*xue rou you qing zhi pin*) have a special resonance with essence and are often used to replenish essence. In this specific example, Sun Si-Miao recommended *Tu Si Zi* (Cuscutae Semen) and *Wu Wei Zi* (Schisandrae Fructus).

days, under the influence of modern Western medicine, andrology books usually use the term male infertility (*nan xing bu yu zheng*).

Although it is considered a separate disease category on its own, I must mention another Chinese andrological disease category in the context of male infertility—inability to ejaculate (*bu she jing zheng*). Although this is the most common name for this condition, it is also traditionally listed under the headings of nonejaculation of semen (*jing bu xie*) and essence block (*jing bi*). Regardless of the specific name, the chief manifestation of this condition is the normal attainment of erection during sexual activity, but without ejaculation of semen through the urethra. Often, some time later, the man will notice semen in his urine or spontaneous leakage of semen from the urethra some time after orgasm. When we seek to reframe male infertility into its pertinent Chinese andrological disease category, we should remember to also look for insight under these headings. This disease category embodies modern Chinese andrologists' experiences in treating conditions such as retrograde ejaculation, which can be a factor in male infertility.

Disease causes and pathomechanisms

In Chinese medicine, there are several physiological factors that must come together to enable a man to be fertile. He must have adequate kidney essence, his life gate fire must be sufficiently warm to power the engenderment and transformation of kidney essence into semen and sperm, he must have free-flowing liver qi to regulate kidney qi transformation and maintain normal ejaculatory function, he must be free of substantial obstructions such as phlegm and blood stasis so that the seminal pathway is sufficiently patent to allow normal ejaculation, he must be free of damp-heat and heat toxins in the essence chamber that might otherwise scorch and decoct the semen and damage the sperm, and he must have adequate qi and blood to ensure the constant cultivation of later heaven essence which can be stored in the kidney and can supplement early heaven essence. In clinical practice, men usually become infertile because they have a failure in two or more of these physiological aspects of their fertility.

It is important to note that prior to the past few decades—during which the modern clinical specialty of Chinese andrology truly flowered—male infertility was most often seen as a problem of kidney essence vacuity and debility of life gate fire. Prior to this modern period of development, there were relatively few sources which reflected a sophisticated understanding of the role of repletion disease causes and pathomechanisms in male infertility. We now know that damp-heat, phlegm, and blood stasis are extremely important factors in the development of male infertility, and we can deliver our patients mature treatment strategies that fully take them into account.

• Natural endowment insufficiency or acquired constitutional debility and weakness of kidney essence

The kidney stores essence and governs growth and reproduction. The kidney stores both early heaven essence (endowed by one's parents) and later heaven essence (acquired from water and grain essence). Essence serves as the most substantial and foundational raw material which can be differentiated into various other physiological substances necessary for normal functioning of the human body, including qi, blood, fluids, and semen and sperm.[12] This means that the quantity and quality of one's sperm is directly dependent on the quantity and quality of one's essence.

Chapter 1 of *Su Wen* (*Plain Questions*) states: "At two times eight [*i.e.*, 16 years of age in men], kidney qi [*i.e.*, essence] is effulgent and heavenly tenth (*tian gui*) arrives, essential qi flows downward and yin and yang are in harmony; [hence], there is the ability to have a child." This quote reveals that once kidney essence reaches a state of abundance, heavenly tenth—the substance which endows humans with their reproductive capacity—flows downward into the thoroughfare (*chong mai*) and conception vessels (*ren mai*) and creates fertility. It follows then that when a male is either born with an insufficient natural endowment of early heaven essence, or when he suffers a disease or adopts habits which significantly waste his supply of stored kidney essence (a combination of early heaven and later heaven essence), heavenly tenth ceases to flow and he either never attains or he loses his fertility. In modern clinical practice, we understand that this pathomechanism can lead to decreased seminal volume, low sperm density (total sperm count), abnormal morphology, and increased seminal viscosity and liquefaction time.

• Life gate fire debility with vacuous and cold essential qi
Normally life gate fire (*ming men zhi huo*)[13] provides the warmth and activation for the entire body and especially for the sexual, reproductive, and urinary functions of the kidney. When life gate fire is sufficient, it catalyzes the transformation of kidney essence into kidney qi, and encourages the engenderment and transformation of semen and sperm. In the modern clinical practice of Chinese andrology, it ensures that sperm are adequately and properly formed and sufficiently motile, and that the seminal fluid is not overly "cold" and therefore too dilute and watery.

Some authors reason that the liquefaction of semen is powered by kidney yang and cite decreased liquefaction time in patterns of kidney yang vacuity (Chen and Jiang, 2000, p. 397). Kidney essence and life gate fire may be damaged by excessive sexual activity (especially at a young age) including excessive masturbation. Over a long period of time, kidney qi and kidney yang are affected, the essence chamber is damaged, and the clinical picture of "vacuous and cold essential qi" (*jing qi xu leng*) emerges. This essentially means that there is kidney yang vacuity with clinical manifestations of sexual and/or reproductive disease. Hence, when there is debility of life gate fire, there may be yang wilt or other sexual dysfunction, and infertility due to either increased seminal volume, low sperm density, delayed liquefaction time, abnormal morphology, or decreased sperm motility.

---

[12] I have been intrigued in recent years by the resonance between the Chinese concept of essence in the human body and the emerging Western understanding of stem cells.

[13] Life gate fire (*ming men zhi huo*) refers to the warmth and activation and therefore life promoting action provided by kidney yang.

• Turbid phlegm and static blood obstructing the essence pathway
Constitutional spleen qi vacuity and excessive consumption of sweets, greasy-fried, and fatty foods lead to splenic movement and transformation failure. This results in the accumulation of water-damp and in food stagnation, which become depressed and then either singly or mutually congeal into phlegm. This blocks the essence pathway and forms a significant obstruction to normal male sexual and reproductive function. Hence, this pathomechanism may cause decreased seminal volume, decreased sperm density, increased liquefaction time, inability to ejaculate, or abnormal morphology.

As a yin evil—and thus as a source of obstruction to the movement and transformation of other yin aspects of the human body—phlegm depression leads to blood depression. The joining of phlegm and blood stasis is described as a "mutual binding of phlegm and blood stasis," or simply as "phlegm-stasis" (*tan yu*). Although static blood may have its origins in phlegm depression, it may also arise independently of it through the blood-decocting power of heat, or through trauma, surgery, or the entrance of enduring illness into the network vessels.[14] Whatever its origins, static blood—either alone or in concert with phlegm—is a formidable barrier to male fertility in that it may block the penis and the essence chamber and pathway, and may thereby interfere with the normal formation and distribution of semen and sperm. This can lead to inability to ejaculate, abnormal morphology, decreased seminal volume and density, increased seminal viscosity and increased liquefaction time, as well as to decreased motility.

• Liver depression and qi stagnation
The liver governs free coursing of all qi, blood, and fluids within the human body. Its channel skirts around the genitals and thus free flow within the liver viscus and its associated channels and tissues is necessary in order for the penis and the essence pathway to function normally. Normal erection—which is of course a prerequisite to ejaculation and delivery of sperm—requires free-flowing liver qi, and patency of the essence pathway is similarly dependent on liver's free-coursing. Because it fails to provide free coursing, depressed liver qi can cause male infertility by causing a decrease in the production of sperm. Or, by resulting in an inability to ejaculate and hence to a lack of distribution of semen and sperm, liver depression can cause infertility even in a man with adequate sperm-producing capacity. Enduring anger, resentment, frustration, hatred, and unfulfilled desires can lead to liver depression and very often to its natural outcome: depressed fire. When heat enters the essence chamber, it scorches semen and sperm and decocts blood; hence, it may cause decreased seminal volume, increased viscosity, prolonged liquefaction time, decreased sperm density, and abnormal morphology.

• Damp-heat pouring downward
When a man has poor dietary habits such as overconsumption of alcohol, greasy-

---

[14] This concept is usually attributed to Ye Tian-Shi and summarized under the dictum "enduring diseases enter the network vessels."

fried foods, fatty foods, and sweets, his splenic movement and transformation of both water and grain and water-damp becomes impaired. This leads to the collection of water-damp and food stagnation which become depressed over time and transforms heat. Dampness and heat then mutually contend and pour downward from the center burner to the lower burner. Damp-heat acts as a significant obstructive factor in normal male sexuality and fertility. When damp-heat enters the essence chamber, it scorches essence and obstructs the essence pathway, and can result in premature ejaculation, hematospermia, decreased seminal volume, increased viscosity and prolonged liquefaction time, abnormal morphology, decreased sperm density, or inability to ejaculate. Further, when lower burner damp-heat obstructs qi and blood flow to the penis, yang wilt results.

• Dual vacuity of qi and blood

To understand the connection between qi and blood to essence, it is helpful to first understand the dictum "the liver and kidney share the same source." Although explained in greater detail in Book 1, Chapter 4 on viscera-bowel physiology, most pertinent to our current discussion here is the fact that surplus liver blood can be stored in the kidney as essence. This is often also summarized under the heading that later heaven and early heaven mutually transform into one another. If surplus liver blood can be transformed into essence and stored in the kidney, it can supplement early heaven essence and make it more abundant. The more essence stored in the kidney, the more raw material there is for the engenderment, nourishment, and activation of sperm. It follows that those with an abundance of qi and blood would have adequate essence and would be more fertile than those with insufficient qi and blood. Thus, in male infertility, qi and blood vacuity always appears in concert with kidney essence vacuity and so leads to the same sperm abnormalities as those discussed above. Common causes of qi and blood vacuity include constitutional vacuity, dietary irregularities, and overtaxation.

Pattern discrimination and treatment_____

1. Kidney yin vacuity

Signs: Low seminal volume, low sperm density, prolonged semen liquefaction time, and high levels of abnormal morphology, soreness and weakness of the lumbus and knees, dizzy head and tinnitus, signs of sexual dysfunction including either seminal emission, premature ejaculation, frequent erections, or inability to ejaculate, insomnia and forgetfulness, vexing heat in the five hearts, night sweats, dry mouth and throat, thin emaciated physique, pain in the heels,[15] dry stools, red tongue with scanty fur or lack of fur, fine rapid pulse.

Treatment principles: Enrich yin and supplement the kidney, replenish essence and engender sperm

---

[15] This reflects insufficient nourishment to the kidney channel. From my personal experience, this sign is fairly common in such patients. I also find that fairly consistently patients with kidney yin vacuity exhibit a physical concavity in the area of *Tai Xi* (KI-3), the source point of the kidney channel.

Guiding formulas: Modified *Wu Zi Yan Zong Wan* (Five-Seed Progeny Pill) plus *Zuo Gui Yin* (Left-Restoring [Kidney Yin] Beverage)

Ingredients:
> *Tu Si Zi* (Cuscutae Semen), 15g
> *Gou Qi Zi* (Lycii Fructus), 15g
> *Fu Pen Zi* (Rubi Fructus), 15g
> *Shu Di Huang* (Rehmanniae Radix Praeparata), 15g
> *Shan Zhu Yu* (Corni Fructus), 10g
> *Wu Wei Zi* (Schisandrae Fructus), 10g
> *Shan Yao* (Dioscoreae Rhizoma), 10g
> *Fu Ling* (Poria), 10g
> *Che Qian Zi* (Plantaginis Semen), 20g
> *Gan Cao* (Glycyrrhizae Radix), 3g

Modifications: For patients with premature ejaculation and seminal emission, add *Duan Long Gu* (Mastodi Ossis Fossilia Calcinata), 15g, *Duan Mu Li* (Ostreae Concha Calcinata), 15g, *Jin Ying Zi* (Rosae Laevigatae Fructus), 10g, and *Wu Wei Zi* (Schisandrae Fructus), 10g, to help kidney qi to secure essence. For decreased sperm density and motility accompanied by qi and essence-blood vacuity, add *Huang Qi* (Astragali Radix), 15g, *Dang Shen* (Codonopsis Radix), 15g, *Mai Men Dong* (Ophiopogonis Radix), 10g, *He Shou Wu* (Polygoni Multiflori Radix), 15g, and *Lu Lu Tong* (Liquidambaris Fructus), 10g, to supplement spleen qi, nourish yin, enrich kidney essence, and free the seminal pathway. For prolonged liquefaction time, add *Xuan Shen* (Scrophulariae Radix), 12g, *Mai Men Dong* (Ophiopogonis Radix), 10g, *Tian Men Dong* (Asparagi Radix), 10g, *Sheng Di Huang* (Rehmanniae Radix Exsiccata seu Recens), 15g, and *Zhi Mu* (Anemarrhenae Rhizoma), 10g, to further supplement kidney yin, replenish essence, and engender fluid. For hyperactive ministerial fire due to kidney yin vacuity, add *Zhi Mu* (Anemarrhenae Rhizoma), 10g, *Huang Bai* (Phellodendri Cortex), 10g, *Han Lian Cao* (Ecliptae Herba), 10g, *Nu Zhen Zi* (Ligustri Lucidi Fructus), 12g, and *Mu Dan Pi* (Moutan Cortex), 10g, to clear heat, drain fire, and nourish yin. For detriment and damage to kidney essence, add *Huang Jing* (Polygonati Rhizoma), 10g, and medicinals with an affinity to flesh and blood[16] such as *Gui Ban Jiao* (Testudinis Carapacis et Plastri Gelatinum), 10g, *Lu Jiao Jiao* (Cervi Cornus Gelatinum), 10g, Hominis Placenta (*Zi He Che*), 6g, and Cordyceps (*Dong Chong Xia Cao*), 2 grams of a 5:1 extract twice per day. For concurrent damp-heat in the lower burner, use *Zhi Bai Di Huang Wan* (Anemarrhena, Phellodendron, and Rehmannia Pill) as the base formula, and add *Che Qian Zi* (Plantaginis

---

[16] Medicinals with an affinity to flesh and blood are medicinals generally produced from animal by-products. Although this treatment method can be traced back to the *Nei Jing* (*Inner Canon*), Ye Tian-Shi, in his Qing dynasty text, *Lin Zheng Zhi Nan Yi An* (*A Clinical Guide with Case Histories*) succinctly stated it in the following way: "Essence and blood have form. [Therefore do not], use grasses and wood—substances which lack feeling—in order to supplement and boost [them]; their qi does not correspond [to essence and blood]."

Semen), 15g, *Cang Zhu* (Atractylodis Rhizoma), 12g, *Bi Xie* (Dioscoreae Hypoglaucae seu Semptemlobae Rhizoma), 12g, and *Tu Fu Ling* (Smilacis Glabrae Rhizoma), 10g.[17] If there is hematospermia due to frenetic heat scorching the network vessels in the seminal pathway, use *Zhi Bai Di Huang Wan* (Anemarrhena, Phellodendron, and Rehmannia Pill) plus *Dan Shen* (Salviae Miltiorrhizae Radix), 10g, *Chi Shao* (Paeoniae Radix Rubra), 10g, *Di Yu Tan* (Sanguisorbae Radix Carbonisata), 10g, and *Bai Mao Gen* (Imperatae Rhizoma), 12g, to enrich yin and to clear heat, cool blood, and stanch bleeding.

2. Kidney yang vacuity

Signs: Clear cold semen,[18] low sperm motility, low sperm vitality, prolonged liquefaction time, weak ejaculation with decreased intensity of orgasm, low libido, yang wilt, premature ejaculation, coldness and weakness of lumbus and knees, aversion to cold and cold limbs, listlessness of essence-spirit, fatigued spirit and lack of strength, somber-white facial complexion, a sensation of cold and dampness in the anterior yin region, long clear urination, frequent nocturia, pale enlarged tongue with white moist fur, sinking fine forceless pulse (*ruo mai*) which is noticeably weak in the cubit position.

Treatment principles: Supplement the kidney and warm yang, replenish essence

Guiding formulas: Modified *You Gui Wan* (Right-Restoring [Life Gate] Pill) and *Wu Zi Yan Zong Wan* (Five-Seed Progeny Pill)

Ingredients:
> *Fu Zi* (Aconiti Radix Lateralis Praeparata), 6g
> *Rou Gui* (Cinnamomi Cortex), 6g
> *Shu Di Huang* (Rehmanniae Radix Praeparata), 10g
> *Shan Yao* (Dioscoreae Rhizoma), 12g
> *Shan Zhu Yu* (Corni Fructus), 12g
> *Lu Jiao Jiao* (Cervi Cornus Gelatinum), 6g
> *Du Zhong* (Eucommiae Cortex), 15g
> *Gou Qi Zi* (Lycii Fructus), 15g
> *Dang Gui* (Angelicae Sinensis Radix), 12g
> *Wu Wei Zi* (Schisandrae Fructus), 10g
> *Fu Pen Zi* (Rubi Fructus), 10g
> *Tu Si Zi* (Cuscutae Semen), 15g
> *Rou Cong Rong* (Cistanches Herba), 10g
> *Xian Mao* (Curculiginis Rhizoma), 10g
> *Yin Yang Huo* (Epimedii Herba), 12g

---

[17] In cases where damp-heat is prominent, it is prudent to first emphasize damp-heat clearing and to gradually increase one's emphasis on enriching yin. When prostatitis is suspected, use the protocols discussed in Prostatitis: Book 2, Chapter 1.

[18] Clear cold semen means that the semen is watery, dilute, and cold to the touch. This corresponds to the dictum from *Nei Jing* (*Inner Canon*) which states that "All watery, clear, and dilute discharges are ascribed to cold."

Modifications: For low libido, yang wilt, and dilute semen, add *Yang Qi Shi* (Actinolitum), 10g, and *Jiu Cai Zi* (Allii Tuberosi Semen), 10g, to further supplement the kidneys and invigorate yang. For low sperm motility, add *Ren Shen* (Ginseng Radix), 10g, and *Huang Qi* (Astragali Radix), 15g, to supplement the spleen and boost qi. For delayed liquefaction of semen, add *Gan Jiang* (Zingiberis Rhizoma), 6g, to assist yang qi transformation. For patients who also have premature ejaculation or seminal efflux, add *Lian Xu* (Nelumbinis Stamen), 10g, and *Duan Long Gu* (Mastodi Ossis Fossilia Calcinata), 15g, to secure essence. For inability to ejaculate, add *Zi Shi Ying* (Fluoritum), 10g, and *Wang Bu Liu Xing Zi* (Vaccariae Semen), 12g, to further invigorate yang and free the essence gate.

3. Dual vacuity of spleen and kidney qi and insufficiency of heart and liver blood

Signs: Dilute semen, low sperm density, low sperm motility and vitality, decreased libido, yang wilt and premature ejaculation, nonlustrous facial complexion, physical weakness, abdominal distention and loose stools, soreness and limpness of the lumbus and knees, listlessness of essence-spirit, palpitations and fearful throbbing, insomnia with copious dreams, poor memory and dizzy head and eyes, low appetite and torpid intake, laziness to speak and shortness of breath, pale nails, pale tongue with scanty fur, deep fine or soft pulse.

Treatment principles: Boost qi and supplement the spleen, nourish and enrich blood, supplement the kidneys and replenish essence

Guiding formulas: Modified *Yu Lin Zhu* (Unicorn-Rearing Pill) and *Shi Quan Da Bu Tang* (Perfect Major Supplementation Decoction)

Ingredients:
    Ren Shen (Ginseng Radix), 15g
    Chao Bai Zhu (Atractylodis Macrocephalae Rhizoma Frictum), 15g
    Fu Ling (Poria), 12g
    Bai Shao (Paeoniae Radix Alba), 12g
    Dang Gui (Angelicae Sinensis Radix), 12g
    Shu Di Huang (Rehmanniae Radix Praeparata), 12g
    Chuan Xiong (Chuanxiong Rhizoma), 10g
    Tu Si Zi (Cuscutae Semen), 15g
    Gou Qi Zi (Lycii Fructus), 15g
    Shan Yao (Dioscoreae Rhizoma), 15g
    Shan Zhu Yu (Corni Fructus), 12g
    Du Zhong (Eucommiae Cortex), 15g
    Lu Jiao Jiao (Cervi Cornus Gelatinum), 10g
    Hua Jiao (Zanthoxyli Pericarpium), 3g
    Huang Qi (Astragali Radix), 30g
    Rou Gui (Cinnamomi Cortex), 6g
    Zhi Gan Cao (Glycyrrhizae Radix cum Liquido Fricta), 3g

Modifications: For markedly low sperm motility, add *Yin Yang Huo* (Epimedii Herba), 15g, and *Ba Ji Tian* (Morindae Officinalis Radix), 15g, to further supplement the kidneys and improve the motility of sperm. For low sperm density, add *He Shou Wu* (Polygoni Multiflori Radix), 12g, *Huang Jing* (Polygonati Rhizoma), 10g, and *Nu Zhen Zi* (Ligustri Lucidi Fructus), 12g, to supplement the kidneys, nourish blood, and engender essence. For inability to ejaculate, add *Shi Chang Pu* (Acori Tatarinowii Rhizoma), 6g, and *Wu Gong* (Scolopendra), 1g, to free the seminal pathway and open the lower orifice. For delayed liquefaction of semen, add *Wu Mei* (Mume Fructus), 6g, *He Zi* (Chebulae Fructus), 6g, and *Sheng Gan Cao* (Glycyrrhizae Radix Cruda), 3g, to engender fluid through the combination of sweet and sour flavors. For more pronounced heart blood vacuity and insomnia, add *Suan Zao Ren* (Ziziphi Spinosi Semen), 15g, *Yuan Zhi* (Polygalae Radix), 10g, and *Ye Jiao Teng* (Polygoni Multiflori Caulis), 10g.

4. Damp-heat pouring downward

Signs: Thicker yellow semen, nonliquefaction or prolonged liquefaction of semen, high levels of white blood cells or pus in the semen, low seminal volume, high quantity of dead sperm in the semen, low sperm motility, possible delayed ejaculation, priapism, or inability to ejaculate, a sensation of distention and pain in the genitals after sexual activity, short reddish urine with a scorching sensation and possible pain in the penis, a tendency to have an overly warm and moist genital area with possible genital malodor, swollen itchy genitals and a tendency to have moist, red, and warm skin outbreaks in the inguinal and testicular region, soreness and heaviness in the lumbus, heavy sensation in the legs, generalized fatigue and lack of strength, heaviness of the head, heart vexation and dry mouth with desire for cool fluids, unsmooth bowel movements, red tongue with yellow slimy fur, and a slippery stringlike rapid pulse.

Treatment principles: Clear and disinhibit dampness and heat, disperse swelling and resolve toxicity

Guiding formulas: Modified *Long Dan Xie Gan Tang* (Gentian Liver-Draining Decoction) and *Bi Xie Shen Shi Tang* (Fish Poison Yam Dampness-Percolating Decoction)

Ingredients:
    Long Dan Cao (Gentianae Radix), 10g
    Huang Bai (Phellodendri Cortex), 10g
    Tong Cao (Tetrapanacis Medulla), 10g
    Huang Qin (Scutellariae Radix), 10g
    Shan Zhi Zi (Gardeniae Fructus), 10g
    Mu Dan Pi (Moutan Cortex), 10g
    Ze Xie (Alismatis Rhizoma), 10g
    Fu Ling (Poria), 10g
    Dang Gui (Angelicae Sinensis Radix), 10g
    Bi Xie (Dioscoreae Hypoglaucae seu Semptemlobae Rhizoma), 15g

    Che Qian Zi (Plantaginis Semen), 12g
    Yi Yi Ren (Coicis Semen), 20g
    Sheng Di Huang (Rehmanniae Radix Exsiccata seu Recens), 15g

Modifications: If there is pus and/or white blood cells in the semen, add *Tu Fu Ling* (Smilacis Glabrae Rhizoma), 12g, *Pu Gong Ying* (Taraxaci Herba), 10g, and *Jin Yin Hua* (Lonicerae Flos), 12g, to clear heat and resolve toxicity. For decreased sperm motility, add *Shan Zha* (Crataegi Fructus), 12g, *Dan Shen* (Salviae Miltiorrhizae Radix), 10g, *Cang Zhu* (Atractylodis Rhizoma), 10g, and *Lu Lu Tong* (Liquidambaris Fructus), 6g, to disinhibit dampness and transform turbidity, and to free the network vessels. For patients with blood in the semen, add *Da Ji* (Cirsii Japonici Herba seu Radix), 10g, *Xiao Ji* (Cirsii Herba), 10g, *Bai Mao Gen* (Imperatae Rhizoma), 10g, and *Han Lian Cao* (Ecliptae Herba), 10g, to clear heat and cool the blood and stop bleeding. For patients with bound stool or unsmooth bowel movements, add *Zhi Ke* (Aurantii Fructus), 6g, and *Da Huang* (Rhei Radix et Rhizoma), 6g, to free the bowels and conduct out stagnation. For patients who also have kidney qi vacuity, add *Tu Si Zi* (Cuscutae Semen), 15g, and *Fu Pen Zi* (Rubi Fructus), 10g, to supplement kidney qi and secure essence.

5. Congelation and stagnation of phlegm turbidity

Signs: Low seminal volume, low sperm density and motility, low sperm vitality, inability to ejaculate, testicular hardness, swelling, and pain, dizziness of the head and eyes, oppression in the chest and upflow nausea, heavy cumbersome limbs, copious sputum, heart palpitations, an overweight body, an enlarged tongue with white slimy fur, and a sinking slippery pulse.

Treatment principles: Transform phlegm and rectify qi, dissipate binds and free the network vessels

Guiding formula: Modified *Cang Fu Dao Tan Wan* (Atractylodes and Cyperus Phlegm-Abducting Pill)

Ingredients:
    Cang Zhu (Atractylodis Rhizoma), 12g
    Xiang Fu (Cyperi Rhizoma), 12g
    Chen Pi (Citri Reticulatae Pericarpium), 10g
    Ban Xia (Pinelliae Rhizoma), 10g
    Zhi Shi (Aurantii Fructus immaturis), 10g
    Fu Ling (Poria), 12g
    Bai Zhu (Atractylodis Macrocephalae Rhizoma), 12g
    Ze Xie (Alismatis Rhizoma), 12g
    Che Qian Zi (Plantaginis Semen), 15g
    Lu Lu Tong (Liquidambaris Fructus), 6g
    Zhe Bei Mu (Fritillariae Thunbergii Bulbus), 12g
    Zhi Gan Cao (Glycyrrhizae Radix cum Liquido Fricta), 3g

Modifications: For patients with spleen qi vacuity, combine with *Liu Jun Zi Tang* (Six Gentlemen Decoction) and *Huang Qi* (Astragali Radix), 15g. For patients with nonliquefaction of semen, add *Xuan Shen* (Scrophulariae Radix), 10g, *Xing Ren* (Armeniacae Semen), 6g, and *Sheng Mu Li* (Ostreae Concha Cruda), 15g, to help qi to transform semen. For low sperm motility, add *Yi Yi Ren* (Coicis Semen), 20g, and *Shan Zha*, 10g, to transform turbidity and open the orifices. For retrograde ejaculation, add *Niu Xi* (Achyranthis Bidentatae Radix), 12g, and *Wang Bu Liu Xing Zi* (Vaccariae Semen), 12g, to move and disinhibit the lower orifice. For a cold and damp sensation in the scrotum accompanied by lesser abdominal pulling pain, add *Li Zhi He* (Litchi Semen), 6g, *Wu Yao* (Linderae Radix), 10g, and *Yan Hu Suo* (Corydalis Rhizoma), 10g. For white turbid penile discharge, combine with *Bi Xie Fen Qing Yin* (Fish Poison Yam Clear-Turbid Separation Beverage). For patients who also have liver depression, add *Yu Jin* (Curcumae Radix), 10g, and *Chai Hu* (Bupleuri Radix), 6g, to course the liver and rectify the qi.

Liu Jun Zi Tang (Six Gentlemen Decoction)

> *Ren Shen* (Ginseng Radix), 10g
> *Bai Zhu* (Atractylodis Macrocephalae Rhizoma), 12g
> *Fu Ling* (Poria), 12g
> *Ban Xia* (Pinelliae Rhizoma), 10g
> *Chen Pi* (Citri Reticulatae Pericarpium), 10g
> *Zhi Gan Cao* (Glycyrrhizae Radix cum Liquido Fricta), 6g

Bi Xie Fen Qing Yin (Fish Poison Yam Clear-Turbid Separation Beverage)

> *Yi Zhi Ren* (Alpiniae Oxyphyllae Fructus), 9g
> *Chuan Bi Xie* (Dioscoreae Hypoglaucae seu Semptemlobae Rhizoma), 9g
> *Shi Chang Pu* (Acori Tatarinowii Rhizoma), 9g
> *Wu Yao* (Linderae Radix), 9g

6. Blood stasis obstruction

Signs: A scrotum that feels like a bag of worms (indicating varicocele), a sensation of distention, heaviness and pain of the scrotum and perineum, pain along the course of the essence pathway during ejaculation, low sperm density, low sperm motility, high rate of sperm abnormalities, high levels of red blood cells in the semen, sinking pain in the testes, fixed lesser abdominal pain, a long disease history with periods of relapse and remission, purple lips, purple tongue with purple spots, a sinking rough pulse or a fine rough pulse.

Treatment principles: Quicken the blood and transform stasis, free the essence

Guiding formula: Modified *Xue Fu Zhu Yu Tang* (House of Blood Stasis-Expelling Decoction)

Ingredients:
> *Chai Hu* (Bupleuri Radix), 10g
> *Zhi Ke* (Aurantii Fructus), 6g

Niu Xi (Achyranthis Bidentatae Radix), 10g
Tao Ren (Persicae Semen), 10g
Hong Hua (Carthami Flos), 10g
Chi Shao (Paeoniae Radix Rubra), 10g
Dang Gui (Angelicae Sinensis Radix), 10g
Chuan Xiong (Chuanxiong Rhizoma), 10g
Lu Lu Tong (Liquidambaris Fructus), 6g
Dan Shen (Salviae Miltiorrhizae Radix), 15g
Wang Bu Liu Xing Zi (Vaccariae Semen), 15g
San Leng (Sparganii Rhizoma), 10g
E Zhu (Curcumae Rhizoma), 10g

Modifications: For patients with mutual binding of phlegm and blood stasis (phlegm-stasis), add *Chen Pi* (Citri Reticulatae Pericarpium), 10g, *Ban Xia* (Pinelliae Rhizoma), 10g, *Gua Lou* (Trichosanthis Fructus), 12g, and *Yi Yi Ren* (Coicis Semen), 20g, to fortify the spleen and transform phlegm. When binding depression of liver qi leads to blood stasis, add *Qing Pi* (Citri Reticulatae Pericarpium Viride), 10g, and *Xiang Fu* (Cyperi Rhizoma), 12g, to move qi. When cold in the liver channel leads to blood stasis, add *Chuan Lian Zi* (Toosendan Fructus), 10g, *Xiao Hui Xiang* (Foeniculi Fructus), 10g, and *Wu Yao* (Linderae Radix), 10g, to warm the liver channel and dissipate cold. When depressed heat brews in the liver channel, decocts blood and leads to blood stasis, add *Shan Zhi Zi* (Gardeniae Fructus), 10g, and *Mu Dan Pi* (Moutan Cortex), 10g, to clear heat from depression. When blood stasis transforms heat and scorches essence and leads to low seminal volume and density, add *Huang Bai* (Phellodendri Cortex), 10g, *Wang Bu Liu Xing Zi* (Vaccariae Semen), 15g, *Gui Ban* (Testudinis Carapax et Plastrum), 15g, and *Bie Jia* (Trionycis Carapax), 15g, to clear heat, transform stasis and engender essence. For inability to ejaculate, add *Wu Gong* (Scolopendra), 1g, and *Lu Feng Fang* (Vespae Nidus), 6g, to free the essence gate and pathway. For patients with yang wilt, add *Ba Ji Tian* (Morindae Officinalis Radix), 15g, *Wu Gong* (Scolopendra), 1g, *She Chuang Zi* (Cnidii Fructus), 12g, and *Zi Shi Ying* (Fluoritum), 10g, to support the yang and rouse that which has wilted. For pronounced pain during ejaculation, add *Hu Po* (Succinum), 2g, powdered and swallowed with the strained decoction, *Pu Huang* (Typhae Pollen), 10g, and *Yan Hu Suo* (Corydalis Rhizoma), 12g, to free the essence pathway and relieve pain. If enduring blood stasis transforms heat which rots healthy tissue and forms an abscess, combine with *Wu Wei Xiao Du Yin* (Five-Ingredient Toxin-Dispersing Beverage), to clear heat and resolve toxicity, and disperse the abscess.

Wu Wei Xiao Du Yin (Five-Ingredient Toxin-Dispersing Beverage)

Jin Yin Hua (Lonicerae Flos), 20g
Ye Ju Hua (Chrysanthemi Indici Flos), 15g
Pu Gong Ying (Taraxaci Herba), 15g
Zi Hua Di Ding (Violae Herba), 15g
Zi Bei Tian Kui (Begoniae fimbristipulatae Herba), 15g

7. Cold stagnating in the liver channel

Signs: Clear and cold semen, distention, swelling, and pain in the testes, sagging, distention, and pain in the lesser abdomen which worsens after sexual activity, dampness and coldness of the scrotum which worsens when exposed to cold and is accompanied by retraction and pain of the scrotum, occasional feelings of generalized exhaustion, soreness and pain of the lumbus, somber white facial complexion, generalized aversion to cold and especially cold feet and legs, pale tongue with tooth marks and a thin white fur, stringlike tight or stringlike moderate pulse.

Treatment principles: Warm the liver and dissipate cold, warm the liver channel and move qi

Guiding formula: Modified *Nuan Gan Jian* (Liver-Warming Brew)

Ingredients:
    Rou Gui (Cinnamomi Cortex), 6g
    Xiao Hui Xiang (Foeniculi Fructus), 10g
    Wu Yao (Linderae Radix), 10g
    Dang Gui (Angelicae Sinensis Radix), 10g
    Fu Ling (Poria), 12g
    Sheng Jiang (Zingiberis Rhizoma Recens), 3 slices
    Gou Qi Zi (Lycii Fructus), 15g
    Hu Lu Ba (Trigonellae Semen), 10g
    Ba Ji Tian (Morindae Officinalis Radix), 15g

Modifications: For patients with pulling pain in the lesser abdomen and more pronounced coldness and dampness of the scrotum, add *Li Zhi He* (Litchi Semen), 10g, *Ju He* (Citri Reticulatae Semen), 10g, and *Yan Hu Suo* (Corydalis Rhizoma), 15g, to further warm the liver channel and relieve pain. For binding depression of liver qi with rib-side pain and distention, add *Chuan Lian Zi* (Toosendan Fructus), 10g, *Xiang Fu* (Cyperi Rhizoma), 12g, and *Mei Gui Hua* (Rosae Rugosae Flos), 10g, to course the liver and rectify the qi and relieve pain. When cold congeals the blood and causes blood stasis, add *Niu Xi* (Achyranthis Bidentatae Radix), 12g, and *Wu Ling Zhi* (Trogopteri Faeces), 10g, to transform stasis and free the network vessels.

Acumoxa therapy

Main points: *Ming Men* (GV-4), *Yao Yang Guan* (GV-3), *Guan Yuan* (CV-4), *Zhong Ji* (CV-3), *San Yin Jiao* (SP-6), *Shen Shu* (BL-23), *Zhi Shi* (BL-52), *Tai Xi* (KI-3), *Zu San Li* (ST-36)

Vacuity patterns

For kidney yin vacuity, add *Qi Hai* (CV-6) and *Da He* (KI-12)

For kidney yang vacuity, add moxa on *Ming Men* (GV-4) and *Guan Yuan* (CV-4), and also add *Pi Shu* (BL-20), *Qi Hai* (CV-6), and *Bai Hui* (GV-20)

For qi and blood vacuity, add *Qi Hai* (CV-6), *Shan Zhong* (CV-17), *Pi Shu* (BL-20), *Wei Shu* (BL-21), *Ge Shu* (BL-17), *Shang Ju Xu* (ST-37), *Xia Ju Xu* (ST-39), and *Da Zhu* (BL-11)[19]

Repletion patterns

For damp-heat pouring downward, add *Tai Bai* (SP-3), *Feng Long* (ST-40), *Pi Shu* (BL-20), *Li Gou* (LV-5), *Yin Lian* (LV-11), and *Xing Jian* (LV-2)

For blood stasis obstruction, add *Shang Ju Xu* (ST-37), *Xia Ju Xu* (ST-39), *Da Zhu* (BL-11), *Ge Shu* (BL-17), *Tai Chong* (LV-3), *Qu Gu* (CV-2), *Yin Lian* (LV-11), *Xing Jian* (LV-2), and *Da Dun* (LV-1)

For cold stagnating in the liver channel, add *Tai Chong* (LV-3) and *Qu Quan* (LV-8), and moxa *Guan Yuan* (CV-4), *Yin Jian* (LV-11), *Ming Men* (GV-4), *Gan Shu* (BL-18), and *Shen Shu* (BL-23)

Experiential formulas

Scanty semen due to kidney vacuity and blood stasis

Wang (1997) provides a self-composed formula called *Sheng Jing Tang* (Essence-Engendering Decoction) for the treatment of kidney vacuity and blood stasis with scanty semen. The ingredients are as follows:
He Shou Wu (Polygoni Multiflori Radix), 10g
Lu Feng Fang (Vespae Nidus), 10g
Lu Xian Cao (Pyrolae Herba), 10g
Tu Si Zi (Cuscutae Semen), 15g
Gou Qi Zi (Lycii Fructus), 15g
She Chuang Zi (Cnidii Fructus), 15g
Yin Yang Huo (Epimedii Herba), 10g
Huang Jing (Polygonati Rhizoma), 15g
Dan Shen (Salviae Miltiorrhizae Radix), 20g

Low sperm motility due to kidney yang vacuity and waning of life gate fire

Luo (1990) reports on his positive clinical experiences with his own formula called *Wen Shen Yi Jing Wan* (Kidney-Warming Essence-Boosting Pill) for treating low sperm motility due to kidney yang vacuity and waning of life gate fire. The ingredients are as follows:
Pao Tian Xiong (Aconiti Tuber Laterale Tianxiong Praeparatum), 180g
Shu Di Huang (Rehmanniae Radix Praeparata), 180g
Tu Si Zi (Cuscutae Semen), 480g
Lu Jiao Shuang (Cervi Cornu Degelatinatum), 120g
Bai Zhu (Atractylodis Macrocephalae Rhizoma), 480g
Rou Gui (Cinnamomi Cortex), 30g

---

[19] ST-37, ST-39, and BL-11 are points of the sea of blood and therefore can be used for all blood disorders.

Instructions: All the ingredients should be ground together into a fine powder and mixed evenly with honey to form small pills. Six grams should be taken twice per day.

Liver depression, blood stasis, and qi vacuity

Qi *et al.* (1988) discussed a formula called *Tong Jing Jian Jia Wei* (Added Flavors Essence-Freeing Brew) for the treatment of male infertility due to liver depression, blood stasis, and qi vacuity. The ingredients are:

Dan Shen (Salviae Miltiorrhizae Radix), 15g
E Zhu (Curcumae Rhizoma), 15g
Chuan Niu Xi (Cyathulae Radix), 15g
Chai Hu (Bupleuri Radix), 10g
Sheng Mu Li (Ostreae Concha Cruda), 30g
Sheng Huang Qi (Astragali seu Hedysari Radix Cruda), 20g

Modifications: For more pronounced signs of liver channel stagnation, including a unilateral sagging of the scrotum with distention and pain and stringlike pulse, add *Ju Ye* (Citri Reticulatae Folium), 10g, *Ju He* (Citri Reticulatae Semen), 10g, *Li Zhi He* (Litchi Semen), 15g, and *Xiao Hui Xiang* (Foeniculi Fructus), 10g. For signs of damp-heat in the liver channel such as dampness and itchiness of the scrotum and yellowish-red urine, add *Che Qian Zi* (Plantaginis Semen), 15g, *Zhi Mu* (Anemarrhenae Rhizoma), 10g, and *Huang Bai* (Phellodendri Cortex), 10g. For more pronounced signs of qi vacuity such as a sensation of the scrotum and testes sagging downward and exhaustion of essence-spirit, add *Dang Shen* (Codonopsis Radix), 10g, and *Bai Zhu* (Atractylodis Macrocephalae Rhizoma), 10g. For patients with yang vacuity signs such as cold extremities and cold sensations of the genitals, add *Shu Fu Zi* (Aconiti Radix Lateralis Conquita), 10g, and *Gui Zhi* (Cinnamomi Ramulus), 10g. For yin vacuity with signs such as dry mouth and red tongue, and vexing heat in the five hearts, add *Sheng Di Huang* (Rehmanniae Radix Exsiccata seu Recens), 15g, *Bai Shao* (Paeoniae Radix Alba), 10g, and *Zhi Bie Jia* (Trionycis Carapax cum Liquido Frictus), 10g.

Nonliquefaction of semen due to kidney yin vacuity

He and Zhou (1997) report on Jin Wei-Xin's experience treating nonliquefaction of semen due to kidney yin vacuity with a formula called *Ye Hua Tang* (Humor-Transforming Decoction). The ingredients are:

Zhi Mu (Anemarrhenae Rhizoma), 9g
Huang Bai (Phellodendri Cortex), 9g
Tian Hua Fen (Trichosanthis Radix), 9g
Chi Shao (Paeoniae Radix Rubra), 9g
Bai Shao (Paeoniae Radix Alba), 9g
Mai Men Dong (Ophiopogonis Radix), 9g
Sheng Di Huang (Rehmanniae Radix Exsiccata seu Recens), 12g
Shu Di Huang (Rehmanniae Radix Praeparata), 12g
Xuan Shen (Scrophulariae Radix), 12g
Gou Qi Zi (Lycii Fructus), 12g

Yin Yang Huo (Epimedii Herba), 12g
Che Qian Cao (Plantaginis Herba), 12g
Dan Shen (Salviae Miltiorrhizae Radix), 30g

Preventive measures and lifestyle modification

I. Maintain psychological wellness

In three treasures theory, in order for essence to be engendered, the spirit must be abundant and harmonious. Therefore, men with infertility should be encouraged to express their feelings and not to repress them so that their liver and heart qi will flow freely. As a result, the spirit can more effectively engender essence, and qi can guarantee that essence flows freely.

2. Avoid exposing the testes to excessive heat

Since normal spermatogenesis requires a slightly cooler temperature than one's core temperature, natural selection has guaranteed that the testes hang in the scrotum in which the temperature is on average one-half degree lower. Therefore, it is advisable for men with infertility to avoid exposing the testes to excessive heat. In modern terms, this means avoiding taking hot baths and sitting in the Jacuzzi, avoiding the use of tight-fitting briefs in favor of either no underwear or boxer shorts, and treating any febrile disease promptly and completely.

3. Eat a balanced, light, and clear diet

Eating a balanced, light, and clear diet consists of eating lots of fresh vegetables and fruits, legumes, whole grains, small amounts of lean meats and seafood, and avoiding excessive amounts of fats, sweets, and spicy-hot foods. A light diet enhances the flow of qi and blood to the penis by nourishing the viscera and bowels and the anterior yin region, and by avoiding the accumulation of dampness, phlegm, and heat. On the contrary, fats and sweets encourage the collection of dampness, phlegm, and heat in the anterior yin. These evils damage essence, thus causing or exacerbating infertility. Eating spicy-hot foods in moderation—especially in colder climates and by men with constitutional yang vacuity—can be beneficial by warming the anterior yin region and hence can improve sperm motility and spermatogenesis. Excessive consumption of spicy-hot foods, however, can scorch and damage essence, and lead to the formation of evil heat in the interior, which damages sperm. Over time and if severe, this heat can consume kidney yin-essence and lead to infertility.

In addition to eating a generally healthful diet, it is wise for men to periodically eat foods that are especially known to supplement kidney essence and enhance their fertility. These include oysters, sea cucumber, abalone, shitake mushrooms, shrimp, scallops, walnuts, chestnuts, Chinese chives, venison, lamb, goat, and turtle.

4. Maintain regular sexual activity

It is well-documented that men who have infrequent sexual activity have a lower percentage of motile sperm. From the perspective of Chinese andrology, regular sexual activity is important to maintain free flow of qi, blood, and essence, and to maintain fertility. The longer semen and sperm remain in the essence chamber and the testes, the greater is the risk that they will be subjected to the damaging effects of evil heat, dampness, phlegm, and blood stasis. Essence that has remained in these areas for too long, then, can become vanquished essence. Of course, excessive sexual activity can damage essence and lead to infertility through other pathomechanisms.

5. Prevent and treat deep-lying damp-heat, heat, and heat toxin

Deep-lying damp-heat, heat, and toxin diseases, when present for a long time, represent a major threat to male fertility. Heat and heat toxin scorches semen and sperm, and damp-heat scorches and obstructs semen and adversely affects the formation, morphology, viability, and motility of sperm. In terms of Western medicine, these conditions correlate with chronic infections and inflammatory conditions, including chronic prostatitis, sexually-transmitted diseases including *Chlamydia*, pharyngitis, and periodontal disease. Hence, we should treat these conditions completely and effectively.

Representative Chinese Research

Warming and supplementing spleen and kidney, nourishing blood, and replenishing essence

Chen and Xi (1998) report on the effectiveness of a formula called *Wen Bu Yang Xue Tian Jing Tang* (Warming and Supplementing, Blood-Nourishing, and Essence-Replenishing Decoction), which they modified according to the pattern, in the treatment of 25 cases of male infertility. The main ingredients consisted of:

   Shan Zhu Yu (Corni Fructus), 15g
   Tu Si Zi (Cuscutae Semen), 15g
   Dang Shen (Codonopsis Radix), 15g
   Shan Yao (Dioscoreae Rhizoma), 20g
   Shu Di Huang (Rehmanniae Radix Praeparata), 20g
   Bai Zhu (Atractylodis Macrocephalae Rhizoma), 10g
   Dang Gui (Angelicae Sinensis Radix), 10g
   Yin Yang Huo (Epimedii Herba), 10g
   Bai Ji Tian (Morindae Officinalis Radix), 10g
   Suo Yang (Cynomorii Herba), 10g

Modifications: For patients with yang wilt and premature ejaculation, add *Shu Fu Zi* (Aconiti Radix Lateralis Conquita), 8g, *Rou Gui* (Cinnamomi Cortex), 3g, and *Lu Rong* (Cervi Cornu Pantotrichum), 6g. For patients with seminal efflux and/or incontinence of urine, add *Jin Ying Zi* (Rosae Laevigatae Fructus), 15g, and *Bu Gu Zhi* (Psoraleae Fructus), 15g. For palpitations and shortness of breath, add *Bai Zi Ren* (Platycladi Semen), 15g, *Wu Wei Zi* (Schisandrae Fructus), 15g, and *Zi He Che* (Hominis Placenta), 20g. For inability to ejaculate, add *Lu Lu Tong* (Liquidambaris Fructus), 15g, and *Chuan Shan Jia* (Manitis Squama), 15g. [20]

Results: In this study, one packet of medicine was used per day, and one month comprised one treatment course. Twenty-five men with a history of three or more years of unprotected intercourse participated in the study and their semen was abnormal for one or more of the following values: sperm density; sperm motility and; seminal liquefaction time. Among them, 23 cases were cured (as measured by disappearance of symptoms, completely normal semen analysis after treatment, and successful pregnancy), and 2 cases had no results (as measured by no successful treatment even after 1–1½ years of treatment.

Supplementing the kidney and engendering essence

Li (2003) used a formula called *Bu Shen Sheng Jing Tang* (Kidney-Supplementing Essence-Engendering Decoction) to treat 105 cases of male infertility. All cases had a semen analysis (SA), which exhibited 20 million or fewer sperm per ml, and/or less than 50% sperm motility, and exhibited vacuity signs such as dizziness of head and tinnitus, soreness and limpness of the lumbus and knees, exhaustion, and nonlustrous facial complexion. The ingredients of the formula were:

Tu Si Zi (Cuscutae Semen), 15g
Sha Yuan Ji Li (Astragali Complanati Semen), 15g
Chu Shi Zi (Broussonetiae Fructus), 15g
Shan Zhu Yu (Corni Fructus), 15g
Ze Xie (Alismatis Rhizoma), 15g
Dang Gui (Angelicae Sinensis Radix), 15g
Shu Di Huang (Rehmanniae Radix Praeparata), 20g
Dan Shen (Salviae Miltiorrhizae Radix), 20g
Fu Ling (Poria), 15g
Ba Ji Tian (Morindae Officinalis Radix), 20g
Shan Yao (Dioscoreae Rhizoma), 30g
Jiu Cai Zi (Allii Tuberosi Semen), 12g

Results: One packet per day for one month comprised one treatment course. The majority of patents had 3–6 treatment courses. Among the 105 cases, 62 cases were cured (either successful pregnancy during or after treatment, normal semen analysis and disappearance of clinical symptoms), 39 cases experienced some positive effect (either normal semen analysis or improvement in or disappearance of clinical symptoms), and 4 cases had no effect (no positive change in semen analysis and no improvement in clinical symptoms).

Using a modification of *Wu Zi Yan Zong Wan* (Five-Seed Progeny Pill)

Xu (2003) treated 153 cases of male infertility with a modification of *Wu Zi Yan Zong Wan* (Five-Seed Progeny Pill). The ingredients were:

---

[20] *Chuan Shan Jia* comes from the pangolin, which is a threatened or endangered species. Although farmed sources are available, the pedigree of any given shipment is difficult to establish; hence, I personally do not use it. I include it here because it was used in this research formula. Consider substituting other medicinals such as *E Zhu* (Curcumae Rhizoma).

Tu Si Zi (Cuscutae Semen), 30g
Gou Qi Zi (Lycii Fructus), 30g
Fu Pen Zi (Rubi Fructus), 15g
Yin Yang Huo (Epimedii Herba), 15g
Che Qian Zi (Plantaginis Semen), 10g
Huang Qi (Astragali Radix), 10g
Dang Shen (Codonopsis Radix), 10g
Bai Zhu (Atractylodis Macrocephalae Rhizoma), 10g
Dang Gui (Angelicae Sinensis Radix), 10g
Shu Di Huang (Rehmanniae Radix Praeparata), 10g
Shan Yao (Dioscoreae Rhizoma), 10g
Shan Zhu Yu (Corni Fructus), 6g
Wu Wei Zi (Schisandrae Fructus), 6g

Modifications: For low sperm motility accompanied by qi vacuity signs, increase the dosage of *Huang Qi* to 20–30g, and the dosage of *Bai Zhu* and *Dang Shen* to 15g. For patients with blood vacuity, increase the dosage of *Dang Gui* to 15g, and add *E Jiao* (Asini Corii Colla), 6g. For yin vacuity, add *Zhi Mu* (Anemarrhenae Rhizoma), 10g, *Mai Men Dong* (Ophiopogonis Radix), 10g, and *He Shou Wu* (Polygoni Multiflori Radix), 10g.

Results: One packet per day for 21 days comprised one treatment course. Among the 153 cases treated, after 1–5 treatment courses, 111 cases were cured (disappearance of clinical symptoms, normal semen analysis including greater than 70% sperm motility and normal morphology, less than or equal to 30 minutes liquefaction time, and/or successful pregnancy during the treatment course), 18 cases had some good results but did not meet the specified criteria for cure, and 12 cases had no results after 5 courses of treatment. The overall amelioration rate was 92.1%.

Using a modification of *Liu Wei Di Huang Wan* (Six-Ingredient Rehmannia Pill) and *Wu Wei Xiao Du Yin* (Five-Ingredient Toxin-Dispersing Beverage)

He and Guo (2003) used a combination of *Liu Wei Di Huang Wan* and *Wu Wei Xiao Du Yin* to treat 45 cases of male infertility. The ingredients were:
Sheng Di Huang (Rehmanniae Radix Exsiccata seu Recens), 20g
Shu Du Huang (Rehmanniae Radix Praeparata), 20g
Shan Yao (Dioscoreae Rhizoma), 30g
Huang Qi (Astragali Radix), 30g
Mu Dan Pi (Moutan Cortex), 10g
Shi Chang Pu (Acori Tatarinowii Rhizoma), 10g
Ye Ju Hua (Chrysanthemi Indici Flos), 10g
Fu Ling (Poria), 15g
Niu Xi (Achyranthis Bidentatae Radix), 15g
Pu Gong Ying (Taraxaci Herba), 18g
Zi Hua Di Ding (Violae Herba), 18g
Che Qian Zi (Plantaginis Semen), 18g
Yin Yang Huo (Epimedii Herba), 18g

Modifications: For patients with yang wilt, remove *Pu Gong Ying*, *Zi Hua Di Ding*, and *Ye Ju Hua*, and add *Shu Fu Zi* (Aconiti Radix Lateralis Conquita). For yin vacuity, remove *Yin Yang Huo* and add *Nu Zhen Zi* (Ligustri Lucidi Fructus) and *Han Lian Cao* (Ecliptae Herba).

Results: Among the 45 cases treated, 15 cases were cured (successful pregnancy during treatment), 20 cases had good results (after 3–5 months of treatment had yet to have successful pregnancy, but showed improvements in semen analysis such that sperm density increased to at least 20 million per ml and sperm motility was greater than 50%), 9 cases had some effect (slight improvements in sperm density and/or motility), and 1 case had no results (no improvements in semen analysis or other symptoms after treatment).

Treating nonliquefaction of semen by nourishing kidney yin

Fu and Huang (2002) used a formula called *Zi Yin Hua Jing Tang* (Yin-Enriching Essence-Transforming Decoction) to treat 38 cases of male infertility due to nonliquefaction of semen. The ingredients were:

Shan Zhu Yu (Corni Fructus), 10g
Zhi Mu (Anemarrhenae Rhizoma), 10g
Mu Dan Pi (Moutan Cortex), 10g
Fu Ling (Poria), 10g
Han Lian Cao (Ecliptae Herba), 10g
Huang Bai (Phellodendri Cortex), 10g
Shan Zha (Crataegi Fructus), 15g
Gou Qi Zi (Lycii Fructus), 15g
Zhi Gui Ban (Testudinis Carapax et Plastrum cum Liquido Frictus), 20g
Zhi Bie Jia (Trionycis Carapax cum Liquido Frictus), 20g
Sheng Di Huang (Rehmanniae Radix Exsiccata seu Recens), 20g
He Shou Wu (Polygoni Multiflori Radix), 20g
Hei Zhi Ma (Sesami Semen Nigrum), 30g
Mai Ya (Hordei Fructus Germinatus), 50g
Shui Zhi (Hirudo), 3g, powdered and taken mixed with the strained
    decoction

Modifications: For patients with qi vacuity and blood stasis, add *Huang Qi* (Astragali Radix), *Ren Shen* (Ginseng Radix), *San Qi* (Notoginseng Radix), *Dang Gui* (Angelicae Sinensis Radix), and *Chi Shao* (Paeoniae Radix Rubra). For kidney qi vacuity and sexual dysfunction, add *Du Zhong* (Eucommiae Cortex), *Ba Ji Tian* (Morindae Officinalis Radix), *Bu Gu Zhi* (Psoraleae Fructus), and *Tu Si Zi* (Cuscutae Semen). For binding depression of liver qi, add *Chai Hu* (Bupleuri Radix) *Yu Jin* (Curcumae Radix), and *Chuan Lian Zi* (Toosendan Fructus). For mutual binding of phlegm and blood stasis, add *Tao Ren* (Persicae Semen), *Dan Shen* (Salviae Miltiorrhizae Radix), *Hong Hua* (Carthami Flos), *Zhe Bei Mu* (Fritillariae Thunbergii Bulbus), and *Tu Bie Chong* (Eupolyphaga/Steleophaga). For patients with damp-heat pouring downward, add *Pu Gong Ying* (Taraxaci Herba), *Yi Yi Ren* (Coicis Semen), *Bi Xie* (Dioscoreae Hypoglaucae seu Semptemlobae Rhizoma), and *Che Qian Zi* (Plantaginis Semen).

All the patients in the study had semen liquefaction times exceeding 60 minutes, sticky and scanty semen, low rates of sperm motility, and also had definite signs of kidney yin vacuity including dizziness of the head and eyes, soreness and limpness of the lumbus and knees, tinnitus, copious dreaming with dream emissions, vexation and heat of the five hearts, night sweating, dry mouth and throat, and a fine rapid pulse. One packet of medicine per day for 90 days comprised one treatment course. The majority of patients completed 2 courses of treatment. While under treatment, patients were advised to: 1) refrain from eating spicy-hot foods; 2) regulate their sexual life and; 3) take a warm sitz bath daily.

Results: Among the 38 cases enrolled in the study, 29 cases were cured (semen liquefaction time of 30 minutes or less, successful pregnancy, and either disappearance or improvement in all the clinical signs), 5 cases had some results (semen liquefaction time reduced to 40 minutes or more, some improvements in other semen analysis values, and improvement in the clinical signs), and 4 cases had no results (no changes in semen liquefaction time and no improvement in clinical signs). The total amelioration rate was 89.5%.

Clearing heat and drying dampness

Wu (2000) treated 151 cases of autoimmune infertility with a formula called *Qing Shi Jie Ning Tang* (Dampness-Clearing Congelation-Resolving Decoction). The ingredients were:

> *Long Dan Cao* (Gentianae Radix), 3g
> *Huang Lian* (Coptidis Rhizoma), 2g
> *Fu Ling* (Poria), 10g
> *Nu Zhen Zi* (Ligustri Lucidi Fructus), 10g
> *Tu Si Zi* (Cuscutae Semen), 10g
> *Mu Dan Pi* (Moutan Cortex), 10g
> *Cang Zhu* (Atractylodis Rhizoma), 10g
> *Ren Shen* (Ginseng Radix), 10g
> *Lu Jiao* (Cervi Cornu), 10g
> *Liu Yi San* (Six-to-One Powder), 15g

Results: All the patients enrolled in the study had two or more years of unprotected intercourse without a successful pregnancy and their semen analysis revealed antisperm antibodies. One packet of medicinals per day for three months comprised one treatment course. Among the 151 cases treated, 34 were cured (used the medicine for 3–6 months, had reversal of antisperm antibody finding, and a successful pregnancy within one year of commencing treatment), 34 cases had some effect (used the medicine for 3–6 months, had reversal of the antisperm antibody finding, but still had not had a successful pregnancy within one year of commencing treatment), and 84 cases had no effect.

Acumoxa therapy

Supplementing the kidneys

Tao (1985) used *Guan Yuan* (CV-4), *Zhong Ji* (CV-3), *Tai Xi* (KI-3), and *Zhao*

Hai (KI-6) with even supplementation and even draining to treat 12 cases of male infertility. After obtaining the qi, he used 2–3 moxa cones on the needles. After needling these points, the investigator either warmed *Hui Yin* (CV-1) with a moxa stick or massaged it for 30 minutes. One treatment course consisted of daily treatment for twenty days; each treatment course was followed by a six-day rest period.

Results: None of the patients received any oral medicine during the study period. All of the subjects showed improvements in sperm density and motility, though the study did not give specifics. Tao reported that all of the subjects' wives subsequently became pregnant.

Chen and Xi (1998) treated 45 cases of male infertility due to low sperm density with two groups of acumoxa points which were modified according to symptoms. The first group of points consisted of: *Tai Xi* (KI-3), *San Yin Jiao* (SP-6), *Guan Yuan* (CV-4), *Shen Shu* (BL-23), and *Fu Liu* (KI-7), and the second group consisted of: *Zhao Hai* (KI-6), *Yin Ling Quan* (SP-9), *Qi Hai* (CV-6), *Zhi Shi* (BL-52), and *Di Ji* (SP-8).

Modifications: For patients with insomnia, add *Bai Hui* (GV-20) and *Nei Guan* (PC-6). For spleen-stomach vacuity-weakness, add *Zu San Li* (ST-36). For yang wilt, add *Ci Liao* (BL-32), and moxa *Ming Men* (GV-4). The reporters specified that when they needled *Guan Yuan* and *Qi Hai*, they strove to cause a distending needle sensation to refer down to the genital region, and to cause an erection. They gave one treatment per day and switched between groups of points. Ten days comprised one treatment course and there was a one-week rest period between each course.

Results: Twenty-two cases were cured, 13 cases had good results, 13 cases had fair results, 6 cases had some results, and 4 cases had no result, for a total amelioration rate of 91.1%. No specific parameters for evaluating effectiveness were provided.

Acumoxa therapy for nonliquefaction of semen

Liu (1990) treated 32 cases of nonliquefaction of semen with one group of acumoxa points that were varied according to the pattern. The main points consisted of: *Guan Yuan* (CV-4), *Zhong Ji* (CV-3), *Shen Shu* (BL-23), and *San Yin Jiao* (SP-6).

Modifications: For kidney yin vacuity, Liu used supplementing needle technique and added *Zhao Hai* (KI-6) and *Shen Men* (HT-7). For damp-heat pouring downward, he used draining needle technique, and added *Ci Liao* (BL-32), *Hui Yin* (CV-1) or *Qu Gu* (CV-2), *Yin Ling Quan* (SP-9), and *Feng Long* (ST-40). Patients were treated daily and 10 days comprised one treatment course. After one treatment course, all patients underwent a repeat semen analysis. For those with prostatitis, a repeat prostate exam was first performed and was compared to pretreatment results. If the prostate exam was normal, then a repeat semen analysis was performed; if the prostate exam was abnormal, patients rested for one week and received another treatment course.

Results: Among the 32 patients treated, 26 cases were cured (81.25%) and 6 cases had good results (18.75%).

Acumoxa therapy for low sperm motility

Tao (1987) observed the effects of acumoxa therapy on sperm motility in 26 cases. Among the subjects, 17 had pretreatment sperm motility rates between 10–20%, 8 cases had 30–60%, and 1 case had 70%. The age of the subjects ranged from 26–34 years, and they had been having unprotected intercourse for 1–6 years without successful pregnancy. The points used were: *Guan Yuan* (CV-4), *Zhong Ji* (CV-3), *Zu San Li* (ST-36), *Tai Xi* (KI-3), and *Zhao Hai* (KI-6). After obtaining qi, 2–3 moxa cones were applied to all the needles. Also, the investigator used a moxa stick to warm *Hui Yin* (CV-1), or he used finger pressure to massage it for 30 minutes. Treatment was given once per day.

Results: After completing an unspecified number of treatment courses, a repeat semen analysis showed improvements in sperm motility rates of 40% or greater in 11 cases, and 20% or greater in 5 cases. By the completion of treatment, 7 cases had already had a successful pregnancy.

Representative Case Studies

Static blood obstructing the network vessels

Wang (1997) reports a case of male infertility in a 26-year old man due to blood stasis obstructing the network vessels. The patient had been married for 2.5 years and still had not had a successful pregnancy. His wife had been fully evaluated and female infertility was completely ruled out. Hence, the patient was referred to Dr. Wang for treatment.

The patient's main symptoms were: occasional feeling of distention in his left testicle; a feeling of coldness and heaviness in his testes; irascibility and; dampness in the genital area. There was neither any urinary frequency, urgency, pain, or turbidity, nor any aching soreness of the lumbus and knees extending into the genital region; further, there were no abnormalities of sexual function. His tongue was red with white fur, and his pulse was stringlike. Physical examination of his external genitalia showed second degree distention of the left spermatic cord, but no other abnormalities. Semen analysis revealed a seminal volume of 2.5 ml, sperm density of 8 million/ml, milky-white semen, 20% motility rate, normal liquefaction time, 25% abnormal morphology, and 0–1 million WBC/ml. The Western medical diagnosis was varicocele.

Dr. Wang's diagnosis was static blood obstructing the network vessels and his treatment principle was to quicken the blood and transform stasis and to boost the kidneys and engender essence. He prescribed the following formula:

    Dan Shen (Salviae Miltiorrhizae Radix), 15g
    Pu Huang (Typhae Pollen), 10g
    Yi Mu Cao (Leonuri Herba), 15g
    Wang Bu Liu Xing (Vaccariae Semen), 15g
    Yi Yi Ren (Coicis Semen), 15g
    Lu Lu Tong (Liquidambaris Fructus), 15g
    Dang Gui (Angelicae Sinensis Radix), 10g
    Xu Duan (Dipsaci Radix), 10g
    Che Qian Zi (Plantaginis Semen), 15g
    Tu Si Zi (Cuscutae Semen), 10g
    Gou Qi Zi (Lycii Fructus), 10g
    Wu Wei Zi (Schisandrae Fructus), 10g
    Rou Cong Rong (Cistanches Herba), 10g
    Shu Di Huang (Rehmanniae Radix Praeparata), 15g
    Bai Ji Li (Tribuli Fructus), 15g

Results: Wang did not indicate what the results of treatment were, but this is a case which models how a modern Chinese andrology specialist approaches the problem of varicocele.

Insufficiency of kidney essence with low sperm density, vitality, and motility

Qi (1987) treated a case of male infertility in a 29 year-old male with a four-year history of unprotected intercourse and no successful pregnancy. Semen analysis revealed a sperm density of 21 million/ml, 15% motility rate, and a low percentage of live sperm (unspecified). In the past, he had used vitamin E without any positive effect. Examination of the external genitalia was normal. His tongue was pale red and the fur was thin white; the pulse was fine.

Dr. Qi's diagnosis was insufficiency of kidney essence and his treatment principle was to supplement the kidneys and strengthen essence. He used *Qiang Jing Jian* (Essence-Strengthening Brew). The ingredients are as follows:
    Chao Lu Feng Fang (Vespae Nidus Frictus), 15g
    Yin Yang Huo (Epimedii Herba), 15g
    Rou Cong Rong (Cistanches Herba), 10g
    Dang Gui (Angelicae Sinensis Radix), 10g
    Shu Di Huang (Rehmanniae Radix Praeparata), 15g
    Xu Duan (Dipsaci Radix), 10g
    Gou Ji (Cibotii Rhizoma), 10g
    Suo Yang (Cynomorii Herba), 10g
    Sha Yuan Ji Li (Astragali Complanati Semen), 15g
    He Shou Wu (Polygoni Multiflori Radix), 15g
    Zhi Huang Jing (Polygonati Rhizoma Praeparata), 15g
    Lu Jiao (Cervi Cornu), 10g

Results: After taking 14 packets of this prescription, Dr. Qi added *Bai Zi Ren* (Platycladi Semen), 10g, and he prescribed another 14 packets. A repeat semen analysis at that time revealed 33 million/ml, and 60% motility rate. Before long, his wife became pregnant and she gave birth to their child.

Yin vacuity, dampness, and blood stasis

Deng (2000) reports on a case of male infertility in a 28 year-old male. The patient had been having unprotected intercourse for more than three years with no successful pregnancy. The semen analysis revealed thick ashen white semen, seminal volume of 2.5 ml, a pH of 8.0, 90 minutes liquefaction time, 65 million/ml, 60% motility rate, and low rate of vitality (specifics not provided). The tongue was red and the fur was thin yellow. The pulse was stringlike slippery. The Western diagnosis was male infertility due to nonliquefaction of semen.

Dr. Deng's treatment principle was to enrich yin and clear heat and to disinhibit dampness and transform stasis. He prescribed the following formula:

   Tian Hua Fen (Trichosanthis Radix), 20g
   Sheng Di Huang (Rehmanniae Radix Exsiccata seu Recens), 15g
   Mai Men Dong (Ophiopogonis Radix), 15g
   Zhi Mu (Anemarrhenae Rhizoma), 10g
   Huang Bai (Phellodendri Cortex), 5g

Results: The patient took one packet per day for 50 days. A repeat semen analysis was completely normal and three months later his wife became pregnant.

Low sperm motility due to spleen and kidney vacuity and insufficiency of essence-blood

He (2003) treated a case of low sperm motility in a 32 year-old male. The patient had been having unprotected intercourse for more than three years with no successful pregnancy. His wife had been fully examined and no abnormalities had been discovered that would interfere with her fertility. He reported normal sexual function and no history of chronic disease, and did not drink alcohol or smoke cigarettes. His tongue was pale and small with a thin white fur, and his pulse was sinking. The results of the semen analysis were as follows: 32 million/ml; seminal volume of 3 ml; semen liquefaction time of 27 minutes and; a sperm motility rate of 17%. The Western medical diagnosis was low sperm motility.

Dr. He's Chinese medical diagnosis was spleen and kidney vacuity and insufficiency of essence-blood, and he prescribed a variation of his research formula called *Huo Jing Chong Zi Tang* (Sperm-Quickening Seed-Planting Decoction). The ingredients were:

   Huang Qi (Astragali Radix), 30g
   Sang Shen (Mori Fructus), 30g
   Yin Yang Huo (Epimedii Herba), 30g
   Tu Si Zi (Cuscutae Semen), 15g
   Xian Mao (Curculiginis Rhizoma), 15g
   Gou Qi Zi (Lycii Fructus), 15g
   Lu Jiao Jiao (Cervi Cornus Gelatinum), 15g, dissolved into the strained
      decoction

Shan Zhu Yu (Corni Fructus), 12g

Rou Cong Rong (Cistanches Herba), 12g

Shui Zhi (Hirudo), 5g, powdered and taken mixed with the strained decoction

Gan Cao (Glycyrrhizae Radix), 10g

Zi He Che (Placenta Hominis), 15g, powdered and swallowed with the strained decoction

Results: After taking the prescription for 4 weeks, a repeat semen analysis was completely normal. After taking the formula for another 3 weeks, his wife became pregnant.

Acumoxa therapy for low sperm vitality

Shi (2001) reports a case of a 34 year-old male with infertility who had been having unprotected intercourse for over 7 years with no successful pregnancy. Semen analysis revealed: seminal volume of 3 ml; sperm vitality rate of 10% and; a low rate of forward-moving sperm. Additional signs included: somber-white facial complexion; despondent essence-spirit; fatigued cumbersome body; cold limbs; aversion to cold; soreness and limpness of the lumbus and knees; a pale fat tongue with tooth marks and; a fine slow weak pulse.

The diagnosis was kidney yang vacuity and life gate fire debility. The treatment principle was to warm the kidneys and invigorate yang. Two groups of points were used: 1) *Ming Men* (GV-4), *Shen Shu* (BL-23), *Zhi Shi* (BL-52), and *Tai Xi* (KI-3) and; 2) *Guan Yuan* (CV-4), *Qi Hai* (CV-6), *Zu San Li* (ST-36), and *San Yin Jiao* (SP-6). Treatment with one or the other group of points was given once per day. The patient was advised to avoid intercourse during the treatment course to preserve his kidney qi.

Results: After two months of daily treatment, the patient's sleep and appetite improved. A repeat semen analysis showed improvements in sperm density, motility, and vitality, but had still not reached normal levels. After two more months of treatment, a third semen analysis was completely normal. Treatment was discontinued, but the patient was advised to treat himself at home by using a moxa stick on *Guan Yuan* (CV-4) and *Qi Hai* (CV-6) for 20 minutes a day. Six months later, his wife became pregnant.

Peyronie's Disease

Western Medicine

Peyronie's disease—first described by the French surgeon Francois Gigot de la Peyronie in 1743—is characterized by the formation of a fibrous plaque (most often on the dorsum of the penis) within the tunica albuginea of the cavernous sheaths of the penis that usually results in painful and bent erections. The main issues for the patient include: 1) inability to have normal sexual intercourse due to a misshaped erection; 2) pain during erection; 3) varying degrees of erectile dysfunction and; 4) relationship tension created by sexual dysfunction. Though the exact causative mechanism is unclear, the predominant opinion is that Peyronie's disease is caused by either chronic penile inflammation as a result of autoimmune disorders, abnormal collagen deposition in collagen diseases, or isolated or repeated penile trauma. Rarely, it may arise as a side effect of beta-blockers. Risk factors include decreased penile elasticity due to aging, genetic predisposition, and Dupuytren's contracture.[1]

Depending on the location of the lesion, the erect penis of a man with Peyronie's disease will bend in a different direction. For example, lesions on the dorsum of the penis result in a downward-bending erection, lesions on the ventral portion of the penis result in an upward-bending erection, and bilateral lesions (more rare) result in an indented and shortened penis.

Peyronie's disease is distinguished from congenital penile curvature by two facts: that it is acquired and by the degree of curvature and angle. Further, congenital curvature is a benign condition that usually does not prevent normal intercourse because the shaft of the erect penis remains straight enough for normal intromission. In the early stages of Peyronie's disease (during the first 12–18 months), there is often pain with erection. In the later stages, however, pain may resolve, but varying degrees of erectile dysfunction are usually present due to fibrosis within the sinusoidal spaces of the corpus cavernosa that interferes with normal penile tumescence.

---

[1] Dupuytren's contracture is characterized by the formation of a cord-like fibrous band across the palm of the hand that tends to cause the fingers to contract.

Diagnosis

• *Physical examination*

Physical examination reveals a band of fibrous tissue on the shaft of the penis, that is usually on the dorsum, but it may be located on other parts of the penile shaft, and can even be present in more than one location. Patients and their physicians can usually palpate the lesion on either a flaccid or erect penis, but at times erections must be induced by injectable medications in the office for complete evaluation.

• *Ultrasound*

In some cases, ultrasound imaging is used to verify the presence of penile fibrous plaques and to differentiate them from other lesions. Some researchers feel that there may be many more cases of otherwise undetected Peyronie's disease among patients with erectile dysfunction (Amin *et al.*, 1993).

Treatment

• *Watchful waiting*

Since some cases of Peyronie's disease improve spontaneously over time, physicians may adopt a watchful waiting approach for the first several months to see if it will resolve spontaneously. When symptoms persist over a period of months or are severe, especially when there is pain or an abnormal penile angle to the point of discomfort during intercourse, doctors usually adopt a more active treatment approach.

• *Non-surgical treatments*

1. Colchicine

Because of the presumed connection between Peyronie's disease and chronic penile inflammation, some urologists use oral colchicine to reduce penile collagen deposition for patients with Peyronie's.

2. Potassium aminobenzoate (POTABA)

POTABA is a prescription-only form of vitamin B-complex that has antifibrotic properties. Weidner *et al.* (2005) concluded that although POTABA does not change existing lesions, it may slow the progression of an existing disease.

3. Intralesional injections

Drugs such as interferon-alpha-2a or 2b, verapimil, or collagenase injected directly into the penile lesions appear to have some benefit for patients with Peyronie's diseases. Trost *et al.* (2007) report that interferon has been widely shown to be effective. In a recent study, intralesional verapimil injections appeared to show a reduction in penile curvature in 18% of patients and disease stabilization in 60% of patients. The patients in the study received six injections of verapimil directly into the penile lesions at an interval of every two weeks (Bennett *et al.*, 2007).

• Surgery

Surgery should be the last resort for patients who do not respond to more conservative forms of treatment, and for patients who have had severe symptoms for at least one year (Gelbard, 2005). The risks of surgery for Peyronie's disease include penile shortening, as well as decreased penile sensation and tumescence.

There are four main surgical methods used for Peyronie's disease including plaque excision, plaque incision with saphenous vein graft, nesbit plication, and penile prosthesis. Plaque excision consists of surgical removal of the fibrous plaque and replacement of the affected area with normal tissue from the pubic region. In plaque incision, the surgeon makes many cuts within the lesion in order to allow for normal straightening during erection and then covers them with a graft from the saphenous vein. Through nesbit plication the surgeon seeks to cancel the bending effect by plicating (gathering) or removing tissue on the opposite side of the penis. Finally, an implanted solid or inflatable biocompatible plastic penile prosthesis may be used as a means of straightening and increasing the rigidity of the penis (Mayo, 2005).

Western Complementary Medicine

• Vitamin E

Vitamin E may have some benefit for preventing and treating early stage Peyronie's disease, though urologists generally feel that it is not particularly helpful for those with more advanced disease (Mayo, 2005).

Chinese Medicine

Disease discrimination

Peyronie's disease is obviously a Western medical disease category. Only very few Chinese andrology texts I have referenced even have a chapter on Peyronie's disease. The ones that do generally name this condition using Western medical terms in Chinese. These texts invariably correlate Peyronie's disease with what is presumably a Chinese andrological disease category, namely yin stem phlegm node (*yin jing tan he*). However, they uncharacteristically do not give any classical references for these specific terms, and I have been unable to find any Chinese literature accessible under these specific headings using the tools I have available to me. Barring an even more extensive search, my current conclusion is that these are actually new terms that have resulted from the integration of Chinese and Western medicine in modern Chinese andrology.

However, we can find premodern discussions of the term phlegm node (*tan he*) in the external medicine (*wai ke*) literature. For example, in its chapter on scrotal abscess (*nang yong*), *Wai Ke Li Lie* (*Rationale and Examples in External Medicine*),[2]

---

[2] *Wai Ke Li Lie* was written by Wang Ji in 1519, during the Ming dynasty.

states: "A weak man has a phlegm node at the root of the penis somewhat like a large bean; with taxation it becomes swollen and painful." Further, in its chapter on flowing phlegm (*liu tan*), *Wai Zheng Yi An Hui Bian* (*Collected Case Studies of External Patterns*)[3] states: "Phlegm obstructed within the skin but outside the membranes, with copious qi but scant flesh, with neither blood nor flesh pus transformation, and having form that can be palpated is called phlegm lump (*tan kuai*), phlegm pouch (*tan bao*), phlegm node (*tan he*), or phlegm scrofula (*tan li*)."

In any case, modern Chinese andrologists offer disease causes and pathomechanisms, as well as pattern discriminations for Peyronie's disease and base these on Chinese medical theory for conditions such as phlegm node and combine it with theory relating to the function, relationships, and location of the penis according to Chinese medicine.

Disease causes and pathomechanisms

• Binding depression of liver qi
The liver channel skirts the genitals, liver free-coursing moves the blood, the liver governs the sinews (including the ancestral sinew), and the liver regulates the activity of the affect-mind. Enduring depression, resentment, and other forms of affect-mind damage make the liver lose its ability to course and discharge and to orderly reach; this leads to binding depression of liver qi. When binding depression of liver qi endures, blood becomes static and fluids collect within the penis; over time they congeal into a phlegm node.

• Liver-kidney yin vacuity
The liver channel skirts the genitals and the kidneys govern the anterior yin. Either because of natural endowment insufficiency, constitutional vacuity, or overtaxation, liver and kidney yin become vacuous. Liver and kidney yin vacuity leads to hyperactive ministerial fire. When this fire endures, it decocts blood and fluids into a phlegm node on the penis.

• Spleen and kidney yang vacuity
The spleen governs movement and transformation of water-damp. The kidney governs water as well as the anterior yin region. Either due to natural endowment or constitutional spleen and kidney yang vacuity, to dietary irregularities damaging the spleen, or to overtaxation, splenic movement and transformation failure ensues, and the kidney lacks warmth and power to govern water metabolism. This results in the formation of dampness, phlegm, and water-rheum, which collects in the penis and over time forms a phlegm node. Further, when there is spleen and kidney yang vacuity, there is a lack of warmth and power for moving blood; hence, blood becomes static and gathers within the ancestral sinew.

• Traumatic injury to the penis
When the penis is injured by trauma, qi and blood within the channels and

---

[3] *Wai Zheng Yi An Hui Bian* was written by Yu Jing He in 1894, during the Qing dynasty.

network vessels become obstructed. Over time, fluids also become obstructed and phlegm forms. Hence, penile trauma leads to qi stagnation, blood stasis, and phlegm congelation within the channels and network vessels of the penis.

Pattern discrimination

1. Congelation and binding of turbid phlegm with qi stagnation and blood stasis

Signs: Plaques and lumps or narrow strips of hardened areas along the body of the penis of indefinite number and size, and that feel like hardened bone when pressed, marked pain and pulling sensation with erection, repressed and depressed affect-mind, distention and pain of the chest and rib-side, sagging distention in the testes, dark tongue with possible stasis macules, and a sinking rough or sinking stringlike pulse.

Treatment principles: Course the liver and quicken the blood, transform phlegm and dissipate binds

Guiding formulas: Modified *Chai Hu Shu Gan San* (Bupleurum Liver-Coursing Powder) with *Tao Hong Si Wu Tang* (Peach Kernel and Carthamus Four Agents Decoction)

Ingredients:
> *Chai Hu* (Bupleuri Radix), 10g
> *Bai Shao* (Paeoniae Radix Alba), 12g
> *Zhi Ke* (Aurantii Fructus), 10g
> *Xiang Fu* (Cyperi Rhizoma), 12g
> *Qing Pi* (Citri Reticulatae Pericarpium Viride), 10g
> *Yan Hu Suo* (Corydalis Rhizoma), 12g
> *Chuan Lian Zi* (Toosendan Fructus), 12g
> *Li Zhi He* (Litchi Semen), 6g
> *Chuan Xiong* (Chuanxiong Rhizoma), 10g
> *Tao Ren* (Persicae Semen), 10g
> *Hong Hua* (Carthami Flos), 12g
> *Dang Gui Wei* (Angelicae Sinensis Radicis Extremitas), 12g
> *Kun Bu* (Laminariae/Eckloniae Thallus), 12g
> *Hai Zao* (Sargassum), 12g

Modifications: When depressed liver qi transforms fire, add *Mu Dan Pi* (Moutan Cortex), 9g, and *Zhi Zi* (Gardeniae Fructus), 9g.

2. Yin vacuity with phlegm fire

Signs: Slightly reddish node or nodes on the dorsum of the penis, slight pain with erection, generalized low-grade heat effusion, night sweats, dry mouth and throat, tinnitus, soreness and limpness of the lumbus and knees, small red tongue with either scanty fur or slimy yellow fur, fine rapid pulse

Treatment principles: Enrich yin and downbear fire, transform phlegm and dissipate binds

Guiding formulas: Modified *Da Bu Yin Wan* (Major Yin Supplementation Pill) and *Xiao He Wan* (Node-Dispersing Pill)

Ingredients:

Shu Di Huang (Rehmanniae Radix Praeparata), 12g
Bie Jia (Trionycis Carapax), 15g, predecocted
Gui Ban (Testudinis Carapax et Plastrum), 15g, predecocted
Huang Bai (Phellodendri Cortex), 10g
Zhi Mu (Anemarrhenae Rhizoma), 10g
Yan Ju Hong (Citri Reticulatae Exocarpium Rubrum Salsa), 10g
Chi Fu Ling (Poria Rubra), 10g
Lian Qiao (Forsythiae Fructus), 6g
Huang Qin (Scutellariae Radix), 6g
Shan Zhi Zi (Gardeniae Fructus), 6g
Ban Xia (Pinelliae Rhizoma), 10g
Xuan Shen (Scrophulariae Radix), 10g
Mu Li (Ostreae Concha), 15g, predecocted
Tian Hua Fen (Trichosanthis Radix), 12g
Jie Geng (Platycodonis Radix), 10g
Gua Lou (Trichosanthis Fructus), 12g
Bai Jiang Can (Bombyx Batryticatus), 6g

Modifications: For marked night sweats, add *Yin Chai Hu* (Stellariae Radix), 6g, *Di Gu Pi* (Lycii Cortex), 15g, and *Wu Wei Zi* (Schisandrae Fructus), 6g.

3. Spleen and kidney yang vacuity with phlegm-dampness and blood stasis

Signs: Either one or many small lumps along the penis that feel like soft bone, penile pain or pulling sensation during erection, low libido, yang wilt, obesity, fatigue and lack of strength, a tendency to have sticky sputum and nasal snivel, slimy tongue fur, and sinking stringlike slippery pulse.

Treatment principles: Supplement the spleen and boost the kidneys, transform phlegm and dissipate binds, and quicken the blood and transform stasis

Guiding formulas: Modified *Er Chen Tang* (Two Matured Ingredients Decoction) with *Huo Luo Xiao Ling Dan* (Network-Quickening Miraculous Effect Elixir)

Ingredients:

Ban Xia (Pinelliae Rhizoma), 12g
Chen Pi (Citri Reticulatae Pericarpium), 12g
Fu Ling (Poria), 15g
Zhi Gan Cao (Glycyrrhizae Radix cum Liquido Fricta), 6g
Tu Si Zi (Cuscutae Semen), 12g

Gui Zhi (Cinnamomi Ramulus), 6g
Bai Jie Zi (Sinapis Albae Semen), 6g
Hai Zao (Sargassum), 12g
Kun Bu (Laminariae/Eckloniae Thallus), 12g
Ru Xiang (Olibanum), 10g
Mo Yao (Myrrha), 10g
Dan Shen (Salviae Miltiorrhizae Radix), 20g
Hong Hua (Carthami Flos), 12g
Dang Gui (Angelicae Sinensis Radix), 12g
Tao Ren (Persicae Semen), 10g
E Zhu (Curcumae Rhizoma), 10g
Chi Shao (Paeoniae Radix Rubra), 12g

Modifications: For marked spleen vacuity with fatigue and sloppy stools, add *Dang Shen* (Codonopsis Radix), 15g, *Bai Zhu* (Atractylodis Macrocephalae Rhizoma), 15g, *Huang Qi* (Astragali Radix), 20g, and *Shan Yao* (Dioscoreae Rhizoma), 20g.

Acumoxa therapy

Main points: *Qu Gu* (CV-2), *Zhong Ji* (CV-3), *San Yin Jiao* (SP-6), *Guan Yuan* (CV-4), *Da He* (KI-12), *Feng Long* (ST-40), *Jian Shi* (PC-5), *Tian Jing* (SJ-10)

For binding depression of liver qi, add *Tai Chong* (LV-3), *Li Gou* (LV-5), and *Qu Quan* (LV-8)

For liver-kidney yin vacuity, add *Tai Xi* (KI-3), *Gan Shu* (BL-18), and *Shen Shu* (BL-23)

For spleen and kidney yang vacuity, add moxa on *Pi Shu* (BL-20), *Shen Shu* (BL-23), *Ming Men* (GV-4), and *Guan Yuan* (CV-4)

Experiential formulas

Transforming phlegm

Liu and Liu (2001) report on Liu Hui-Min's experience treating Peyronie's disease by using a specially-prepared formula made with the following medicinals:

Ban Xia (Pinelliae Rhizoma), 24g
Ju Hong (Citri Reticulatae Exocarpium Rubrum), 30g
Ju Luo (Citri Fructus Fasciculus Vascularis), 18g

Instructions: Grind all the medicinals into a fine powder and place in a glass jar with 250 ml of *Bai Jiu* (Granorum Spiritus Incolor). Seal the jar and soak for 7 days. Shake several times per day during the soaking period. After 7 days, strain the medicinal juice and add it to 500 ml of steamed distilled water. Place in a clay pot and boil for several minutes. Cool to room temperature, stir in 5 grams of potassium iodide, and store in a glass bottle. Shake before using and take 2 ml mixed with 3 ml of water three times per day.

External treatments

1. Mix equal parts of a finely powdered modification of *Yu Shu Dan* (Jade Pivot Elixir) and *Er Bai San* (Two White Ingredients Powder) with vinegar to achieve the consistency of a thick paste and apply directly to the affected areas of the penis once a day (Revised from Tan and Tao, 1999). The ingredients are:

   Shan Ci Gu (Cremastrae seu Pleiones Pseudobulbus)
   Wu Bei Zi (Galla Chinensis)
   Da Ji (Cirsii Japonici Herba seu Radix)
   Mu Li (Ostreae Concha)
   Bai Jiang Can (Bombyx Batryticatus)
   Tian Nan Xing (Arisaematis Rhizoma)
   Bei Mu (Fritillariae Bulbus)
   Gui Zhi (Cinnamomi Ramulus)
   Bing Pian (Borneolum)

2. Make a steam wash using 30 grams of *Luo De Da* (Centellae Herba)[4] and steam the affected area once per day (Guo *et al.*, 1999).

Preventive measures and lifestyle modification

1. Maintain a positive and relaxed mental outlook

The main cause of Peyronie's disease is phlegm binding in the penis. The main cause of binding depression of liver qi is affect-mind damage, and liver free coursing is responsible for maintaining the smooth flow of qi and fluids throughout the entire body. Thus, to prevent and treat this disease it is vital to maintain the orderly reaching of liver qi by limiting stress, expressing emotions as they arise, and maintaining a positive mental outlook.

2. Avoid penile trauma

As established previously, trauma to the penis leads to stagnation of qi, collection of phlegm, and stasis of blood in the penis. During treatment of Peyronie's disease or to prevent it, penile trauma should be avoided. Sources of penile trauma can include cycling with an especially hard seat, rough sex, and sports injuries.

Representative Chinese Research

Transforming stasis and dissipating binds

Wei (1994) treated 23 cases of Peyronie's disease with a formula called *Hua Yu San Jie Tang* (Stasis-Transforming Bind-Dissipating Decoction). After cooking and drinking the medicine as usual, the subjects were also asked to cook it a third time for use as a steam wash on the penis. The ingredients are as follows:

---

[4] *Luo De Da* is used in this case to quicken the blood, disperse swelling, and relieve pain.

Huang Qi (Astragali Radix), 15g
Dan Shen (Salviae Miltiorrhizae Radix), 12g
Shan Zhu Yu (Corni Fructus), 12g
Sang Shen Zi (Mori Fructus), 12g
Dang Gui (Angelicae Sinensis Radix), 10g
Niu Xi (Achyranthis Bidentatae Radix), 10g
Chi Shao (Paeoniae Radix Rubra), 10g
Chai Hu (Bupleuri Radix), 10g
Xiang Fu (Cyperi Rhizoma), 10g
Ru Xiang (Olibanum), 9g
Mo Yao (Myrrha), 9g
E Zhu (Curcumae Rhizoma), 9g
Li Zhi He (Litchi Semen), 9g
Fu Ling (Poria), 9g
Chuan Xiong (Chuanxiong Rhizoma), 9g
Ju He (Citri Reticulatae Semen), 9g
Zhi Shi (Aurantii Fructus immaturis), 9g
Gan Cao (Glycyrrhizae Radix), 3g

Results: Among the 23 cases treated, 19 were cured and 4 had some results.

Supplementing spleen qi, enriching liver and kidney yin, transforming stasis, and transforming phlegm and dissipating binds

Wang, Liu, and Chen *et al.* (2003) reported on the treatment of 18 cases of Peyronie's disease with a formula called *Shen Qi Gui Shao San Jie Tang* (Ginseng, Astragalus, Chinese Angelica, and Peony Bind-Dissipating Decoction). The ingredients are as follows:

Huang Qi (Astragali Radix), 15g
Dang Shen (Codonopsis Radix), 12g
Bu Gu Zhi (Psoraleae Fructus), 12g
Sang Shen Zi (Mori Fructus), 12g
Gou Qi Zi (Lycii Fructus), 12g
Dang Gui (Angelicae Sinensis Radix), 10g
Niu Xi (Achyranthis Bidentatae Radix), 10g
Chi Shao (Paeoniae Radix Rubra), 10g
Chen Pi (Citri Reticulatae Pericarpium), 10g
Xiang Fu (Cyperi Rhizoma), 10g
Gan Cao (Glycyrrhizae Radix), 10g
Chai Hu (Bupleuri Radix), 9g
Fu Ling (Poria), 9g
Chuan Xiong (Chuanxiong Rhizoma), 9g
Li Zhi He (Litchi Semen), 9g
Zhi Shi (Aurantii Fructus immaturis), 9g
Zi Su Geng (Perillae Caulis), 9g

Results: Eight cases were cured, as measured by complete disappearance of any penile nodules and erectile bending. Four cases had good results, as measured by reduction of penile nodules and improvement of erectile bending. Six cases had no result, as measured by no improvement in either penile nodules or erectile bending.

Integrated Chinese-Western medicine

Zong (1991) reports on 21 cases of Peyronie's disease treated with integrated Chinese-Western medicine.

Chinese treatment

One packet of the formula below was boiled in water once per day for 30 minutes, and was administered orally six days a week with a rest on the seventh day.

San Leng (Sparganii Rhizoma), 15g
E Zhu (Curcumae Rhizoma), 15g
Tao Ren (Persicae Semen), 15g
Hong Hua (Carthami Flos), 15g
Chen Pi (Citri Reticulatae Pericarpium), 15g
Hou Po (Magnoliae Officinalis Cortex), 15g
Huang Qi (Astragali Radix), 20g
Kun Bu (Laminariae/Eckloniae Thallus), 20g
Bai Shao (Paeoniae Radix Alba), 30g
Hai Zao (Sargassum), 10g
Gan Cao (Glycyrrhizae Radix), 10g
Tu Bie Chong (Eupolyphaga/Stereophaga), 6g
Shui Zhi (Hirudo), 6g

Western treatment

The Western medical treatment consisted of oral administration of 4 mg of chlorpheniramine, three times per day, and 25mg of indomethacin, three times per day. Additionally, the researchers wrapped a strong but loose nylon sock soaked in about 1 ml of a solution of 1% procaine/2–3 ml around the penis once a week.

Results: Seven days comprised one treatment course. Subjects completed between 10–13 treatment courses. All patients were completely cured as defined by: 1) either the disappearance or shrinkage of the penile lesions to less than 0.5 cm; 2) no abnormal sensations accompanying erection; 3) no sexual dysfunction and; 4) disappearance or 85% reduction of any erectile deformity.

Andropause

Western Medicine

Andropause (male climacteric; testosterone deficiency syndrome) refers to a collection of endocrine, somatic, and psychic changes experienced by men in middle age and beyond, including sexual dysfunction, loss of muscle mass and function, decreased bone density, physical frailty, gain in fat mass, cognitive impairment, and loss of body hair. These signs are speculated to be due to declining androgen levels associated with aging. It is important to note, however, that some authorities do not accept andropause as a distinct clinical entity but rather consider these symptoms as a normal part of the male aging process, except when a definitive diagnosis of hypogonadism (testicular failure) can be established (Tancredi et al, 2005). Such cases would be characterized by clinically and chemically demonstrable low levels of testosterone, rather than characteristically low-normal age-related levels.

This suggests that rather than automatically perceiving decreased androgen levels in aging men as a pathological process, physicians should work toward understanding gradually decreasing levels as a physiological part of aging while they also remain alert for men whose androgen levels decrease abruptly or more drastically, as is the case in primary and secondary hypogonadism. The logical clinical conclusion is that when a man presents with andropausal signs and no abnormal decrease in androgens can be identified, he should be encouraged to adopt a healthier diet, increase his exercise levels, seek alternative and complementary modalities, and decrease stress levels—all of which can help to compensate for some aging-related changes—rather than commence androgen replacement therapy (ART). However this remains somewhat controversial.

The term "male menopause," as used by Diamond (1997), is a misnomer because men do not have a menstrual period that pauses or stops at middle age. However, the term evolved out of the perception that men—like women—undergo observable alterations in their quality of life at middle age. The more recent understanding of andropause as a clinical entity also potentially provides a physiological model for understanding the psychological changes some men experience at middle age which have previously been organized under the heading of "male mid-life crisis." This includes behaviors such as abruptly leaving a long-term relationship in search of younger sexual and romantic partners, buying an attractive sports car, as well as feelings of lost career opportunities, regrets, and of being a failure in life.

Handelsman and Liu (2005) suggest that at least part of the enthusiasm generated about andropause in the last ten years is rooted in the profit motives of pharmaceutical companies who are hoping to boost the sales of androgen replacement therapy (ART). They draw an analogy between the previous heyday of estrogen replacement therapy for menopausal women and the current trend toward the use of ART for aging men. They further suggest that the risks of ART in the majority of so-called andropausal men (those who are not truly hypogonadal) probably outweighs the benefits in most cases. Of course, this is also the case with hormone replacement therapy for most menopausal women. Additionally, Handelsman (2006) reports that the sales of testosterone have increased twenty-fold in the U.S. since 1990, whereas they have not changed in Europe or Australia during the same period. He attributes the change to U.S. pharmaceutical companies' direct marketing of testosterone products to the public. Hence, physicians are advised to be cautious about jumping on the andropause bandwagon, and to reserve ART for andropausal men who have a definitive case of hypogonadism.

Diagnosis

The diagnosis of andropause is somewhat unclear since it is not universally accepted as a bonafide clinical entity. Currently, the most careful physician will reserve the diagnosis of andropause for symptomatic older men with demonstrable hypogonadism and will manage men with low-normal serum androgen levels more conservatively with lifestyle modifications as stated above.

Serum androgen levels

A normal serum testosterone level is >350 ng/dl, and a borderline low level is 200–350 ng/dl. The definitive standard for establishing true hypogonadism (failure of the testes to produce adequate testosterone) is a serum testosterone level below 200 ng/dl. In cases of hypogonadism, the current accepted therapeutic goal is to restore the serum testosterone level to the mid-normal range. What is not clear yet, however, is when to use ART for men with borderline low levels and when not to use it.

Although age-related decline in testosterone levels involves other structures, including the hypothalamus and the pituitary, it is mainly thought to be due to testicular failure (hypogonadism). (Fauci *et al.*, 1998) A number of studies—most notably the Baltimore Longitudinal Study of Aging and the Massachusetts Male Aging Study—have concluded that testosterone levels normally decline as men age. This decline begins at about age 30 and steadily continues from mid-life at a rate of about 1% per year. These studies also suggest that about 4% of men between the ages of 40 and 70 have a serum testosterone level <150 ng/dl.

Androgen Deficiency in Aging Males (ADAM) questionnaire

The ADAM questionnaire was developed by Morley *et al.* (2000) as a quick screening method for determining which male patients require laboratory evaluation for hypogonadism. While it is a useful tool that is able to identify hypogonadal males, a recent study concluded that it cannot definitively establish hypogonadism and hence cannot replace laboratory evaluation (Tancredi *et al.*, 2005). A positive answer to either question 1 or 7 below, or any three of the remaining questions necessitates further evaluation of serum androgen levels by a physician.

1. Do you have a decrease in strength and/or endurance?
2. Do you have a lack of energy?
3. Do you have a decrease in your sex drive (libido)?
4. Are you more sad and/or grumpy than usual?
5. Have you lost height?
6. Have you noticed a decreased enjoyment in life?
7. Have you noticed a recent deterioration in your ability to play sports?
8. Has there been a recent deterioration in your work performance?
9. Are your erections less strong?
10. Are you falling asleep after dinner?

Treatment

Men with primarily sexual manifestations of andropause—especially erectile dysfunction (ED)—who are not clearly hypogonadal, should seek nonhormonal treatment for ED. On this note, we may recall that less than 10% of men with ED have it because of decreased androgen levels.[1] Similarly, andropausal men who primarily complain of lower urinary tract symptoms (LUTS) due to prostate disorders should seek nonhormonal treatment for those conditions.

Androgen replacement therapy (ART)

According to Fauci *et al.* (1998), some studies have shown that testosterone replacement therapy can positively affect some of the symptoms experienced by andropausal men such as sexual dysfunction, bone density loss, decreased strength, loss of muscle mass, and cognitive difficulties. According to Handelsman (2006), it is not yet clear and will not be for at least a decade, however, whether the risks of long-term androgen replacement ther-

---

[1] See Book 2, Chapter 4 on ED for further discussion.

apy (*i.e.*, possible increased risk of prostate cancer or cardiovascular disease) outweigh the potential benefits. At this point, most sources agree that testosterone replacement therapy should be reserved for aging men with established hypogonadism.

General lifestyle modifications

• *Increase exercise levels*

Increasing exercise levels for aging men can be very helpful in reducing weight, limiting bone loss, improving aerobic capacity, and in decreasing stress that may accompany andropausal changes.

• *Improve dietary habits*

As an increase in fat mass and decrease of muscle mass are associated with andropause, adopting a low-fat diet is clearly indicated for andropausal men. Further, a recent study (Kaplan, 2007) has shown that increased waist circumference in men is associated with increased pelvic symptoms including lower urinary tract symptoms (LUTS) and sexual dysfunction. It follows logically that a diet that supports weight loss would have beneficial sexual effects for overweight andropausal men.

• *Psychotherapy*

When men present with andropausal symptoms without correspondingly low androgen levels or demonstrably hypogonadal andropausal men struggle with psychological manifestations of their condition, including depression, anxiety, irritability, and insomnia, psychotherapy or psychiatric therapy may be helpful. The focus should be on helping men to adapt to normal age-related changes in themselves, by developing a sense of self-esteem that is not solely linked to youthful vigor. Emphasis on the unique value of life experience—including knowledge and professional skills that they have acquired over decades and can pass on to the next generation—is often useful. At times, mentoring younger people can be of aid in promoting this mindset.

Western Complementary Medicine

• *Dehydroepiandrosterone (DHEA)*

A precursor to testosterone, DHEA is produced by the adrenal glands. It is widely available over the counter as a supplement and is used as a means of reducing andropausal symptoms and marketed as an alternative to pharmacological ART. According to Sahelian (2007), evidence from human studies suggests that DHEA may be useful for andropausal men because it has modest benefits in increasing bone mass, improving insulin sensitivity and blood vessel function in middle-aged men, reducing the risk of cardiovascular disease, and improving cognitive function. The recommended dosage range varies widely, from 5mg per day to more than 100mg per day. It is wise to begin at the most conservative dose and progress upward from there if necessary. Side effects may include acne, increased sweat odor, scalp itching, irritability and restlessness, hair thinning or hair loss, and according to Sahelian and Borken (1998), palpitations and heart arrhythmias.

• *Tribulus terrestris*[2]

An herbal medicine used by many cultures for centuries (including in Chinese medicine as *Bai Ji Li*), a standardized extract of tribulus terrestris has recently become popular as a libido-enhancing supplement in the West. This is partially based on findings in rat studies in which administration of tribulus terrestris extract increased sexual behavior and intracavernous pressure both in normal and castrated rats. The investigators posited that these effects were probably due to the androgen-increasing property of tribulus terrestris. According to Sahelian (2007), there is yet to be clear evidence that tribulus terrestris use leads to long-term increases in androgen levels, but anecdotal reports abound. Normal dosage ranges for the 40% saponin standardized extract range from 250mg–750mg per day.

• *Pregnenolone*

A hormone naturally present in the human body, pregnenolone can be converted into progesterone, testosterone, DHEA, or other steroid hormones. This product is less well-researched than DHEA and tribulus terrestris, but a preliminary study suggested that it may "antagonize certain acute effects of benzodiazepines and may enhance arousal via antagonist or inverse agonist actions at the benzodiazepine/GABA(A) receptor complex" (Meieran *et al.*, 2004). It is sometimes recommended to andropausal men as a means of improving cognitive function. Dosages range from 5–30mg per day.

Chinese Medicine

Disease discrimination

There is no specific corresponding disease category for andropause in the premodern literature of Chinese medicine. However, recent Chinese andrology texts universally contain a chapter on a disease called male climacteric syndrome (*nan xing geng nian qi zong he zheng*), which is categorized in Western medical terms and then discriminated into Chinese patterns. However, although the traditional literature lacks a specific disease category for andropause, it is rich in detailed discussions of the effects of aging on men's health embedded in disease categories such as vacuity taxation (*xu lao*), insomnia, palpitations, yang wilt, fatigue, and depression pathocondition (*yu zheng*). From our understanding of the symptoms andropausal men experience, we can see the logic in using the traditional literature pertaining to these disease categories as the theoretical repository for determining the disease causes, pathomechanisms, and treatment of andropause.

Disease causes and pathomechanisms

The locus classicus for understanding the cycles of men's lives as viewed by Chinese medicine is chapter 1 of *Su Wen* (*Plain Questions*),[3] which states: "When a male is eight years old, his kidney qi is replete and development of

---

[2] See Book 1, Chapter 6 on andrology and note the frequency with which *Bai Ji Li* (Tribuli Fructus) is used in herbal formulas to treat yang wilt.

[3] *Su Wen* is the first section of *Huang Di Nei Jing* (*Yellow Emperor's Inner Canon*), which was written in the 1st century CE.

his teeth continues. At two times eight, heavenly tenth[4] flows, essential qi overflows and drains, yin and yang are harmonious, and he can produce children. At three times eight, kidney qi is completely balanced, the sinews and bones are powerful and strong, and the true teeth develop to their utmost. At four times eight, the sinews and bones flourish [and are] exuberant, and the flesh is full and vigorous. At five times eight, kidney qi is debilitated, the hair falls out, and the teeth are desiccated. At six times eight, yang qi is debilitated above, the face is parched, and the hair at the temples turns gray. At seven times eight, liver qi is debilitated, the sinews are unmovable, heavenly tenth is exhausted, essence is scant, the kidney viscus is debilitated, and the bodily form is completely exhausted. At eight times eight, the teeth and hair fall out."

From analyzing this passage, we see that the main issue in the aging of men is debilitation of kidney essential qi, in this context meaning all physiological aspects of the kidneys including kidney essence, kidney yin, and kidney yang (qi). From clinical practice, it is evident that all age-related problems men experience can usually be explained in large part by kidney vacuity. Although there are various causes and varieties of this kidney vacuity, it is kidney vacuity just the same.

In another important passage in chapter 5 of *Su Wen* (*Plain Questions*), it states: "[In] the fortieth year, yin qi is naturally [depleted] by half, [being] depleted by living. [In] the fiftieth year, the body becomes heavy, and the ears and eyes are no [longer] sharp. [In] the sixtieth year, there is yin wilt, qi is greatly debilitated, the nine orifices are inhibited, there is vacuity below and repletion above, with discharge of both snivel and tears."

It is evident from this passage that at forty years of age, yin is depleted by half simply as a result of the normal aging process. Here we also see that early Chinese medical literature reveals an awareness of the progressive weakening of men's bodies as they age; this perspective is very useful for treating andropause.

In addition to kidney vacuity, binding depression of liver qi also plays an important role in the disease causes and pathomechanisms of andropause. Using five-phase theory, we can understand this as debilitation of water failing to engender wood. In terms of viscera-bowel theory, the liver and kidney share the same source. Hence, when kidney yin is vacuous, liver yin becomes vacuous, and when kidney yang is vacuous, liver yang becomes vacuous. If liver yin becomes insufficient and liver yin is not enriched, liver qi fails to course and discharge and becomes depressed. Similarly, if kidney yang is debilitated, liver yang becomes debilitated in turn; as a result, the liver lacks adequate power for coursing and discharge and becomes depressed.

---

[4] According to Wiseman and Feng (1998), heavenly tenth (*tian gui*) is that which the development of the human body, sexual function, and the ability to reproduce depends.

• Insufficiency of kidney yin

Kidney yin may be vacuous due to a variety of factors including the natural aging process, natural endowment insufficiency, bedroom taxation, overwork, excessive intake of warm supplementation, and enduring hyperactive heart fire caused by depression of the seven affects.

Because water and fire benefit each other, under normal conditions kidney yin enriches heart yin and vice versa. However, when kidney yin becomes debilitated, ministerial fire (kidney fire) becomes hyperactive and agitates the sovereign fire (heart fire). Therefore, we often see evidence not only of kidney yin vacuity and hyperactive ministerial fire in these patterns, but also of heart yin vacuity and hyperactive sovereign fire, which may be described as "noninteraction of the heart and kidneys."

Because kidney yin serves as the material foundation for liver yin-blood, once kidney yin becomes vacuous, liver yin-blood usually also becomes insufficient. Owing to the physiologically yang nature of the liver ("the liver is yin in body and yang in function") bestowed upon it by the warmth and activity of ministerial fire, when liver yin becomes insufficient, liver yang becomes hyperactive and ascends upward unchecked by liver yin. So, in clinical practice, andropausal men with kidney yin vacuity often also have hyperactive ascendancy of liver yang due to liver-kidney yin vacuity.[5]

• Debilitation of kidney yang

Kidney yang becomes debilitated as a result of aging itself, or due to natural endowment or constitutional vacuity of yang, bedroom taxation, enduring seminal efflux, excessive intake of cold raw foods or cold medicinals, or yang vacuity of other organs—most notably the spleen and heart—that eventually affect the kidneys. Because "where there is lack of yang, cold arises," interior cold is the natural outcome of kidney yang vacuity and is usually part of the clinical picture.

Kidney yang is the root of yang for the entire body, and spleen yang is especially reliant on kidney yang for warmth and activation, in clinical practice, andropausal men with kidney yang vacuity usually also have spleen yang vacuity.

In physiological circumstances, kidney yang warms the heart yang and heart yang in turn warms the kidney yang. It is the fires of these two viscera that are primarily responsible for warming and activating all physiological activities in the human body. So, when kidney yang-fire is debilitated, heart yang-fire wanes. Many andropausal men with kidney yang vacuity present with signs and symptoms of debilitated heart fire.

---

[5] For further discussion of this physiological relationship between the liver and kidneys, see Book 1, Chapter 4 on viscera-bowel physiology in andrology.

• Dual vacuity of kidney yin and yang

As Zhang Jing-Yue established in the Ming dynasty, "Kidney yin and yang are mutually rooted." Once one becomes vacuous, the other tends to also become vacuous. For example, when yin is vacuous, there is lack of foundation for the formation of yang, and when yang is vacuous, there is no power for engendering yin. It is perhaps more common to see these two pathomechanisms together rather than separate, and this scenario is extremely common in andropausal men.

• Kidney essence depletion and vacuity

Kidney essence is the raw material for the formation of all other substances within the body and is the material foundation from which qi is engendered. As men age, the quantity of essence left stored in the kidneys gradually declines. This is often caused by insufficient natural endowment or direct depletion of kidney (early heaven) essence by bedroom taxation, overwork, and dietary irregularities, but it is also caused by spleen vacuity failing to engender later heaven essence that would normally be banked up in the kidneys,[6] and by insufficiency of liver blood that would normally be transformed into kidney essence when needed.

The kidney stores essence, and essence serves as the material foundation for marrow and blood, and is therefore the source for semen and sperm. Therefore, the main andropausal pathomechanisms related to kidney essence vacuity center around insufficiency of essence to engender marrow to fill the bones, brain ("sea of marrow"), and sense organs, insufficient blood to nourish and enrich the entire body, and lack of raw material for the formation of semen and sperm.

• Heart-spleen dual vacuity

As a result of aging, overtaxation, natural endowment insufficiency or constitutional vacuity of qi, spleen qi becomes vacuous. Spleen qi is the later heaven source for the engenderment and transformation of qi and blood. Hence, when spleen qi is vacuous and weak, it does not adequately move and transform the essence of water and grain. Consequently, there is no material foundation for engendering qi and blood. When blood is vacuous, the heart is undernourished and unable to store the spirit or to govern the activity of the affect-mind.

• Binding depression of liver qi

The liver and kidneys share the same source, meaning that liver and kidney yang mutually warm each other, liver and kidney yin mutually enrich each other, and that liver blood and kidney essence mutually transform.[7] As men age and their kidneys weaken, the liver can be affected in of all the following

---

[6] For further discussion of this physiological relationship between the spleen and kidneys, see Book 1, Chapter 4 on viscera-bowel physiology in andrology.

[7] For further discussion of this physiological relationship between the liver and kidneys, see Book 1, Chapter 4 on viscera-bowel physiology in andrology.

ways: 1) kidney yin fails to enrich liver yin; 2) kidney yang fails to warm the liver yang and; 3) kidney essence fails to transform into liver blood. While each of these scenarios has its own unique set of pathomechanisms, for the purposes of our current discussion, they all can cause the liver to fail in its ability to orderly reach and course and discharge; the pathological result is binding depression of liver qi.

Chapter 54 of *Ling Shu* (*Magic Pivot*) states: "[In] the fiftieth year, liver qi becomes debilitated, and the liver leaves[8] [*i.e.*, lobes] become thin." This exhibits a sense of both liver qi and substance becoming weakened as men age, which results in decreased ability of the liver to orderly reach and course and discharge. Also, as revealed earlier in this section, chapter 1 of *Su Wen* states that at seven times eight, liver qi becomes debilitated.

Affect-mind damages the liver and leads to binding depression of liver qi. For andropausal men, this may derive specifically from enduring and unresolved anger and indignation, regrets, and depression and unhappiness. Very often these men will also exhibit signs of the pathomechanism of binding depression of liver qi transforming fire.

Further, once liver qi becomes depressed, it has a tendency to invade the spleen and cause splenic movement and transformation failure. If this endures, dampness forms and over time depressed dampness transforms into phlegm. Also, enduring depressed liver qi readily transforms fire, which decocts dampness into phlegm. The resulting combination of liver depression, phlegm and fire is often categorized under the heading of gallbladder depression with phlegm fire harassing the gallbladder and heart. If this pattern presents without heat and just with gallbladder depression and phlegm, the term gallbladder depression with phlegm harassing is used.

Pattern discrimination

1. Kidney yin vacuity with interior heat

Signs: Emaciation, tidal heat effusion and night sweating, vexation and heat of the five hearts, dry mouth and red cheeks, soreness and limpness of the lumbus and knees, dizzy head and tinnitus, insomnia with copious dreaming, premature ejaculation and seminal efflux, yellowish urine with a heat sensation during urination, dry bound stool, red tender thin tongue with scanty fur, fine rapid pulse.

Treatment principles: Supplement and enrich kidney yin, clear heat and consolidate yin

Guiding formula: Modified *Zhi Bai Di Huang Wan* (Anemarrhena, Phellodendron, and Rehmannia Pill)

---

[8] Early Chinese anatomical descriptions of the viscera, especially the lung and liver use the term leaves (*ye*) to refer to what we now refer to as lobes. Early graphic depictions of these organs depict these organs as having a leaf-life structure.

Ingredients:

Zhi Mu (Anemarrhenae Rhizoma), 10g
Huang Bai (Phellodendri Cortex), 12g
Sheng Di Huang (Rehmanniae Radix Exsiccata seu Recens), 15g
Shan Zhu Yu (Corni Fructus), 10g
Shan Yao (Dioscoreae Rhizoma), 12g
Fu Ling (Poria), 10g
Ze Xie (Alismatis Rhizoma), 10g
Mu Dan Pi (Moutan Cortex), 6g
Gui Ban (Testudinis Carapax et Plastrum), 15g
Bie Jia (Trionycis Carapax), 15g
Wu Wei Zi (Schisandrae Fructus), 6g
Sha Shen (Adenophorae seu Glehniae Radix), 10g
Tian Men Dong (Asparagi Radix), 10g
Mai Men Dong (Ophiopogonis Radix), 6g

Modifications: For patients with prominent night sweats, add *Di Gu Pi* (Lycii Cortex), 15g, *Duan Mu Li* (Ostreae Concha Calcinata), 15g, and *Fu Xiao Mai* (Tritici Fructus Levis), 20g, to further enrich yin, and to constrain sweat. For yang wilt and premature ejaculation, add *Ba Ji Tian* (Morindae Officinalis Radix), 15g, *Rou Cong Rong* (Cistanches Herba), 15g, *Jin Ying Zi* (Rosae Laevigatae Fructus), 12g, and *Tu Si Zi* (Cuscutae Semen), 15g, to supplement kidney qi and secure essence. For more extreme emaciation and dessication of essence-blood, remove *Gui Ban* and replace it with other medicinals with an affinity to flesh and blood such as *Gui Ban Jiao* (Testudinis Carapacis et Plastri Gelatinum), 10g, dissolved into the strained decoction, *Lu Jiao Jiao* (Cervi Cornus Gelatinum), 10g, dissolved into the strained decoction, and *Zhu Gu* (Suis Os), 10g.

For concurrent hyperactive ascendancy of liver yang with dizzy head and eyes, headache, vexation and irascibility, and tinnitus, combine *Zhi Bai Di Huang Wan* with Modified *Zhen Gan Xi Feng Tang* (Liver-Settling Wind-Extinguishing Decoction).

Modified *Zhen Gan Xi Feng Tang*

Huai Niu Xi (Achyranthis Bidentatae Radix), *15g*
Dai Zhe Shi (Haematitum), *30g*, predecocted
Ju Hua (Chrysanthemi Flos), *10g*
Tian Men Dong (Asparagi Radix), *15g*
Xuan Shen (Scrophulariae Radix), *12g*
Bai Shao (Paeoniae Radix Alba), *12g*
Sheng Long Gu (Mastodi Ossis Fossilia Cruda), *15g*
Sheng Mu Li (Ostreae Concha Cruda), *15g*
Gui Ban (Testudinis Carapax et Plastrum), *15g*
Yin Chen (Artemisiae Scopariae Herba), *6g*
Chuan Lian Zi (Toosendan Fructus), *10g*
Sheng Mai Ya (Hordei Fructus Germinatus Crudus), *12g*
Gan Cao (Glycyrrhizae Radix), *6g*

For noninteraction of the heart and kidneys with insomnia and poor memory, palpitations and fearful throbbing, use a combination of *Tian Wang Bu Xin Dan* (Celestial Emperor Heart-Supplementing Elixir) and *Jiao Tai Wan* (Peaceful Interaction Pill) instead.

Modified *Tian Wang Bu Xin Dan* with *Jiao Tai Wan*

Dan Shen (Salviae Miltiorrhizae Radix), 10g
Dang Shen (Codonopsis Radix), 12g
Xuan Shen (Scrophulariae Radix), 12g
Dang Gui (Angelicae Sinensis Radix), 12g
Tian Men Dong (Asparagi Radix), 10g
Mai Men Dong (Ophiopogonis Radix), 12g
Fu Shen (Poria cum Pini Radice), 12g
Wu Wei Zi (Schisandrae Fructus), 10g
Yuan Zhi (Polygalae Radix), 10g
Bai Zi Ren (Platycladi Semen), 10g
Sheng Di Huang (Rehmanniae Radix Exsiccata seu Recens), 15g
Huang Lian (Coptidis Rhizoma), 6g
Rou Gui (Cinnamomi Cortex), 3g

2. Kidney yang debility

Signs: Exhaustion of essence-spirit, somnolence, soreness, coldness, and pain of the lumbus and knees, fear of the cold and a liking for warmth, lack of strength, decreased ability to work, low libido, yang wilt or premature ejaculation, cold genitals and possibly retracted genitals, nocturia, ashen-white facial complexion, slight puffy swelling, pale tender tongue with tooth marks and white fur, sinking fine forceless pulse.

Treatment principles: Warm and supplement kidney yang

Guiding formula: Modified *You Gui Wan* (Right-Restoring [Life Gate] Pill)

Ingredients:
Fu Zi (Aconiti Radix Lateralis Praeparata), 6g
Rou Gui (Cinnamomi Cortex), 3g, powdered and taken mixed with the strained decoction
Shu Di Huang (Rehmanniae Radix Praeparata), 15g
Shan Yao (Dioscoreae Rhizoma), 12g
Shan Zhu Yu (Corni Fructus), 12g
Gou Qi Zi (Lycii Fructus), 15g
Lu Jiao Jiao (Cervi Cornus Gelatinum), 10g, dissolved into the strained decoction
Du Zhong (Eucommiae Cortex), 15g
Tu Si Zi (Cuscutae Semen), 15g
Dang Gui (Angelicae Sinensis Radix), 12g

Modifications: For patients with long clear urination, urinary incontinence, or more prominent nocturia, add *Jin Ying Zi* (Rosae Laevigatae Fructus), 12g, *Wu Wei Zi* (Schisandrae Fructus), and *Fu Pen Zi* (Rubi Fructus), 10g each, to secure kidney qi and restrain urine. For patients with concurrent spleen yang vacuity with sloppy stool, poor appetite, and abdominal distention, remove *Shu Di Huang*, and add *Bu Gu Zhi* (Psoraleae Fructus), 12g, *Hong Ren Shen* (Ginseng Radix Rubra), 10g, *Bai Zhu* (Atractylodis Macrocephalae Rhizoma), 12g, *Fu Ling* (Poria), 12g, and *Rou Dou Kou* (Myristicae Semen), 10g, to warm and supplement the spleen yang. For more prominent low libido, yang wilt or premature ejaculation, add *Yin Yang Huo* (Epimedii Herba), 15g, *Ba Ji Tian* (Morindae Officinalis Radix), 15g, and *Jin Ying Zi* (Rosae Laevigatae Fructus), 12g, to further supplement kidney yang and secure essence.

3. Dual vacuity of kidney yin and yang

Signs: Premature physical debility, low libido, premature ejaculation and yang wilt, soreness and limpness of the lumbus and knees, dizzy head and poor memory, tinnitus, abnormal sorrow and joy, booming heat effusion and sweating, fear of the cold and cold limbs, puffy swelling and sloppy stool, pale tender tongue with white fur, fine rapid pulse.

Treatment principles: Regulate and supplement kidney yin and yang

Guiding formula: Modified *Er Xian Tang* (Two Immortals Decoction)

Ingredients:
Zhi Mu (Anemarrhenae Rhizoma), 6g
Huang Bai (Phellodendri Cortex), 6g
Yin Yang Huo (Epimedii Herba), 15g
Xian Mao (Curculiginis Rhizoma), 15g
Ba Ji Tian (Morindae Officinalis Radix), 15g
Dang Gui (Angelicae Sinensis Radix), 12g

Modifications: For patients with booming heat in the face, add *Zhen Zhu Mu* (Concha Margaritifera), 18g, *Sheng Long Gu* (Mastodi Ossis Fossilia Cruda), 20g, predecocted, *Sheng Mu Li* (Ostreae Concha Cruda), 20g, predecocted, and *Huang Lian* (Coptidis Rhizoma), 6g, to further clear heat and downbear fire. For prominence of abnormal sorrow and joy, add *Zhi Gan Cao* (Glycyrrhizae Radix cum Liquido Fricta), 10g, *Da Zao* (Jujubae Fructus), 10 pieces, and *Fu Xiao Mai* (Tritici Fructus Levis), 15g, to supplement the heart and calm the spirit. For prominence of soreness and limpness of the lumbus and knees, add *Du Zhong* (Eucommiae Cortex), 15g, *Gou Ji* (Cibotii Rhizoma), 12g, and *Sang Ji Sheng* (Loranthi Ramus), 15g, to further supplement the kidneys and to strengthen the sinews and bones. For spleen vacuity and sloppy stool, add *Bai Zhu* (Atractylodis Macrocephalae Rhizoma), 12g, *Fu Ling* (Poria), 12g, and *Bu Gu Zhi* (Psoraleae Fructus), 10g, to fortify the spleen and drain dampness, and to supplement spleen and kidney qi.

4. Kidney essence depletion and vacuity

Signs: General decline in sexual function, infertility, loss of hair and loosening of the teeth, dizzy head and tinnitus, decreased aural and visual acuity, soreness and limpness of the lumbus and knees, poor memory and sudden abstraction of the essence-spirit, torpor of essence-spirit, wilting of the limbs and lack of strength, slow physical movements, pale red tongue, sinking fine forceless pulse.

Treatment principles: Supplement and enrich kidney essence

Guiding formulas: *Liu Wei Di Huang Wan* (Six-Ingredient Rehmannia Pill) plus *Gui Lu Er Xian Gao* (Immortal Tortoise Shell and Deerhorn Glue Paste)

Ingredients:
    Shu Di Huang (Rehmanniae Radix Praeparata), 15g
    Shan Yao (Dioscoreae Rhizoma), 15g
    Shan Zhu Yu (Corni Fructus), 15g
    Ze Xie (Alismatis Rhizoma), 10g
    Mu Dan Pi (Moutan Cortex), 6g
    Fu Ling (Poria), 10g
    Gui Ban Jiao (Testudinis Carapacis et Plastri Gelatinum), 10g, dissolve
        into the strained decoction
    Lu Jiao Jiao (Cervi Cornus Gelatinum), 10g, dissolve into the strained
        decoction
    Gou Qi Zi (Lycii Fructus), 15g
    Ren Shen (Ginseng Radix), 15g

Modifications: For patients with yang wilt, add *Yang Qi Shi* (Actinolitum), 10g, *Yin Yang Huo* (Epimedii Herba), 15g, *Ba Ji Tian* (Morindae Officinalis Radix), 15g, and *Rou Cong Rong* (Cistanches Herba), 12g, to further supplement the kidneys and to raise that which has wilted.

5. Heart-spleen dual vacuity

Signs: Palpitations and fearful throbbing, susceptibility to fright, tendency to doubt and suspicion, insomnia and copious dreaming, poor memory and dizzy head, withered-yellow facial complexion, poor appetite, abdominal distention and sloppy stool, fatigued spirit and lack of strength, pale tender tongue with white fur, fine weak pulse.

Treatment principles: Nourish the heart and calm the spirit, supplement qi and nourish blood

Guiding formula: Modified *Gui Pi Tang* (Spleen-Returning Decoction)

Ingredients:
    Hong Ren Shen (Ginseng Radix Rubra), 10g
    Bai Zhu (Atractylodis Macrocephalae Rhizoma), 12g
    Huang Qi (Astragali Radix), 30g
    Dang Gui (Angelicae Sinensis Radix), 12g
    Fu Shen (Poria cum Pini Radice), 12g
    Suan Zao Ren (Ziziphi Spinosi Semen), 20g
    Yuan Zhi (Polygalae Radix), 12g
    Long Yan Rou (Longan Arillus), 10g
    Ye Jiao Teng (Polygoni Multiflori Caulis), 15g

Da Zao (Jujubae Fructus), 6 pieces
Mu Xiang (Aucklandiae Radix), 6g
Sheng Jiang (Zingiberis Rhizoma Recens), 3 slices
Zhi Gan Cao (Glycyrrhizae Radix cum Liquido Fricta), 6g

Modifications: For hyperactive heart fire leading to more prominent insomnia and copious dreaming, add *Lian Zi Xin* (Nelumbinis Plumula), 3g, *Long Chi* (Mastodi Dentis Fossilia), 15g, *Zhen Zhu Mu* (Concha Margaritifera), 12g, and *Huang Lian* (Coptidis Rhizoma), 3g, to clear heart fire and to settle and calm the spirit. For prominence of a tendency to doubt and suspicion, and depressed essence-spirit, add *Shi Chang Pu* (Acori Tatarinowii Rhizoma), 12g, and *He Huan Pi* (Albizziae Cortex), 15g, to further calm the spirit.

6. Binding depression of liver qi with spleen vacuity

Signs: Repressed and depressed affect-mind or irascibility, fullness and distention of the chest and rib-side, scurrying pain in the rib-side, a tendency to sigh, yang wilt or inability to ejaculate, fullness and distention in the genitals, poor appetite and abdominal distention, sloppy stool, intestinal rumblings and fecal qi (*i.e.*, flatulence), diarrhea with pain that diminishes after passing stool, pale tender tongue with thin white fur, stringlike pulse.

Treatment principles: Course the liver and resolve depression, fortify the spleen

Guiding formula: Modified *Xiao Yao San* (Free Wanderer Powder)

Ingredients:
Chai Hu (Bupleuri Radix), 6g
Mei Gui Hua (Rosae Rugosae Flos), 10g
Zi Su Geng (Perillae Caulis), 12g
Fo Shou (Citri Sacrodactylis Fructus), 10g
Qing Pi (Citri Reticulatae Pericarpium Viride), 6g
Dang Gui (Angelicae Sinensis Radix), 12g
Bai Shao (Paeoniae Radix Alba), 12g
Fu Ling (Poria), 12g
Bai Zhu (Atractylodis Macrocephalae Rhizoma), 12g
Wei Jiang (Zingiberis Rhizoma Tostum), 3 slices
Bo He (Menthae Herba), 6g
Zhi Gan Cao (Glycyrrhizae Radix cum Liquido Fricta), 6g

Modifications: For patients who have liver depression transforming fire, add *Shan Zhi Zi* (Gardeniae Fructus), 6g, and *Mu Dan Pi* (Moutan Cortex), 6g, to clear depressed heat from the liver. For more pronounced fatigue and lack of strength, as well as shortness of breath and laziness to speak, add *Dang Shen* (Codonopsis Radix), 15g, and *Huang Qi* (Astragali Radix), 20g, to supplement the spleen and lung qi. For more prominent painful diarrhea, add *Fang Feng* (Saposhnikoviae Radix), 6g, to awaken the spleen with aroma and upbear the spleen qi. For yang wilt, add *Ba Ji Tian* (Morindae Officinalis Radix), 15g, *Bai Ji Li* (Tribuli Fructus), 12g, and *Wu Gong* (Scolopendra), 1 piece.

7. Gallbladder depression with phlegm harassing

Signs: Vexation and oppression, agitation and irascibility, glomus in the chest and fullness in the rib-side, bitter taste in the mouth, nausea and retching, dizzy head with a sinking heavy sensation, torpid intake and poor appetite, insomnia with copious dreaming, dizziness that upsets balance, a sensation of something stuck in the throat that neither be swallowed nor spit up, obesity, slimy tongue fur, slippery stringlike pulse.

Treatment principles: Clear the gallbladder and rectify qi, transform phlegm and harmonize the stomach

Guiding formula: Modified *Wen Dan Tang* (Gallbladder-Warming Decoction)

Ingredients:
> *Zhu Ru* (Bumbusae Caulis in Taenia), 6g
> *Dan Nan Xing* (Arisaema cum bile), 10g
> *He Huan Pi* (Albizziae Cortex), 12g
> *Ban Xia* (Pinelliae Rhizoma), 10g
> *Zhi Shi* (Aurantii Fructus immaturis), 10g
> *Chen Pi* (Citri Reticulatae Pericarpium), 10g
> *Fu Ling* (Poria), 12g
> *Zhi Gan Cao* (Glycyrrhizae Radix cum Liquido Fricta), 6g

Modifications: For prominence of dizziness that upsets balance, add *Tian Ma* (Gastrodiae Rhizoma), 12g, *Gou Teng* (Uncariae Ramulus cum Uncis), 15g, add at the end, and *Shi Jue Ming* (Haliotidis Concha), 15g, predecocted, to extinguish wind and settle the yang. For prominence of irascibility and insomnia, add *Huang Lian* (Coptidis Rhizoma), 6g, *Shi Chang Pu* (Acori Tatarinowii Rhizoma), 12g, *Hu Po Fen* (Succini Pulvis), 3g, taken mixed with the strained decoction, and *Suan Zao Ren* (Ziziphi Spinosi Semen), 20g, to drain heart fire and calm the spirit. For a feeling as if something is stuck in the throat, add *Hou Po* (Magnoliae Officinalis Cortex), 10g, *Jie Geng* (Platycodonis Radix), 15g, *Zi Su Geng* (Perillae Caulis), 12g, and *Mu Hu Die* (Oroxyli Semen), 6g, to rectify qi and disinhibit the throat.

Acumoxa therapy

Main points: *Tai Xi* (KI-3), *Shen Shu* (BL-23), *Guan Yuan* (CV-4), and *San Yin Jiao* (SP-6)

For kidney yin vacuity with interior heat, add *Zhao Hai* (KI-6), *Ran Gu* (KI-2), *Kun Lun* (BL-60), *Tai Chong* (LV-3), *Hou Xi* (SI-3), and *He Gu* (LI-4)

For hyperactive ascendancy of liver yang, add *Xing Jian* (LV-2), *Tai Chong* (LV-3), *Yang Ling Quan* (GB-34), and *Feng Chi* (GB-20)

For noninteraction of the heart and kidneys, add *Shen Men* (HT-7), *Nei Guan* (PC-6), *Xin Shu* (BL-15), and *Tong Li* (HT-5)

For dual vacuity of spleen and kidney yang, add moxa on the main points and also add *Ming Men* (GV-4), *Pi Shu* (BL-20), and *Zu San Li* (ST-36)

For dual vacuity of kidney yin and yang, add *Ming Men* (GV-4), *Zhong Ji* (CV-3), and *Zu San Li* (ST-36)

For liver depression and spleen vacuity, add *Tai Chong* (LV-3), *He Gu* (LI-4), *Zhang Men* (LV-13), *Qi Men* (LV-14), *Qi Hai* (CV-6), *Dan Zhong* (CV-17), *Zu San Li* (ST-36), *Gan Shu* (BL-18), and *Pi Shu* (BL-20)

For gallbladder depression and phlegm harassing, add *Gan Shu* (BL-18), *Dan Shu* (BL-19), *Qi Hai* (CV-6), *Dan Zhong* (CV-17), *Yang Ling Quan* (GB-34), *Xia Xi* (GB-43), *Xing Jian* (LV-2), *Tai Chong* (LV-3), *Feng Long* (ST-40), *Jian Shi* (PC-5), and *He Gu* (LI-4)

Experiential formulas

Replenishing kidney essence, rectifying the thoroughfare and conception vessels, and regulating yin and yang as the main treatment principles

For andropausal men, Dr. Wang Qi primarily emphasizes replenishing kidney essence, rectifying the thoroughfare and conception vessels, and regulating yin and yang. He then varies this approach according to the pattern in the following ways (Wang, 1997).

For patients who mainly have vexation and agitation, and irascibility, he adds medicinals to course the liver and resolve depression as well as heavy spirit-settling medicinals. For such cases, his base formula is *Chai Hu Jia Long Gu Mu Li Tang* (Bupleurum Decoction Plus Dragon Bone and Oyster Shell), and he varies it in the following ways: 1) for enduring insomnia, he adds *Ye Jiao Teng* (Polygoni Multiflori Caulis), *He Huan Pi* (Albizziae Cortex), and *Zhen Zhu Mu* (Concha Margaritifera), to quiet the spirit and stabilize the mind; 2) for effulgent heart fire and a tongue that is red at the tip, he adds *Lian Zi Xin* (Nelumbinis Plumula) and *Zhen Zhu Mu* (Lophatheri Folium Recens) to clear the heart and drain fire; 3) for rib-side pain, he adds *Yu Jin* (Curcumae Radix) and *Fo Shou* (Citri Sacrodactylis Fructus) to rectify qi and relieve pain and; 4) for poor appetite, he adds *Chao Mai Ya* (Hordei Fructus Germinatus Frictus), *Chao Gu Ya* (Setariae Fructus Germinatus Frictus), *Shan Zha* (Crataegi Fructus), *Zhi Ke* (Aurantii Fructus), and *Shan Yao* (Dioscoreae Rhizoma) to dissolve food and harmonize the stomach.

For patients who mainly have palpitations and poor memory, copious dreaming and susceptibility to fright, and vexation and heat of the five hearts, he adds medicinals that nourish the heart and quiet the spirit. For such cases, he uses *Gan Mai Da Zao Tang* (Licorice, Wheat, and Jujube Decoction) as the base formula, and he adds *Gui Ban* (Testudinis Carapax et Plastrum), *Bie Jia* (Trionycis Carapax), *Mu Li* (Ostreae Concha), *Fu Shen* (Poria cum Pini Radice), and *Yuan Zhi* (Polygalae Radix).

For those who mainly have emotional depression, anxiety, unhappiness, gallbladder vacuity and heart timidity, and a red tongue with slimy fur, he uses a modification of *Wen Dan Tang* (Gallbladder-Warming Decoction) as the main formula to clear the gallbladder and transform phlegm.

Supplementing the liver and kidneys, assisting yang, supplementing qi, and replenishing essence

Dr. Cao Yao-Zhong (1990) uses a formula called *Qian Jian Tang* (Qian[9]-Fortifying Decoction) for treating andropausal men. Its main focus is to supplement the liver and kidneys, assist yang, supplement qi, and replenish essence. He then modifies it according to the pattern (Cao, 1990). The main ingredients are:

> *Sheng Di Huang* (Rehmanniae Radix Exsiccata seu Recens), 30g
> *Gou Teng* (Uncariae Ramulus cum Uncis), 30g, add at the end
> *Yin Yang Huo* (Epimedii Herba), 25g
> *Ba Ji Tian* (Morindae Officinalis Radix), 20g
> *Rou Cong Rong* (Cistanches Herba), 15g
> *Dang Shen* (Codonopsis Radix), 15g
> *Fu Ling* (Poria), 15g
> *Gou Qi Zi* (Lycii Fructus), 15g
> *Che Qian Zi* (Plantaginis Semen), 15g
> *Yin Chen* (Artemisiae Scopariae Herba), 15g
> *Sang Shen Zi* (Mori Fructus), 15g
> *Qing Ban Xia* (Pinelliae Tuber Depuratum), 10g
> *Zi He Che* (Hominis Placenta), 10g
> *Lu Jiao Jiao* (Cervi Cornus Gelatinum), 10g, dissolved into the strained
>   decoction

Modifications: For patients with yang wilt, seminal efflux, or premature ejaculation, increase the dosage of *Lu Jiao Jiao* and *Zi He Che*, and add *Sang Piao Xiao* (Mantidis Ootheca), 15g, and *Yu Biao* (Piscis Vesica Aeris), 10g. For cases that have endured for many years, add *Gui Ban Gao* (Testudinis Carapax et Plastrum Pasta), 15g, *Yu Biao* (Piscis Vesica Aeris), 10g, *Di Bie Chong* (Eupolyphaga seu Steleophaga), 10g, *Sheng Shui Zhi* (Hirudo Cruda), 8g, and *Wu Ji Bai Feng Wan* (Black Chicken and White Phoenix Pill), 1 pill two times a day.

Note: *Wu Ji Bai Feng Wan* is a traditional prepared formula that has different formulations. A common one listed in the *Zhong Yao Zhi Ji Shou Ci* (*Handbook of Processed Chinese Medicinal Formulas*) consists of the following medicinals:

> *Wu Ji* (Galli Gigeriae Nigra), 2kg
> *Shu Di Huang* (Rehmanniae Radix Praeparata), 768g
> *Sheng Di Huang* (Rehmanniae Radix Exsiccata seu Recens), 768g
> *Dang Gui* (Angelicae Sinensis Radix), 432g
> *Ren Shen* (Ginseng Radix), 384g
> *Lu Jiao Jiao* (Cervi Cornus Gelatinum), 384g
> *Bai Shao* (Paeoniae Radix Alba), 384g

---

[9] This character *qian* is the trigram from the *Yi Jing* (*Canon of Change*) that corresponds to heaven and the male principles in the universe.

 Xiang Fu (Cyperi Rhizoma), 384g
 Shan Yao (Dioscoreae Rhizoma), 384g
 Dan Shen (Salviae Miltiorrhizae Radix), 384g
 Bie Jia (Trionycis Carapax), 192g
 Tian Men Dong (Asparagi Radix), 192g
 Chuan Xiong (Chuanxiong Rhizoma), 192g
 Qian Shi (Euryales Semen), 192g
 Sang Piao Xiao (Mantidis Ootheca), 144g
 Duan Mu Li (Ostreae Concha Calcinata), 144g
 Lu Jiao Shuang (Cervi Cornu Degelatinatum), 144g
 Huang Qi (Astragali Radix), 96g
 Yin Chai Hu (Stellariae Radix), 78g
 Gan Cao (Glycyrrhizae Radix), 96g

Preparation: Finely powder all the medicinals, mix with honey and make 9g pills. Take one pill two times per day with boiled water.

Supplementing spleen yang and evenly supplementing kidney yin and yang

Zhu (1990) uses a combination of *Xiao Jian Zhong Tang* (Minor Center-Fortifying Decoction) and *Er Xian Tang* (Two Immortals Decoction) for treating andropausal men. His main treatment principle is to supplement spleen yang as well as kidney yin and yang. His main formula consists of the following medicinals:

 Gui Zhi (Cinnamomi Ramulus), 9g
 Da Zao (Jujubae Fructus), 9g
 Sheng Jiang (Zingiberis Rhizoma Recens), 4.5g
 Gan Cao (Glycyrrhizae Radix), 4.5g
 Yi Tang (Maltosum), 10g
 Xian Mao (Curculiginis Rhizoma), 12g
 Yin Yang Huo (Epimedii Herba), 12g
 Ba Ji Tian (Morindae Officinalis Radix), 12g
 Zhi Mu (Anemarrhenae Rhizoma), 12g
 Gou Qi Zi (Lycii Fructus), 12g
 Huang Bai (Phellodendri Cortex), 12g
 Huang Jing (Polygonati Rhizoma), 12g
 Dang Gui (Angelicae Sinensis Radix), 10g
 Shan Zhu Yu (Corni Fructus), 10g
 Shu Di Huang (Rehmanniae Radix Praeparata), 10g
 Bai Shao (Paeoniae Radix Alba), 10g
 Shan Yao (Dioscoreae Rhizoma), 10g

Preventive measures and lifestyle modification

I. Maintain a regular exercise schedule

It is important for aging men to maintain a healthy level of physical exercise in order to provide a counterbalance to the naturally-occurring decline in kidney essence and heavenly tenth. Traditional Chinese exercises such as *qi gong* and *tai ji chuan* are especially useful because they evolved out of the nourishing life (*yang sheng*) tradition and are therefore particularly targeted towards engendering and preserving essence. This does not mean that nonChinese physical training methods such as yoga, weightlifting, running, etc. are necessarily inferior in this regard. Patients should be encouraged to find what is suitable for their constitutions and lifestyles.

2. Moderate sexual activity

Because bedroom taxation damages kidney essence, and because aging men experience a natural decline in kidney essence, it is wise for men to maintain a moderate sexual life and to avoid excessive expenditures of essence. Traditional Daoist methods of sexual cultivation, if learned from a qualified teacher, can be helpful in this regard, though seminal retention practices should be approached with caution due to the possibility of creating vanquished essence.

3. Maintain a clear bland diet

According to Chinese medicine, a clear bland diet rich in cooked fresh vegetables, whole grains,[10] and moderate amounts of fresh fruit and very lean meats, offers the best chance of maintaining health into old age. This includes the periodic intake of special essence-engendering foods such as abalone, deer meat, wild game, turtle shell and meat, rooster (and other animals') testes, animal liver and kidneys, ox tail, bone marrow, shark fin, sea cucumber, oysters, etc. Also, nuts and seeds are effective at supplementing the spleen and kidneys and engendering essence-blood; this includes walnuts, peanuts, chestnuts, and black sesame seeds. Further, it is wise to avoid excessive intake of alcohol and spicy-hot foods, both of which damage yin and create interior heat when consumed excessively, but can warm the yang and free depression when taken in moderation.

4. Adopt a positive mental outlook and reduce stress

When the affect-mind is smooth, qi and blood flow smoothly and all the viscera and bowels function optimally. When aging men dwell negatively on changes in their bodily functions, reductions in their physical strength and sexual abilities, missed life opportunities, and diminished mental capacities, liver qi becomes depressed. As we have seen, left unchecked this can set all sorts of disease processes into motion. Hence, it is important for andropausal men to see the gradual changes they experience as part of the natural processes of yin and yang, and therefore as a realistic manifestation of growth and decline. However, at the same time, they should continue to expect to remain healthy into their advanced years. The key is to have realistic expectations and to be guided by one's own constitution.

5. Maintain a rhythmic and healthy lifestyle

Aging bodies are less resilient and therefore less tolerant of irregular eating and sleeping habits. Whereas younger men may be able to tolerate a wider degree of variation in daily life rhythm, older men generally do not. For

---

[10] I have admittedly added the word "whole" here based on my understanding of Western nutrition. Strictly speaking, Chinese sources do not say this. However, the importance of having adequate intake of "staple grain" is thickly woven into the traditional Chinese concept of a healthful diet.

example, erratic eating schedules tend to weaken the spleen and stomach and lead to qi, blood, and essence vacuity; this effect is pronounced in middle age, when the spleen and stomach are physiologically weaker than they were in the second decade of life. Further, staying up into the wee hours of the morning on a regular basis damages yin, which is already diminished by half by age forty. Hence, the healthiest option for andropausal men is to maintain a regular schedule of eating and sleeping.

Representative Chinese Research

Chinese herbal medicine

Boosting qi and supplementing the kidneys, nourishing blood and quieting the spirit

Li *et al.* (1992) treated 50 cases of male climacteric syndrome with a formula called *Fu Chun Dan* (Spring Recovery Elixir), which boosts qi and supplements the kidneys, and nourishes blood and quiets the spirit. It consists of the following medicinals:

Gui Ban (Testudinis Carapax et Plastrum), 50g
Lu Jiao Shuang (Cervi Cornu Degelatinatum), 50g
Gou Qi Zi (Lycii Fructus), 50g
Bai He (Lilii Bulbus), 50g
Shu Di Huang (Rehmanniae Radix Praeparata), 50g
Tu Si Zi (Cuscutae Semen), 50g
Ye Jiao Teng (Polygoni Multiflori Caulis), 50g
Shan Yao (Dioscoreae Rhizoma), 50g
Ju Hua (Chrysanthemi Flos), 30g

All the ingredients were ground into powder and mixed with honey to form pills that were taken at a dose of one pill three times per day. Although no specific pill size was provided in the abstract, normally 9 grams is the target weight for pills like these.

Results: Patients were also advised to reduce stress and to moderate their sexual activity. Among the 50 cases treated, 45 cases were cured, and 5 cases had good results. The treatment period ranged from 1–3 months.

Supplementing and boosting the liver and kidneys, quickening the blood and transforming stasis, and settling the heart and quieting the spirit

Ji (1995) treated 80 cases of male climacteric syndrome with a variation of *Liu Wei Di Huang Wan* (Six-Ingredient Rehmannia Pill). The main formula consisted of the following medicinals:

Sheng Di Huang (Rehmanniae Radix Exsiccata seu Recens), 30g
Shan Yao (Dioscoreae Rhizoma), 20g
Shan Zhu Yu (Corni Fructus), 20g
Ze Xie (Alismatis Rhizoma), 15g
Fu Ling (Poria), 15g
Mu Dan Pi (Moutan Cortex), 15g

Gou Qi Zi (Lycii Fructus), 10g
Dang Gui (Angelicae Sinensis Radix), 12g
Yuan Zhi (Polygalae Radix), 12g
Wu Wei Zi (Schisandrae Fructus), 12g
Shi Chang Pu (Acori Tatarinowii Rhizoma), 12g
Long Gu (Mastodi Ossis Fossilia), 12g
Mu Li (Ostreae Concha), 12g
Gan Cao (Glycyrrhizae Radix), 6g

Modifications: For internally-engendered heat from yin vacuity, add *Huang Bai* (Phellodendri Cortex) and *Zhi Mu* (Anemarrhenae Rhizoma). For liver-kidney yin vacuity, add *Ju Hua* (Chrysanthemi Flos) and *Gui Ban* (Testudinis Carapax et Plastrum). For noninteraction of the heart and kidneys, add *Huang Lian* (Coptidis Rhizoma) and *Rou Gui* (Cinnamomi Cortex). For spleen and kidney yang vacuity, add *Yin Yang Huo* (Epimedii Herba) and *Rou Cong Rong* (Cistanches Herba). For emotional depression and susceptibility to anger, add *Bai He* (Lilii Bulbus) and *Bai Tou Weng* (Pulsatillae Radix).

Results: Among the 80 cases treated, 36 were cured, 40 cases had good results, and 4 cases had no result. The total amelioration rate was 94%. During the treatment protocol, patients were asked to avoid smoking and drinking alcohol, eating spicy-hot foods, and to refrain from sexual activity.

Acumoxa therapy

Liu and Liang (1992) treated 25 cases of male climacteric syndrome with acumoxa therapy. They discriminated three patterns: 1) liver-kidney yin vacuity; 2) spleen and kidney yang vacuity and; 3) noninteraction of the heart and kidneys.

For liver-kidney yin vacuity, they supplemented *Tai Xi* (KI-3), *San Yin Jiao* (SP-6), *Gan Shu* (BL-18), and *Shen Shu* (BL-23), and drained *Xing Jian* (LV-2), *Shen Men* (HT-7), and *Nei Guan* (PC-6). For spleen and kidney yang vacuity, they supplemented *Guan Yuan* (CV-4), *Zhong Ji* (CV-3), *Shen Shu* (BL-23), *Pi Shu* (BL-20), *Zu San Li* (ST-36), and *San Yin Jiao* (SP-6). When these patients exhibited loss of appetite, they added *Zhong Wan* (CV-12) and *Tian Shu* (ST-25). Sometimes, they used moxa on *Guan Yuan, Shen Shu,* and *Zu San Li.* For noninteraction of the heart and kidneys, they used neutral needling on *Shen Men* (HT-7), *Nei Guan* (PC-6), *Bai Hui* (GV-20), *Zu San Li* (ST-36), *San Yin Jiao* (SP-6), *Shen Shu* (BL-23), and *Tai Xi* (KI-3). In all cases, treatment was given daily for 20–30 minutes, and 10 days comprised one treatment course.

Results: Of the 25 cases treated, 16 were cured, 7 had good results, and 2 had no result.

Acumoxa and Chinese medicinals combined

Wang (1992) used acumoxa therapy in combination with a Chinese medicinal formula to treat 106 cases of male climacteric syndrome. Patients were needled daily at *He Gu* (LI-4), *Tai Chong* (LV-3), and *San Yin Jiao* (SP-6); 10 days comprised one treatment course. The formula consisted of the following medicinals:

Tian Ma (Gastrodiae Rhizoma), 10g
Gou Teng (Uncariae Ramulus cum Uncis), 30g
Ji Xue Teng (Spatholobi Caulis), 30g
Chuan Niu Xi (Cyathulae Radix), 20g
Ye Jiao Teng (Polygoni Multiflori Caulis), 25g
Sang Ji Sheng (Loranthi Ramus), 15g
Dan Shen (Salviae Miltiorrhizae Radix), 15g
Du Zhong (Eucommiae Cortex), 12g
Chuan Xiong (Chuanxiong Rhizoma), 12g
Dang Gui (Angelicae Sinensis Radix), 12g
Gan Cao (Glycyrrhizae Radix), 3g

Results: Among the 106 cases treated, 93 cases were cured, 6 cases had excellent results, 2 cases had good results, and 3 cases had no result.

Representative Case Studies

Liver and kidney yin vacuity and binding depression of liver qi

Chen and Zhang (1998) report on a case of a 58 year-old andropausal male who had been experiencing yang wilt, depressed essence-spirit, dizzy head, insomnia, a tendency to doubt and suspicion, bad temper, lack of strength, and tidal heat effusion with copious sweating. His serum testosterone level was 250ng/dl. There were no other remarkable features in his medical history. His Western medical diagnosis was male climacteric syndrome, though none of the Western medical treatments he had pursued, including nutritional supplementation, sedatives, and androgen replacement therapy had any salutary effects.

When he came for treatment he had the following signs: red tongue tip and margins and a slightly yellow tongue fur, and his pulse was fine rapid. The Chinese medical diagnosis was yang wilt due to liver-kidney yin vacuity and binding depression of liver qi. The treatment principle was to boost the kidneys and nourish the liver, and to course the liver and open depression. The guiding formula which was varied according to the pattern was *Liu Wei Di Huang Wan* (Six-Ingredient Rehmannia Pill). The ingredients are as follows:
Shu Di Huang (Rehmanniae Radix Praeparata), 40g
Shan Yao (Dioscoreae Rhizoma), 20g
Shan Zhu Yu (Corni Fructus), 20g
Mu Dan Pi (Moutan Cortex), 15g
Fu Ling (Poria), 15g
Ze Xie (Alismatis Rhizoma), 15g
Gou Qi Zi (Lycii Fructus), 15g
Han Lian Cao (Ecliptae Herba), 15g
Nu Zhen Zi (Ligustri Lucidi Fructus), 15g
Ju Hua (Chrysanthemi Flos), 10g
Chai Hu (Bupleuri Radix), 10g
Suan Zao Ren (Ziziphi Spinosi Semen), 10g
Su Xin Hua (Jasmini Officinalis Flos), 5g

The patient took ten packets of this formula and had improved sleep and essence-spirit, many fewer worries, and much less dizziness. The prescription was then modified by removing *Ju Hua*, *Chai Hu*, and *Su Xin Hua*, and by adding *Yin Yang Huo* (Epimedii Herba), 15g, and *Tu Si Zi* (Cuscutae Semen), 15g.

After taking twenty more packets of the formula, the yang wilt greatly improved and his serum testosterone level returned to normal.

Noninteraction of the heart and kidney with frenetic movement of vacuity fire

Li (1984) reported a case of a 45 year-old male surgeon with signs of the traditional disease category vacuity taxation (*xu lao*), which can be logically reframed today as a case of andropause because it occurred in a middle-aged male. His chief complaint was insomnia, which he had for twenty-five years, but it had worsened during the previous six months. When he was a student twenty-five years ago, he developed the habit of studying until midnight. As a result, he began having difficulty falling asleep, copious dreaming, and seminal emission. At that time, he took some sleep-promoting medicine and the problem improved. However, thereafter, after a period of especially hard work and study until late into the night, the insomnia would become worse again, even to the point of not responding to the sleep-promoting medicines.

Three years ago, after some intense mental activity, the insomnia became especially severe and he began not being able to sleep at all throughout the entire night. Further, he developed vexation and heat of the five hearts, dry mouth and throat, irascibility, dizzy head and tinnitus, throbbing of the heart and palpitations, soreness and limpness of the lumbus and knees, low-grade heat sensation and pain in the lumbus, and seminal emission and seminal efflux. All of these symptoms became worse over the following six months, and he subsequently developed additional symptoms including low libido, decreased firmness of his penis, premature ejaculation, dry bound stools, and yellow urine with a heat sensation while urinating. He tried both Western and Chinese treatments without result.

Upon examination, he appeared emaciated, his fingernails were desiccated and nonluxuriant but reddish, and when pressed the reddish color easily dissipated and readily returned. The tongue was thin and somber-old, and red with scanty fur that was peeling off in some areas. The pulse was fine stringlike rapid, and the pulse at the left wrist was notably weak.

The diagnosis was heart and kidney yin vacuity with frenetic movement of vacuity fire, noninteraction of the heart and kidneys, and disquieted heart-spirit. Dr. Li prescribed a variation of *Huang Lian E Jiao Tang* (Coptis and Ass Hide Glue Decoction) combined with *Suan Zao Ren Tang* (Spiny Jujube Decoction). He instructed the patient to take one packet per day in three divided doses, and to take the last dose one-half hour before retiring to bed. He also stressed the importance of not overworking, especially during the evening hours. The ingredients are as follows:

Mai Men Dong (Ophiopogonis Radix), 24g
Sheng Di Huang (Rehmanniae Radix Exsiccata seu Recens), 18g
Huang Lian (Coptidis Rhizoma), 6g

Huang Bai (Phellodendri Cortex), 9g
Yu Zhu (Polygonati Odorati Rhizoma), 15g
Shi Hu (Dendrobii Herba), 15g
He Huan Pi (Albizziae Cortex), 18g
Ye Jiao Teng (Polygoni Multiflori Caulis), 24g
Suan Zao Ren (Ziziphi Spinosi Semen), 18g
Fu Shen (Poria cum Pini Radice), 12g
E Jiao (Asini Corii Colla), 9g, dissolved into the strained decoction
Ji Zi Huang (Galli Vitellus), 10 yolks, stirred into the strained decoction[11]

After taking six packets of this formula, the vexation and heat reduced, and he was able to fall asleep at night. After taking another twelve packets, the heat signs had reduced by about half and he was sleeping much better, but he still had copious dreaming and was easily awakened. After taking another twenty-five packets of a few different variations of essentially the same formula minus *Ji Zi Huang*, all of his symptoms improved greatly. He then took prepared pills of *Liu Wei Di Huang Wan* (Six-Ingredient Rehmannia Pill) and *Zhu Sha An Shen Wan* (Cinnabar Spirit-Quieting Pill) for three months to consolidate the therapeutic effects. Follow up over a three-year period revealed that although he occasionally had a mild bout of insomnia, it would resolve spontaneously without sleep medication.

Kidney essence vacuity and dual vacuity of kidney yin and yang

Wu (1989) treated a case of andropause in a 46 year-old man with the strategy of supplementing kidney essence, as well as kidney yin and yang. The patient reported that for the past year, for no apparent reason, he began to experience irascibility and emotional depression and tension along with dizzy head and eyes, tinnitus, decrease in physical strength, insomnia with copious dreaming, vexation and heat of the five hearts, night sweats, and soreness, lack of strength, and limpness of the lumbus and knees. He consulted a Western doctor who diagnosed him with male climacteric syndrome, and gave him testosterone, vitamin E, and nutritional therapy without any result. His tongue was red with scanty fur and his pulse was stringlike fine. The diagnosis was gradual exhaustion of heavenly tenth (*tian gui*), insufficiency of original qi, kidney yin and yang vacuity, and disharmony of the conception vessel. The treatment principle was to supplement kidney essence and regulate yin and yang. Dr. Wu prescribed a modification of *Er Xian Tang* (Two Immortals Decoction) with the following medicinals:

Xian Mao (Curculiginis Rhizoma), 30g
Yin Yang Huo (Epimedii Herba), 30g
Han Lian Cao (Ecliptae Herba), 30g
Dang Gui (Angelicae Sinensis Radix), 10g
Gan Cao (Glycyrrhizae Radix), 10g
Ba Ji Tian (Morindae Officinalis Radix), 10g

---

[11] This is a rather high dosage. Normally, two or three yolks are used. This may be a typographical error in the source text. It is safer to start with two or three yolks and then increase if the patient needs such an increase and can tolerate it.

Huang Bai (Phellodendri Cortex), 8g
Gou Qi Zi (Lycii Fructus), 20g
Shan Yao (Dioscoreae Rhizoma), 25g

After taking twelve packets of the medicine, the vexation, depression and tension, the insomnia with copious dreaming, and night sweats all greatly diminished. However, he still felt dizzy, had poor memory and tinnitus, and had soreness and limpness of the lumbus and knees. Dr. Wu decided to change the treatment principle to enriching and nourishing liver and kidney yin, and replenishing essence and supplementing marrow. He used a combination of *Er Xian Tang* and *Qi Ju Di Huang Wan* (Lycium Berry, Chrysanthemum, and Rehmannia Pill) as the base formulas; the ingredients are listed below:

Xian Mao (Curculiginis Rhizoma), 10g
Ba Ji Tian (Morindae Officinalis Radix), 10g
Zhi Mu (Anemarrhenae Rhizoma), 10g
Dang Gui (Angelicae Sinensis Radix), 10g
Mu Dan Pi (Moutan Cortex), 10g
Gou Qi Zi (Lycii Fructus), 20g
Shu Di Huang (Rehmanniae Radix Praeparata), 20g
Fu Ling (Poria), 20g
Long Gu (Mastodi Ossis Fossilia), 20g
Huang Bai (Phellodendri Cortex), 8g
Ju Hua (Chrysanthemi Flos), 15g
Yin Yang Huo (Epimedii Herba), 30g
Shan Yao (Dioscoreae Rhizoma), 25g

After eighteen packets of this formula, all the symptoms disappeared. Dr. Wu changed the emphasis of treatment again to emphasize warming and supplementing the spleen and kidneys with a modification of *Huan Shao Dan* (Rejuvenation Elixir) as seen below:

Shan Zhu Yu (Corni Fructus), 10g
Du Zhong (Eucommiae Cortex), 10g
Rou Cong Rong (Cistanches Herba), 10g
Ba Ji Tian (Morindae Officinalis Radix), 10g
Wu Wei Zi (Schisandrae Fructus), 10g
Zhi Yuan Zhi (Polygalae Radix cum Liquido Fricta), 10g
Fu Ling (Poria), 20g
Shu Di Huang (Rehmanniae Radix Praeparata), 20g
Gou Qi Zi (Lycii Fructus), 20g
Shan Yao (Dioscoreae Rhizoma), 25g
Niu Xi (Achyranthis Bidentatae Radix), 15g

After taking six packets of this formula, he was completely cured. Follow-up one year later indicated no recurrence of the symptoms.

Bibliography

Agarwal, A. and Said, T.M., *Carnitines and Male Infertility*. Comment in *Journal of Urology*, 2005. Oct; 174 (4 Pt 1): 1369.

Ahmad, I., Kirshna, M.S., *Hemospermia*. *Journal of Urology*, 2007. May; 177(5): 1613–8.

Amin, Z., Patel, U., and Friedman, E.P. *et al.*, *Colour Doppler and Duplex Ultrasound Assessment of Peyronie's Disease in Impotent Men*. *The British Journal of Radiology*, 1993, 66; 785: 398–402.

Attia, A.M., Al-Inany, H.G., and Proctor, M.L., *Gonadotrophins for Idiopathic Male Factor Subfertility*. *Cochrane Database*, 2007. [Online]. Art. No.: CD005071. DOI: 10.1002/14651858.CD005071.pub.

Balercia, G., Regoli, F., Koverich, A. *et al.*, *Placebo-Controlled Double-Blind Randomized Trial on the use of L-carnitine, L-acetylcarnitine, or Combined L-carnitine and L-acetylcarnitine in Men with Idiopathic Asthenozoospermia*. *Fertility and Sterility*, 2005, Sep; 84(3): 662–71.

Balon, R., *Fluoxetine-Induced Sexual Dysfunction and Yohimbine*. *Journal of Clinical Psychiatry*, 1993. 54(4): 161–162.

Bansal, A.R., Godara, R., and Garg, P., *Cold Saline Enema in Priapism—A Useful Tool for the Underprivileged*. *Tropical Doctor*, 2004. Oct; 34(4): 227–8.

Barry, M.J., and O'Leary, M.P. *et al.*, *The American Urological Association Symptom Index for Benign Prostatic Hyperplasia*. *Journal of Urology*, 1992. 148: 1549.

Beers, M.H., and Berkow, R. (Eds.), *The Merck Manual of Diagnosis and Therapy* (17th Ed.), 1999. New Jersey: Merck Research Laboratories.

Beers, M.H. and Porter, R.S. *et al.* (Eds.), *The Merck Manual of Diagnosis and Therapy* (18th Ed.), 2006. New Jersey: Merck Research Laboratories.

Bennett, N.E., Guhring, P., and Mulhall, J.P., *Intralesional Verapamil Prevents the Progression of Peyronie's Disease*. Urology, 2007. Jun; 69(6): 1181–4.

Bensky, D. and Gamble, A., *Chinese Herbal Medicine: Formulas and Strategies*, 1986. Seattle: Eastland Press.

Bent, S., Kane, C., Shinohara, K., Neuhaus, J., Hudes, E. *et al.*, *Saw Palmetto for Benign Prostatic Hyperplasia*. New England Journal of Medicine, 2006. 354(6): 557–566.

Beta Carotene Cancer Prevention Study Group, *The Effect of Vitamin E and Beta Carotene on the Incidence of Lung Cancer and Other Cancers in Male Smokers*. New England Journal of Medicine, 1994. Apr 14; 330(15): 1029–35.

Bhasin, S. and Jameson, J.L., From *Harrison's Principles of Internal Medicine (16th Ed.)*, 2007. New York: McGraw-Hill.

Boggs, W., *Sexually-Transmitted Pathogens Common in Semen of Infertile Men*. [Online], 2007. Available: www. merckmedicus.com.

Burnett, A.L., *Nitric Oxide in the Penis—Science and Therapeutic Implications From Erectile Dysfunction to Priapism*. Journal of Sexual Medicine, 2006. Jul; 3(4): 578–82.

Campbell, T.C. and Campbell, T.M., *The China Study*, 2005. Dallas, Texas: Benbella Books.

Cao, A.L. *et al.*, *Journal of Chinese Medicine*, 1990. 31(8): 54.

Cao, K.Y., *Nan Xing Xing Gong Neng Zhan Hai Zhi Liao Bao Jian (The Treatment and Prevention of Male Sexual Dysfunction)*, 1990. Beijing: Chinese Medicine Press.

Cao, Y.Z., *Cao Yao Zhong's Qian Jian Tang (Qian-Fortifying Decoction) in the Treatment of 36 Cases of Male Climacteric Syndrome*. Hebei Chinese Medicine, 1990. (2): 34.

Cha, Y.M., In Zhang, F.Q. (Ed.)., *Shou Pi Guo Jia Ming Lao Zhong Yi Xiao Yan Mi Fang Jing Xuan (Selected Efficacious Secret Formulas from Top-Level Famous Old Chinese Doctors)*, 1996. p. 245. People's Republic of China: National Cultural Press Company.

Chang, Q. and Sun, W.T., *Nan Ke Bing: Zui Xin Zhong Yi Zhi Liao (Andrological Diseases: The Latest Chinese Medical Treatments)*, 1997. Beijing: Ancient Chinese Medical Literature Press.

Chen, J.F. (Ed.), *Jin Gui Yao Lue (Essentials of Prescriptions of the Golden Coffer)*, 2000. Beijing: People's Hygiene Press.

Chen, Q.Q. and Zhang, Y.Q., *An Investigation into the Treatment of 124 Cases of Male Climacteric Syndrome with Liu Wei Di Huang Wan (Six-Ingredient Rehmannia Pill)*. New Chinese Medicine, 1998. 30(4): 17.

Chen, S.S., *Chen Shu Sen Yi Liao Jing Yan Ji Cui (A Treasury of Chen Shu Sen's Medical Experience)*, 1989. Beijing: People's Army Medical Press.

Chen, W.S., *Accomplishments of Famous Modern Chinese Medical Andrologists*, 2002. (1): 98.

Chen, X.Y., and Xi, H.H., *The Method of Warming and Supplementing the Spleen and Kidney, Nourishing Blood, and Replenishing Essence in the Treatment of 45 Cases of Male Infertility. New Chinese Medicine*, 1998. 30(5): 38.

Chen, Z.Q. and Jiang, H.S., *Nan Ke Zhuan Bing (Specialty Diseases in Andrology)*, 2002. Beijing: People's Hygiene Press.

Cheung, C.S., *The Management of Prostatitis: Essence Turbidity*, 1992. San Francisco: Harmonious Sunshine Cultural Center.

Cheung, C.S., *Creamy Milky Urine Exudate (Bai Zhuo). Abstract and Review of Clinical Traditional Chinese Medicine*, 1994. 2, April: 12–28.

Choi, H.K., Seong, D.H., and Rha, K.H., *Clinical Efficacy of Korean Red Ginseng for Erectile Dysfunction. International Journal of Impotence Research*, 1995. Sep. 7(3): 181–6.

Clark, L.C., Dalkin, B., Krongrad, A., Combs, G.F. Jr., and Turnbull, B.W. *et al., Decreased Incidence of Prostate Cancer with Selenium Supplementation: Results of a Double-Blind Cancer Prevention Trial. British Journal of Urology*, 1998. May; 81(5): 730–4.

Cohen, A.J. and Bartlick, B., *Ginkgo Biloba for Antidepressant-Induced Sexual Dysfunction. Journal of Sex and Marital Therapy*, 1998. Apr–Jun; 24(2): 139–43.

Corachan, M., Valls, M.E., Gascon, J., Almeda, J., Vilana, R., *Hematospermia: A New Etiology of Clinical Interest. American Journal of Tropical Medical Hygiene*, 1994 May; 50(5): 580–4.

Crouch, J., *Functional Human Anatomy (3rd Ed.)*, 1978. Philadelphia: Lea and Febiger.

Dai, X.H. and Liu, J.H., *Gu Jin Nan Ke Yi An Xuan Bian (Anthology of Premodern and Modern Case Studies in Andrology)*, 1990. Beijing: China Press.

Damone, B. (Speaker), *Four Steps to Diagnosis and Treatment*. (CD recording of a live seminar), 2002. Boulder: Blue Poppy Seminars.

Damone. B. (Speaker), *Returning to the Source: A Deeper Understanding of the Zang-Fu Through Classic Texts*. (CD recording of a live seminar), 2005. Boulder, CO: Blue Poppy Seminars.

Damone, B. (Speaker), *Improving Men's Sexual Health and Reproductive Function with Chinese Medicine*. (CD recording of a live seminar), 2006. Boulder, CO: Blue Poppy Seminars.

Dan, S.J., Chen, Z.H., and Shi, Z.C., *Gu Jin Ming Yi Lin Zheng Jin Jian; Nan Ke Juan (The Clinical Golden Mirror of Ancient and Current Famous Doctors; Andrology Volume)*, 1999. Beijing: China Chinese Medical Press.

de Andrade, E., de Mesquita, A.A. *et al.*, *Study of the Efficacy of Korean Red Ginseng in the Treatment of Erectile Dysfunction. Asian Journal of Andrology*, 2007. Mar; 9(2): 241–4. Epub, 2006. Jul 11.

Deadman, P. and Al-Khafagi, M., *A Manual of Acupuncture*, 1998. England: Journal of Chinese Medicine Publications.

Deng, T.D., *Deng Tie-Dao Lin Chuang Jing Yan Ji Yao* (*Abstracts of Deng Tie Dao's Clinical Experiences*), 1998. p. 223. Beijing: China Medicine and Technology Press.

Deng, Z.H., *Pu Xie Di Huang Tang* (Dandelion, Fish Poison Yam, and Rehmanniae Decoction) *in the Treatment of 94 Cases of Male Infertility. Shanxi Chinese Medicine*, 2000. 21(7): 295.

Diamond, J., *Male Menopause*, 1997. Naperville, IL: Sourcebooks.

Ding, G.D. *et al.* (Eds.), *Zhu Bing Yuan Hou Lun Jiao Zhu* (*The Origin and Indicators of Disease Annotated*), 1991. Beijing: People's Science and Technology Press.

DiPaola, R.S., Zhang, H., Lambert, G.H., Meeker, R., Licitra, E. *et al.*, *Clinical and Biologic Activity of an Estrogenic Herbal Combination (PC-SPES) in Prostate Cancer. New England Journal of Medicine*, 1998. Sep 17; 339(12): 785–91.

Dong, J.H. (Ed.), *Xian Dai Zhong Guo Ming Zhong Yi Yi An Jing Hua* (*The Quintessence of Case Studies* [From] *Modern China's Famous Chinese Medical Doctors*), 1990. Beijing: Beijing Press.

El-Nashar, A. and Shamloul, R., *Antibiotic Treatment Can Delay Ejaculation in Patients with Premature Ejaculation and Chronic Bacterial Prostatitis. The Journal of Sexual Medicine*, 2007. Mar; 4(2): 491–6.

Eskenazi, B., and Kidd, S.S. *et al.*, *Antioxidant Intake is Associated with Semen Quality in Healthy Men. Human Reproduction*, 2005. Apr; 20(4): 1006–12. Epub, 2005. Jan 21.

Fan, J.M., *Chinese Medical Treatment of Male Infertility*. Unpublished lecture notes from conference proceedings, 2004. San Diego, CA.

Fan, W.J., *Chinese Medicine Journal*, 1989. 30(4): 46.

Fauci, A., Braunwald, E., Martin, J. *et al.* (Eds.), *Harrison's Principles of Internal Medicine* (14th Ed.), 1998. New York: McGraw-Hill.

Fu, Y.C. and Huang, W.L., *Zi Yin Hua Jing Tang* (Yin-Enriching Essence-Transforming Decoction) *in the Treatment of 38 Cases of Infertility Due to Non-Liquefaction of Semen. Jiangsu Chinese Medicine*, 2002. 23(5): 21.

Gao, X.S., *Zhong Yi Nan Ke Zheng Zhi Lei Cui* (*A Collection of Chinese Andrological Patterns and Treatment*), 1994. Tianjin: Tianjin Science and Technology Press.

Gauthaman, K. and Adaikan, P.G., *Effect of Tribulus Terrestris on Nicotinamide Adenine Dinucleotide Phosphate-Diaphorase Activity and Androgen Receptors in Rat Brain. Journal of Ethnopharmacology*, 2005. 96(1–2): 127–32.

Gelbard, M., *Peyronies.org: Information for Patients and Health Care Providers*. [Online], 2005. Available: http://www.peyronies.org/index.htm.

Giovannucci, E., Rimm, E.B., Colditz, G.A., Stampfer, M.J., Ascherio, A. *et al., A Prospective Study of Dietary Fat and Risk of Prostate Cancer. Journal of the National Cancer Institute*, 1993. Oct 6; 85(19): 1571–9.

Goldman, L. and Ausiello, D. (Eds.), *Cecil Textbook of Medicine*, (22nd Ed.), 2004. Philadelphia: W.B. Saunders.

Greene, H., Johnson, W., and Lemcke, D., *Decision-Making in Medicine: An Algorithmic Approach* (2*nd* Ed.), 1998. St. Louis: Mosby.

Gu, F.J., Deng, W., and Zhang, Z., *Observing the Efficacy of Using Old Chinese Doctor Zhang Zheng-Yuan's Zao Xie Tang (Premature Ejaculation Decoction) to Treat 85 Cases of Premature Ejaculation*, 1996. *Hebei Chinese Medicine*; 18(6): 41.

Guo, R.L. (Ed.), *Shi Yong Nan Xing Ji Bing Zhen Duan Zhi Liao Xue (Practical Diagnosis and Treatment of Diseases of Men)*. 1999. Beijing: People's Army Medical Press.

Handelsman, D.J, and Liu, P.Y., *Andropause: Invention, Prevention, Rejuvenation. Trends in Endocrinology and Metabolism*, 2005. Mar; 16(2): 39–45.

Handelsman, D.J., *Testosterone: Use, Misuse and Abuse. Medical Journal of Australia*, 2006. 185 (8): 436–439.

He, Q.H. and Zhou, S., *Qian Bing Zhen Liao Yao Lan (An Exhibition of the Essentials of Diagnosis and Treatment of a Thousand Diseases)*, 1997. Beijing: World Book Press Company.

He, W.X., *Jiangsu Chinese Medicine*, 1989. 10(3): 25.

He, X.Y. and Guo, H. J., *Liu Wei Di Huang Wan* (Six-Ingredient Rehmannia Pill) and *Wu Wei Xiao Du Yin* (Five-Ingredient Toxin-Dispersing Beverage) *in the Treatment of 45 Cases of Male Infertility. Jiangsu Chinese Medicine*, 2003. 24(5): 31.

He, Y.X. *A Clinical Investigation of Huo Jing Chong Zi Tang* (Sperm-Quickening Seed-Planting Decoction) *for the Treatment of 168 Cases of Male Infertility due to Low Sperm Motility. Jiangxi Chinese Medicine*, 2003. 34(9): 28.

Hong, B, Ji, Y.H., Hong, J.H., Nam, K.Y., Ahn, T.Y., *A Double-Blind Crossover Study Evaluating the Efficacy of Korean Red Ginseng in Patients with Erectile Dysfunction: A Preliminary Report. Journal of Urology*, 2002. Nov; 168(5): 2070–3.

Hoole, A. *et al., Patient Care Guidelines for Nurse Practitioners*. 1999. Philadelphia: Lippincott.

Hosseini, S.R., *Does a Constriction Ring Alter Ejaculation Latency?* British Journal of Urology, 2007. May 29; [Epub ahead of print].

Hua, L.C., *Experience in the Diagnosis and Treatment of Prostatic Hyperplasia. New Chinese Medicine*, 1986. 3, 54.

Huang, X.W. and Bai, L.S. (Eds.), *Nan Ke Bing Qi Nan Wan Zheng Te Xiao Lia Fa (Special Treatment Methods for Rare and Difficult Andrological Diseases)*, 2004. Beijing: Science and Technology Literature Press.

Huang, Q.J. and Zhan, F.R., *Zhen Jiu Bian Zheng Zhi Liao Xue* (*Acumoxa: Pattern Discrimination and Treatment*), 1999. Beijing: China Medicine and Technology Press.

Huang, M.X. *et al., Combined Chinese-Western Medicine in the Treatment of 103 Cases of Urinary Retention Due to Benign Prostatic Hyperplasia. Guiyang Journal of Chinese Medicine*, 1994. 1: 25.

Ji, Y.H., *Zhejiang Journal of Chinese Medicine*, 1994. 29(7): 305.

Ji, Y.H., *Jiangxi Chinese Medicine*, 1995. 26(4): 16.

Kaplan, S., Reported by *Reuters Health Information*, [Online], 2007. Available: www.medscape.com/viewarticle/557098.

Kasper, D.L., Braunwald, E., and Fauci, A., *et al.* (Eds.), *Harrison's Principles of Internal Medicine (16th Ed.)*, 2007. New York: McGraw-Hill.

Kesskes-Ammar, L., Feki-Chakroun, N. *et al., Archives of Andrology*, 2003. Mar–Apr; 49(2): 83–94.

Kessoupoulu, E., Powers, H.J., and Sharma, K.K. *et al., Fertility and Sterility*, 1995. Oct; 64(4): 825–31.

Levin, E.I., *Vacuum-Constriction Therapy in Association of Erectile Dysfunction and Premature Ejaculation. Urologiia*, 2002. Nov–Dec; (6): 37–41.

Li, G. and Tian, J.B. (Eds.), *Nan Ke Bing Zhen Zhi Jue Zhao* (*Mastery of the Diagnosis and Treatment of Andrological Diseases*), 2002. Hebei: Hebei Science and Technology Press.

Li, F.D., *Qinghai Journal of Medicine*, 1990. (4): 15.

Li, G.L., Li, Y.D., and Li, S.W., *An Investigation into the Treatment of 11 Cases of Hematospermia with Acumoxa Therapy. Gansu Chinese Medicine*, 1994. 7(5): 24–25.

Li, J.S., *Bu Shen Sheng Jing Tang* (Kidney-Supplementing Essence-Engendering Decoction) *in the Treatment of 105 Cases of Male Infertility. Journal of the Henan College of Chinese Medicine*, 2003. 18(4): 77.

Li, R. and Song, N.G. (Eds.), *Nan Xing Bing Dan Yan Fang Da Quan* (*Compendium of Experiential Formulas for Men's Diseases*), 1998. Beijing: China Chinese Medical Press.

Li, S.B. and Liu, Y.J. *et al.*, *Nan Xing Xing Gong Neng Zhan Ai Yu Bu Yu Zhen Liao Er Bai Wen (Two-Hundred Questions on Male Sexual Dysfunction and Male Infertility)*, 2004. Beijing: Study Center Press.

Li, Y.C. *et al.* (Eds.), *Zhong Yi Da Ci Dian (The Great Dictionary of Chinese Medicine)*, 1975. Beijing: Peoples' Hygiene Press.

Li, Z.W. *et al.*, *Jiangxi Chinese Medicine*, 1992. 13(129): 417.

Liang, J.B., In Zhang, F.Q. (Ed.), *Shou Pi Guo Jia Ming Lao Zhong Yi Xiao Yan Mi Fang Jing Xuan (Selected Efficacious Secret Formulas from Top-Level Famous Old Chinese Doctors)*, 1996. p. 451. People's Republic of China: National Cultural Press Company.

Liang, N.J., In Mi Y.E. (Ed.), *Shou Pi Guo Jia Ming Lao Zhong Yi Xiao Yan Mi Fang Jing Xuan (Selected Efficacious Secret Formulas from Top-Level Famous Old Chinese Doctors [Sequel])*, 1999. p.267. Beijing: China Today Press.

Liu, C.Q., *Zhejiang Journal of Chinese Medicine*, 1992. (9): 399.

Liu, H.E., Wang, W.P., and Hu, W.L., *The Treatment of 28 Cases of Chronic Prostatitis with Acupuncture and Moxa. The Journal of the Changchun College of Chinese Medicine*, 2002. 18: 24.

Liu, J., *Shanxi Journal of Chinese Medicine*, 1990. 6(6): 15.

Liu, J., *Jiangsu Chinese Medicine*, 1990. 11(2): 23.

Liu, J. and Liang, S.Y., *Acumoxa Therapy in the Treatment of 25 Cases of Male Climacteric Syndrome. Jiangsu Chinese Medicine*, 1992. (2): 26.

Liu, L.F. and Liu, D.G., *Zhong Yi Nan Ke Yi Nan Za Zheng Zhen Liao Bei Yao (Essential Diagnosis of Difficult and Complicated Andrological Diseases with Chinese Medicine)*, 2001. Beijing: People's Army Medical Press.

Liu, Z., *Experience Treating One Case of Rigid Yang. Journal of the Chengdu College of Chinese Medicine*, 1994. 17(4): 37.

Long, T., *Zhang Shou Rui's Experience Treating Premature Ejaculation. Shandong Chinese Medicine Journal*, 1998. 17(8): 362.

Luo J. H. and Zhang X. Z., *An Investigation Into the Use of Pen Yan Ling (Pelvic Inflammatory Magic Medicine) Enema as the Primary Treatment for Chronic Non-Bacterial Prostatitis. Journal of Andrology*, 1998. 4: 62–63.

Luo, Y. K., *Luo Yuan-Kai Yi Lun Ji (Collected Medical Treatises of Luo-Yuan Kai)*, (1st Ed.). 1990. Beijing: Peoples Hygiene Press.

Ma, Y.J. and An, C.C., *Zhong Xi Yi Jie He Nan Ke Xue (Andrology: Integrated Chinese-Western Medicine)*. 2001. Beijing: Chinese Medical Press.

Maciocia, G., *The Practice of Chinese Medicine*. 1994. Edinburgh: Churchill Livingstone.

Mayo Clinic Staff, *Mayo Clinic.com. Men's Health; Peyronie's Disease*. [On-line], 2005. Available: www.mayoclinic.com.

McConnell, J.D., Roehrborn, C.G., Bautista, O.M., Andriole, G.L., Dixon, C.M. (for the Medical Therapy of Prostatic Symptoms (MTOPS) Research Group), *The Long-Term Effect of Doxazosin, Finasteride, and Combination Therapy on the Clinical Progression of Benign Prostatic Hyperplasia. New England Journal of Medicine*, 2003. 349: 2387–98.

McKay, D., *Nutrients and Botanicals for Erectile Dysfunction: Examining the Evidence. Alternative Medicine Review*, 2004. Mar; 9(1): 4–16.

Meieran, S.E., Reus, V.I., Webster, R., Shafton, R., and Wolkowitz, O.M., *Chronic Pregnenolone Effects in Normal Humans: Attenuation of Benzodiazepine-Induced Sedation. Psychoneuroendocrinology*, 2004. 29(4):486–500.

Messina, M.J., Persky, V., Setchell, K.D., and Barnes, S., *Soy Intake and Cancer Risk: a Review of the In Vitro and In Vivo Data. Nutrition in Cancer*, 1994. 21(2): 113–31.

Morley, J.E., Charlton, E., Patrick, P. *et al.*, *Validation of a Screening Questionnaire for Androgen Deficiency in Aging Males. Metabolism*, 2000. Sep; 49(9): 1239–42.

Mou, L.M., *Experience in the Treatment of Enduring Erection. Beijing Chinese Medicine*, 1994. 9(5): 55.

Ni, Y.T. and Damone, R., *Zhu Dan-Xi's Treatment of Diseases of the Spleen and Stomach. Journal of Chinese Medicine*, 1992. 40.

Ni, Y.T., *Navigating the Channels of Traditional Chinese Medicine*, 1996. San Diego: Oriental Medicine Center.

Nickel, J.C., Downey, J., Feliciano, A.E. Jr. *et al.*, *Merck Medicus: Best Practice of Medicine*. [Online]. Available: www.merckmedicus.com.

O'Connor, J., and Bensky, D., *Acupuncture: A Comprehensive Text*, 1984. Seattle: Eastland Press.

Omu, A.E., Al-Bader, A.A., Dashti, H., and Oriowo, M.A., *Magnesium in Human Semen: Possible Role in Premature Ejaculation. Archives of Andrology*, 2001. Jan–Feb; 46(1): 59–66.

Pan, X.Z. and Shao, Z.S., *A Preliminary Exploration of Treating Chronic Prostatitis as Insufficiency of the Liver and Kidney. Shanxi Chinese Medicine*, 1995. 16: 453–454. Reprinted in Chen, Z.Q. and Jiang, H.S., 2000. pp. 25–26.

Peng, J.Z. (Ed.), *Zhong Guo Gu Jin Yi An Jing (Essential Anthology of Premodern and Modern Case Studies in Chinese Medicine)*, 1998. Beijing: Academy Press. Reprinted in Chen, Z.Q. and Jiang, H.S., 2000. pp. 18–19.

Peng, X.X. *et al.*, *Huo Xue Tong Lin Tang* (*Blood Quickening Strangury-Freeing Decoction*) *and Ion Therapy in the Treatment of 50 Cases of Benign Prostatic Hyperplasia*. *Liaoning Chinese Medicine Journal*, 1993. 7, 23.

Penson, D.F., *Benign Prostatic Hyperplasia* (*BPH*). *Merck Medicus*: *Best Practice of Medicine* [Online], 2001. Available: www.merckmedicus.com.

Pollan, M., *The Omnivore's Dilemma*: *A Natural History of Four Meals*, 2006. Waterville, Me: Thorndike Press.

Potts, J.M. and Fynn, N., *Merck Medicus*: *Best Practice of Medicine*, [Online]. Available: www.merckmedicus.com. Also in Zermann, D.H., Ishigooka, M., Doggweiler, R. *et al.*, *Chronic Prostatitis*: *A Myofascial Pain Syndrome? Infectious Urology*, 1999. 12: 84–88.

Priviero, F.B. and Leite, R. *et al.*, *Neurophysiological Basis of Penile Erection*. *Acta Pharmacalogica Sinica*, 2007. Jun; 28 (6): 751–5.

Pryor, J., Akkus, E. and Alter, G. *et al.*, *Priapism*. *Journal of Sexual Medicine*, 2004. Jul; 1(1): 116–20.

Qi, G.C., *A Clinical Discussion of Qiang Jing Jian* (Essence-Strengthening Brew) *in the Treatment of Seminal Abnormalities*. *Hebei Chinese Medicine*, 1987. (5): 21.

Qi, G.C. *et al.*, *The Journal of Integrated Chinese-Western Medicine*, 1988. 8(10): 626.

Qian, J., *Shanghai Journal of Chinese Medicine*, 1990. (4): 23.

Qiao, A.L., *Journal of Integrated Chinese-Western Medicine*, 1986. 6(9): 566.

Qin, B.W. *et al.*, *Zhong Yi Lin Chuang Bei Yao* (*Essential Clinical Chinese Medicine*), 1989. Beijing: People's Hygiene Press

Qin, B.W., *A Qin Bo-Wei Anthology*. (Chace, C. and Zhang, T., Trans.), 1997. Brookline, Massachusetts: Paradigm Publications.

Qin, C.G., *Modified Long Dan Xie Gan Tang* (*Gentian Liver-Draining Decoction*) *for Treating Abnormal Erection*. *Sichuan Chinese Medicine*, 1989. (2): 25.

Qin, Y.F., *A Deeper Understanding of the Chinese Medical Disease Causes and Pathomechanisms of Prostatitis*. *Journal of Andrology*, 1999. 5: 239–241.

Qiu, M.L. (Ed.), *Shi Yong Zhen Jiu Xue* (*Practical Acumoxa*), 2000. Beijing: People's Army Medical Press.

Qu, X.Y. and Guo, T.M. (Eds.), *Nan Ke Bing Yan Fang* (*Effective Formulas for Andrological Diseases*), 2005. Guangzhou: Guangdong Science and Technology Press.

Ren, L.J. *et al.*, *Chinese Acumoxa*, 1991. 11(5): 15.

Ripoll, E. and Mahowald, D., *Hatha Yoga Therapy Management of Urologic Disorders*. *World Journal of Urology*, 2002. Nov; 20(5): 306–9. Epub, 2002. Oct 24.

Rowland, D.L., Patrick, D.L., Rothman, M., and Gagnon, D.D., *The Psychological Burden of Premature Ejaculation. Journal of Urology*, 2007. Mar; 177(3): 1065–70.

Rozzati, R., Reddy, P.P., Reddanna, P., and Mujtaba, R., *Role of Environmental Estrogens in the Deterioration of Male Factor Fertility. Fertility and Sterility*, 2002. Dec; 78(6): 1187–94.

Sadeghi-Negad, H. and Jackson, I., *New-Onset Priapism Associated with Ingestion of Terazosin in an Otherwise Healthy Man. Journal of Sexual Medicine*, 2007. Apr 19; [Epub ahead of print].

Sahelian, R., Borken, S., *Dehydroepiandrosterone and Cardiac Arrhythmia. Annals of Internal Medicine*, 1998. Oct; 129(7): 588.

Sahelian, R., *Tribulus Terrestris*. [Online], 2007. Available: http://www.raysahelian.com/tribulus.html.

Salem, E.A. *et al.*, *Tramadol HCL has Promise in On-Demand Use to Treat Premature Ejaculation. Journal of Sexual Medicine*, 2007. Mar 14; [Epub ahead of print].

Salonia, A. *et al.*, *A Prospective Study Comparing Paroxetine Alone Versus Paroxetine Plus Sildenafil in Patients with Premature Ejaculation. Journal of Urology*, 2002. Dec; 168(6): 2486–9.

Scheid, V., *Chinese Medicine in Contemporary China; Plurality and Synthesis*, 2002. Durham and London: Duke University Press.

Schiff, J.D. and Mulhall, J. (2006). *Hematospermia*. [Online]: available at http://www.emedicine.com/med/topic3466.htm

Schlossberg, D., *Current Therapy of Infectious Disease (2nd Ed.)*. 2001. St Louis: Saunders.

Screponi, E. *et al.*, *Prevalence of Chronic Prostatitis in Men with Premature Ejaculation. Urology*, 2001. Aug; 58(2): 198–202.

Shi, Q. L., *External Treatment of Penile Swelling and Pain. New Chinese Medicine*, 2002. 34(5): 46.

Shi, X.M. *et al.* (Eds.), *Zhen Jiu Zhi Liao Xue (Acumoxa Therapy)*. 2001. Beijing: People's Hygiene Press.

Shi, Y.G. (Ed.), *Dang Dai Ming Yi Lin Chuang Jing Hua: Nan Ke Zhuan Ji (The Quintessence of Modern Famous Doctors' Clinical Experience: Andrology Section)*. 1992. Beijing: Ancient Chinese Medical Texts Press.

Shoskes, D.A., Zeitlin, S.I., Shahed, A. *et al.*, *Quercetin in Men with Category III Chronic Prostatitis: A Preliminary Prospective, Double-Blind, Placebo-Controlled Trial. Urology*, 54: 960–963. Found on *Merck Medicus* [Online], 1999. Available: www.merckmedicus.com.

Sikora, R., Sohn, M.H., Engelke, B. *et al.*, *Randomized Placebo-Controlled Study on the Effects of Oral Treatment with Gingko Biloba Extract in Patients with Erectile Dysfunction. Journal of Urology*, 1998. 159 (suppl 5): 240.

Sobel, J., *Prostatitis. Merck Medicus: Best Practice of Medicine* [Online], 2000. Available: www.merckmedicus.com.

Sotomayer, M., *The Burden of Premature Ejaculation: The Patient's Perspective. Journal of Sexual Medicine*, 2005. May; 2 Suppl 2: 110–4.

Sovak, M., Seligson, A.L., and Konas, M. *et al.*, *Herbal Composition PC-SPES for Management of Prostate Cancer: Identification of Active Principles. Journal of the National Cancer Institute*, 94, 2002. (17): 1275–81.

Tan, X.H. and Tao, D.M. (Eds.), *Zhong Yi Wai Ke Xue* (*Chinese External Medicine*), 1999. Beijing: People's Hygiene Press.

Tancredi, A., Reginster, J.Y., Schleich, F. *et al.*, *Interest of the Androgen Deficiency in Aging Males* (*ADAM*) *Questionnaire for the Identification of Hypogonadism in Elderly Community-Dwelling Male Volunteers. European Journal of Endocrinology*, 2005. 151: 355–360.

Tao, H.M., *New Chinese Medicine*, 1994. 26(6), 39.

Tao, Z.X., *Zhejiang Journal of Chinese Medicine*, 1985. (11): 495.

Tao, Z.X., *First World Academic Conference on Acumoxa Therapy*, 1987.

Thompson, I., *Merck Medicus*; *Best Practice of Medicine*, [Online]. 2002. Available: www.merckmedicus.com.

Trost, L.W., Gur, S. Hellstrom, W.J., *Pharmacological Management of Peyronie's Disease. Drugs*, 2007. 67(4): 527–45.

Unschuld, P., *Medicine in China*; *A History of Pharmaceutics*, 1986. Berkeley: University of California Press.

Van Gulik, R.H., *Sexual Life in Ancient China*, 1961. Leiden, Netherlands: E.J. Brill.

Vardi, M, Nini, A., *Phosphodiesterase Inhibitors for Erectile Dysfunction in Patients with Diabetes Mellitus. The Cochrane Database of Systematic Reviews*, 2007. Art. No.: CD002187. DOI: 10.1002/14651858.CD002187. pub3.

Wang, G.J. *et al.*, *Experience Treating Hematospermia. Sichuan Chinese Medicine*, 1990. (5): 32.

Wang, G.Y., *Nan Xing Bing Zhong Yi Zhen Zhi Jiang Yao* (*Essentials of Diagnosis and Treatment of Chinese Andrological Diseases*), 2000. Beijing: Military Science and Technology Press.

Wang, J.F., Wang, Y.N., and Miao, W.P., *Discussion on the use of Tai Chong* (LV-3) *for the Treatment of Difficult Diseases*. Chinese Acumoxa, 1997. 17(7): 432.

Wang, J.H., *Gu Jing Zhi Xie Tang* (Essence-Securing Discharge-Ending Decoction) *in the Treatment of 56 Cases of Premature Ejaculation*. New Chinese Medicine, 1996. 28(8): 53.

Wang, J.S., *Xu Fu-Song's Discussion of Treating Phlegm in Andrological Diseases.* Jiangxi Chinese Medicine, 1997. 28(3): 4.

Wang, Q., *Wang Qi Nan Ke Xue* (Wang Qi's Andrology), (1ˢᵗ Ed.), 1997. Jiazhou: Henan Science and Technology Press.

Wang, Q., *Wang Qi Lin Chuang Yi Xue Cong Shu* (Wang Qi's Textbook of Clinical Medicine), 2003. Beijing: People's Hygiene Press.

Wang, S.M., Li, G.G., and Zhang, Y.F., *The Treatment of 30 Cases of Chronic Prostatitis with Acumoxa Therapy*. The Chinese Journal of Integrated Chinese-Western Medicine, 2003.

Wang, X.Y. (Ed.), *Zhong Yi Ji Chu Li Lun* (Fundamentals of Chinese Medicine), 2001. Beijing: People's Hygiene Press.

Wang, Y.M., *Yunnan Journal of Chinese Medicine*, 1992. 13(1): 20.

Wang, Z., Liu, B.C., and Chen, B. *et al.*, *The Treatment of 18 Cases of Peyronie's Disease with Chinese Medicinals*. Journal of Chinese Medicine, 2003. 44(1): 51.

Wei, D.Z. *et al.*, *Hebei Chinese Medicine*, 1994. 16(5): 43.

Weidner, W., Hauck, E.W., Schnitker, J., *Potassium Paraaminobenzoate* (POTABA) *in the Treatment of Peyronie's Disease: A Prospective, Placebo-Controlled, Randomized Study*. European Urology, 2005. Apr; 47(4): 530–5; discussion 535–6. Epub, 2005. Jan 13.

Wile, D., *Art of the Bedchamber: The Chinese Sexual Yoga Classics Including Women's Solo Meditation Texts*, 1992. Albany: State University of New York Press.

Wilt, T., Ishani, A., MacDonald, R., Rutks, I., and Stark, G., *Pygeum Africanum for Benign Prostatic Hyperplasia*. The Cochrane Database of Systematic Reviews, 1998. Issue 1. Art. No.: CD001044. DOI: 10.1002/14651858.CD001044.

Wilt, T., MacDonald, R., Ishani, A., Rutks, I., Stark, G., *Cernilton for Benign Prostatic Hyperplasia*. The Cochrane Database of Systematic Reviews, 1998. Issue 3. Art. No.: CD001042. DOI: 10.1002/14651858.CD001042.

Wilt, T., Ishani, A., and MacDonald, R., *Serenoa Repens for Benign Prostatic Hyperplasia*. The Cochrane Database of Systematic Reviews, 2002. Issue 3. Art. No.: CD001423. DOI: 10.1002 / 14651858.CD001423.

Wiseman, N. and Feng, Y., A *Practical Dictionary of Chinese Medicine*, 1998. Brookline, Massachusetts: Paradigm Publications.

Wong, K.C. and Wu, L.T., Originally published in 1932. *History of Chinese Medicine: Being a Chronicle of Medical Happenings in China from Ancient Times to the Present Period, 1985*. Taipei: The Republic of China. Reprinted by Southern Materials Center.

Wong, Y.W., Merkus, H.M., and Thomas, C.M. et. al. (2002). *Fertility and Sterility*, 2002. Mar; 77(3): 491–8.

Wu, B.T., *Experience Treating Male Climacteric Syndrome. Sichuan Chinese Medicine*, 1989. (2): 25.

Wu, J.P. (Series Ed.), *Er Shi Shi Jie Zhong Yi Yao Zui Jia Chu Fang; Nan Ke Juan (The Most Distinguished Chinese Medical Prescriptions of the 21st Century; Andrology Volume)*, 2002. Beijing: Study Center Press.

Wu, S.L., *Qing Shi Jie Ning Tang* (Dampness-Clearing Congelation-Resolving Decoction) *in the Treatment of 151 Cases of Autoimmune Male Infertility. Jiangsu Chinese Medicine*, 2000. 21(6): 27.

Wu, Y. and Fischer, W., *Practical Therapeutics of Traditional Chinese Medicine*, 1997. Brookline, Massachusetts: Paradigm Publications.

Xiao, Z.N., *A Clinical Investigation of 60 Cases of Premature Ejaculation Treated by Long Dan Xie Xin Tang (Gentian Heart-Draining Decoction). Shanghai Journal of Chinese Medicine*, 1998. (7): 6.

Xiao, Z.Q., *Journal of the Guiyang College of Chinese Medicine*, 1988. (6): 44.

Xie, H., *Zhong Yi Yan Jiu Yuan Guang An Men Yi Yuan Bian. Yi Hua Yi Lun Hui Yao (Chinese Medical Research Hospitals: Guang An Men Section. Assembly on Medical Discourse and Treatises)*, 1982. Beijing: People's Hygiene Press.

Xing, X.B., *Xing Xi Bo Yi An Ji (The Collected Case Studies of Xing Xi-Bo)*, 1991. Beijing: People's Army Press. Reported in Chen, Z.Q. and Jiang, H.S., 2000.

Xu, J.Y., *Yang Jie-Bin's Experience Treating Rigid Center. Journal of Chinese Medicine*, 1995. 36(11): 690.

Xu, J. X., *Modified Wu Zi Yan Zong Wan* (Five-Seed Progeny Pill) *in the Treatment of 153 Cases of Male Infertility. Shandong Journal of Chinese Medicine*, 2003. 22(3): 161.

Xuan, W.H., *Sichuan Chinese Medicine*, 1994. 12(8): 35.

Yang, C.S. (Ed.), *Zhen Jiu Zhi Liao Xue (Acumoxa Treatment)*, 1985. Shanghai: Shanghai Science and Technology Press.

Yang, Z.G., Li, P., and Zhu, K. et al., *A Clinical Study on the Treatment of Chronic Prostatitis with Acupuncture*, 1998. Journal of Andrology, 4: 135–137.

Yin, H.H., In Zhang, F.Q. (Ed.) (1996). *Shou Pi Guo Jia Ming Lao Zhong Yi Xiao Yan Mi Fang Jing Xuan* (*Selected Efficacious Secret Formulas from Top-Level Famous Old Chinese Doctors*), 1996. People's Republic of China: National Cultural Press Company.

Yin, H.H. (Ed.), *Zhong Yi Ji Chu Li Lun* (*Fundamentals of Chinese Medicine*), (2nd Ed.), 2006. Beijing: People's Hygiene Press.

Yin, L.X. *et al.*, *The Journal of Practical Chinese Internal Medicine*, 1995. 9(1): 45.

Yuan, F.R. *et al.*, *Hubei Chinese Medicine*, 1995, 17(119): 16.

Yuan, Q. S., *Acumoxa Treatment of One Case of Rigid Center Caused by Injected Papaverine. Shanxi Chinese Medicine*, 1988. (2): 8.

Zhang, D.B. and Zhou, Z.J., *Zhong Yi Nan Xing Bing Xue* (*Chinese Medical Andrological Diseases*), 1998. Shanxi: Shanxi Science and Technology Press.

Zhang, F.Q. *et al.*, *Ming Lao Zhong Yi Xiao Yan Mi Fang Jing Xuan* (*Selected Effective Secret Formulas of Famous Old Chinese Doctors*), 1996. Beijing: Ancient Chinese Medicine Texts Press.(1): 416–417.

Zhang, J.M., *A Clinical Investigation Into the Treatment of Chronic Prostatitis with Chinese Medicinals. Journal of Andrology*, 1999. 5: 59–60.

Zhang, J.T., *Zhong Yi Zhen Liao Te Ji Jing Dian.* (*Essential Classics of Chinese Medical Diagnosis and Treatment with Special Effects*), 1994. Beijing: Ancient Chinese Medicine Texts Press.

Zhang, M., *Gao Ling Long Bi Zhi Yan* (*Advanced Experience Treating Dribbling Urinary Block*). *Sichuan Chinese Medicine*, 1984. 6, 23. Reported in Chen, Z.Q. and Jiang, H.S. (2000).

Zhang, P.Y., Song, J.G., and Gao, Z.W., *A Clinical Investigation of Modified Zhen Gan Xi Feng Tang* (*Liver-Settling Wind-Extinguishing Decoction*) *for Treating 45 Cases of Premature Ejaculation. Shandong Journal of Chinese Medicine*, 2003. 22(5): 274.

Zhang, Q. *et al.*, *Shanghai Journal of Chinese Medicine*, 1985. (5): 4.

Zhang, Z.Y., Wang, Y.S., and Gao, J.H., *Nan Ke Jin Fang* (*Precious Andrology Formulas*), 2001. Hebei: Hebei Science and Technology Press.

Zhang, X.Y. *Che Qian Zi* (*Plantaginis Semen*) *for Pediatric Penile Pain and Swelling. Journal of Chinese Medicine*, 1998. 39(11): 647.

Zheng, C.L., *Jiangsu Chinese Medicine*, 1991. (8): 18.

Zhong, J.H. (Ed.), *Zhong Guo Xian Dai Ming Zhong Yi Yi An Jing Hua* (*The Quintessence of Preeminent Modern Chinese Doctors' Case Studies*), 1997. Beijing: Beijing Press.

Zhou, L. *et al.*, *A Clinical Investigation Into the Treatment of Chronic Prostatitis with Ba Zheng San (Eight Corrections Powder)*. Journal of Andrology, 1998. 5: 138.

Zhu, B.Y., *Four Principles from Experience in the Treatment of Male Climacteric Syndrome*. Shanghai Chinese Medicine, 1990. (2): 25.

Zhu, Q.T., *Xue Jing Tang (Bloody Semen Formula) in the Treatment of Bloody Semen Related to Old Age*. New Chinese Medicine, 2001. 33(5): 43.

Zhu, Z.Y. (Ed.), *Shi Jin Mo Lin Chuang Jing Yan Ji (Collected Clinical Experiences of Shi Jin-Mo)*, 1982. pp. 123–124. Beijing: People's Hygiene Press.

Zong, G. F., *Journal of the Shandong College of Chinese Medicine*, 1991. 15(5): 29–30.

Zou, Y.X., *Zou Yun Xiang Yi An Xuan (Selected Case Studies of Zou Yun-Xiang)*, 1981. Nanjing: Jiangsu Science and Technology Press.

Formula Index

General Index

tion Record), 99, 106, 11
bicycle riding, 152, 164, 191, 302
Bing Ji Sha Zhuan (The Sand Seal of Pathomechanisms), 117
bladder block, 110
bladder channel, 40-42, 46, 126, 128-131, 134, 136, 138, 139, 142, 144, 166, 167
bladder, heat distressing the, 83, 84
bladder outlet obstruction, 178, 191, 203, 207, 293
bladder qi, 41, 42, 46, 73-75, 83, 108, 119-121, 133, 151, 167, 168, 181-183
bladder qi transformation, 41, 42, 46, 73-75, 83, 119-121, 151, 167, 168, 181-183
bladder stones, 178
bleeding diatheses (von Willebrand disease), 291
blood mounting (*xue shan*), 52, 109, 110
blood heat, 151, 152
blood extreme (*xue ji*), 108
blood strangury (*xue lin*), 108, 120, 121
bloody urine (*xue niao*), 207
bloody strangury (*xue lin*), 84, 148, 193, 294
bobble wind (*xiu qiu feng*), 114
bone mass, 354
bone extreme (*gu ji*), 108, 294
bound stool (*bian jie*), 34, 47, 74, 116, 184, 186, 187, 194, 210, 272, 279, 280, 324, 359
brain, 39-42, 50, 140, 358
brewing and binding of dampness, 81
brewing and binding of damp-heat, 82, 115, 151, 170, 171
bulbourethral glands (Cowper's glands), 26
burning and painful micturition, 145

C
calculi, ejaculatory duct, 293
cannabis, 87, 310
caput epididymidis, 24
castration, 6, 54, 206
cauda epididymidis, 24, 25
cavernosa- or (corpora) spongiosum shunt, 275
celibate Daoist men, 106
channel and network vessel theory, 29-31, 33, 34, 76
chaotic qi dynamic, 153

chestnuts, 240, 263, 330, 369
childlessness (*wu zi*), 315
Chinese chives, 240, 263, 330
Chinese andrological disease categories, 7, 79, 85, 90, 97-99, 101, 103, 105, 107, 109, 111, 113, 115, 117, 119, 121, 225, 275
Chlamydia, 91, 309, 310, 331
chlorpheniramine, 350
circumcision, 28
clear sky, 41
clear and turbid, 38, 39, 81, 120, 182
clear-bland (*qing dan*) diet, 191
cloudy turbid urine, 157
cocaine, 87, 208, 274, 310
Colchicine, 342
cold genitals (*yin han*), 9, 103
cold evil, 7, 49, 80, 81, 90, 101, 116, 128, 131, 136, 228, 230
cold mounting (*han shan*), 52
cold semen and infertility (*jing leng wu zi*), 9
collagenase, intralesional injections, 342
conception vessel, 32, 33, 37, 49-53, 55, 117, 126, 128-130, 134, 136, 138, 139, 142, 144, 166, 167, 228, 289, 374
congestive heart failure, 177
constitutional vacuity and natural endowment insufficiency, 80
construction qi (*ying qi*), 15, 37, 39, 41, 60, 226
corpora or cavernosa-spongiosum shunt, 275
corpus epididymidis, 24
corpus cavernosum, 27, 28, 222, 273, 274
corpus spongiosum urethrae, 28
courage, 70
Cowper's glands, (bulbourethral glands), 26
crotch-boring eruption (*chuan dang fa*), 150
crotch-boring sore (*chuan dang fa*), 17
crotch-boring welling-abscess (*chuan dang yong*), 115
cryptorchidism, 314
cystectomy, 221
cystitis, recurrent, 146
cystourethroscopy, 293
cytomegalovirus (CMV), 309
cytotoxic chemotherapeutic agents, 206

CURING DEPRESSION NATURALLY WITH
CHINESE MEDICINE
by Rosa Schnyer & Bob Flaws
ISBN 0-936185-94-5
ISBN 978-0-936185-94-1

CURING FIBROMYALGIA NATURALLY WITH
CHINESE MEDICINE
by Bob Flaws
ISBN 1-891845-09-8
ISBN 978-1-891845-09-3

CURING HAY FEVER NATURALLY WITH
CHINESE MEDICINE
by Bob Flaws
ISBN 0-936185-91-0
ISBN 978-0-936185-91-0

CURING HEADACHES NATURALLY WITH
CHINESE MEDICINE
by Bob Flaws
ISBN 0-936185-95-3
ISBN 978-0-936185-95-8

CURING IBS NATURALLY WITH CHINESE
MEDICINE
by Jane Bean Oberski
ISBN 1-891845-11-X
ISBN 978-1-891845-11-6

CURING INSOMNIA NATURALLY WITH
CHINESE MEDICINE
by Bob Flaws
ISBN 0-936185-86-4
ISBN 978-0-936185-86-6

CURING PMS NATURALLY WITH CHINESE
MEDICINE
by Bob Flaws
ISBN 0-936185-85-6
ISBN 978-0-936185-85-9

DISEASES OF THE KIDNEY & BLADDER
by Hoy Ping Yee Chan, et al.
ISBN 1-891845-37-3
ISBN 978-1-891845-35-6

THE DIVINE FARMER'S MATERIA MEDICA
A Translation of the Shen Nong Ben Cao
translation by Yang Shouz-zhong
ISBN 0-936185-96-1
ISBN 978-0-936185-96-5

DUI YAO: THE ART OF COMBINING
CHINESE HERBAL MEDICINALS
by Philippe Sionneau
ISBN 0-936185-81-3
ISBN 978-0-936185-81-1

ENDOMETRIOSIS, INFERTILITY AND
TRADITIONAL CHINESE MEDICINE:
A Laywoman's Guide
by Bob Flaws
ISBN 0-936185-14-7
ISBN 978-0-936185-14-9

THE ESSENCE OF LIU FENG-WU'S
GYNECOLOGY
by Liu Feng-wu, translated by Yang Shou-zhong
ISBN 0-936185-88-0
ISBN 978-0-936185-88-0

EXTRA TREATISES BASED ON INVESTIGATION
& INQUIRY:
A Translation of Zhu Dan-xi's Ge Zhi Yu Lun
translation by Yang Shou-zhong
ISBN 0-936185-53-8
ISBN 978-0-936185-53-8

FIRE IN THE VALLEY: TCM Diagnosis & Treatment
of Vaginal Diseases
by Bob Flaws
ISBN 0-936185-25-2
ISBN 978-0-936185-25-5

FU QING-ZHU'S GYNECOLOGY
trans. by Yang Shou-zhong and Liu Da-wei
ISBN 0-936185-35-X
ISBN 978-0-936185-35-4

FULFILLING THE ESSENCE:
A Handbook of Traditional & Contemporary
Treatments for Female Infertility
by Bob Flaws
ISBN 0-936185-48-1
ISBN 978-0-936185-48-4

GOLDEN NEEDLE WANG LE-TING: A 20th
Century Master's Approach to Acupuncture
by Yu Hui-chan and Han Fu-ru, trans. by Shuai Xue-zhong
ISBN 0-936185-78-3
ISBN 978-0-936185-78-1

A HANDBOOK OF TCM PATTERNS
& THEIR TREATMENTS
by Bob Flaws & Daniel Finney
ISBN 0-936185-70-8
ISBN 978-0-936185-70-5

A HANDBOOK OF TRADITIONAL
CHINESE DERMATOLOGY
by Liang Jian-hui, trans. by Zhang Ting-liang
& Bob Flaws
ISBN 0-936185-46-5
ISBN 978-0-936185-46-0

A HANDBOOK OF TRADITIONAL
CHINESE GYNECOLOGY
by Zhejiang College of TCM, trans. by Zhang Ting-liang
& Bob Flaws
ISBN 0-936185-06-6 (4th edit.)
ISBN 978-0-936185-06-4

A HANDBOOK OF CHINESE HEMATOLOGY
by Simon Becker
ISBN 1-891845-16-0
ISBN 978-1-891845-16-1

A HANDBOOK of TCM PEDIATRICS
by Bob Flaws
ISBN 0-936185-72-4
ISBN 978-0-936185-72-9

THE HEART & ESSENCE OF DAN-XI'S
METHODS OF TREATMENT
by Xu Dan-xi, trans. by Yang Shou-zhong
ISBN 0-926185-50-3
ISBN 978-0-936185-50-7

HERB TOXICITIES & DRUG INTERACTIONS:
A Formula Approach
by Fred Jennes with Bob Flaws
ISBN 1-891845-26-8
ISBN 978-1-891845-26-0

IMPERIAL SECRETS OF HEALTH & LONGEVITY
by Bob Flaws
ISBN 0-936185-51-1
ISBN 978-0-936185-51-4

INSIGHTS OF A SENIOR ACUPUNCTURIST
by Miriam Lee
ISBN 0-936185-33-3
ISBN 978-0-936185-33-0

INTEGRATED PHARMACOLOGY: Combining Modern
Pharmacology with Chinese Medicine
by Dr. Greg Sperber with Bob Flaws
ISBN 1-891845-41-1
ISBN 978-0-936185-41-3

INTRODUCTION TO THE USE OF
PROCESSED CHINESE MEDICINALS
by Philippe Sionneau
ISBN 0-936185-62-7
ISBN 978-0-936185-62-0

KEEPING YOUR CHILD HEALTHY WITH
CHINESE MEDICINE
by Bob Flaws
ISBN 0-936185-71-6
ISBN 978-0-936185-71-2

THE LAKESIDE MASTER'S STUDY OF THE
PULSE
by Li Shi-zhen, trans. by Bob Flaws
ISBN 1-891845-01-2
ISBN 978-1-891845-01-7

MANAGING MENOPAUSE NATURALLY WITH
CHINESE MEDICINE
by Honora Lee Wolfe
ISBN 0-936185-98-8
ISBN 978-0-936185-98-9

MASTER HUA'S CLASSIC OF THE
CENTRAL VISCERA
by Hua Tuo, trans. by Yang Shou-zhong
ISBN 0-936185-43-0
ISBN 978-0-936185-43-9

THE MEDICAL I CHING: Oracle of the
Healer Within
by Miki Shima
ISBN 0-936185-38-4
ISBN 978-0-936185-38-5

MENOPAIUSE & CHINESE MEDICINE
by Bob Flaws
ISBN 1-891845-40-3
ISBN 978-1-891845-40-6

TEST PREP WORKBOOK FOR THE NCCAOM BIO-
MEDICINE MODULE: Exam Preparation & Study
Guide
by Zhong Bai-song
ISBN 1-891845-34-9
ISBN 978-1-891845-34-5

POINTS FOR PROFIT: The Essential Guide to
Practice Success for Acupuncturists 3rd Edition
by Honora Wolfe, Eric Strand & Marilyn Allen
ISBN 1-891845-25-X
ISBN 978-1-891845-25-3

PRINCE WEN HUI's COOK: Chinese Dietary
Therapy
By Bob Flaws & Honora Wolfe
ISBN 0-912111-05-4
ISBN 978-0-912111-05-6

THE PULSE CLASSIC:
A Translation of the Mai Jing
by Wang Shu-he, trans. by Yang Shou-zhong
ISBN 0-936185-75-9
ISBN 978-0-936185-75-0

THE SECRET OF CHINESE PULSE DIAGNOSIS
by Bob Flaws
ISBN 0-936185-67-8
ISBN 978-0-936185-67-5

SECRET SHAOLIN FORMULAS for the Treatment
of External Injury
by De Chan, trans. by Zhang Ting-liang & Bob Flaws
ISBN 0-936185-08-2
ISBN 978-0-936185-08-8

STATEMENTS OF FACT IN TRADITIONAL
CHINESE MEDICINE   Revised & Expanded
by Bob Flaws
ISBN 0-936185-52-X
ISBN 978-0-936185-52-1

STICKING TO THE POINT 1:
A Rational Methodology for the Step by Step
Formulation & Administration of an Acupuncture
Treatment
by Bob Flaws
ISBN 0-936185-17-1
ISBN 978-0-936185-17-0

STICKING TO THE POINT 2:
A Study of Acupuncture & Moxibustion Formulas
and Strategies
by Bob Flaws
ISBN 0-936185-97-X
ISBN 978-0-936185-97-2

A STUDY OF DAOIST ACUPUNCTURE &
MOXIBUSTION
by Liu Zheng-cai
ISBN 1-891845-08-X
ISBN 978-1-891845-08-6

THE SUCCESSFUL CHINESE HERBALIST
by Bob Flaws and Honora Lee Wolfe
ISBN 1-891845-29-2
ISBN 978-1-891845-29-1

THE SYSTEMATIC CLASSIC OF ACUPUNCTURE
& MOXIBUSTION
A translation of the Jia Yi Jing
by Huang-fu Mi, trans. by Yang Shou-zhong &
Charles Chace
ISBN 0-936185-29-5
ISBN 978-0-936185-29-3

THE TAO OF HEALTHY EATING ACCORDING TO
CHINESE MEDICINE
by Bob Flaws
ISBN 0-936185-92-9
ISBN 978-0-936185-92-7

TEACH YOURSELF TO READ MODERN
MEDICAL CHINESE
by Bob Flaws
ISBN 0-936185-99-6
ISBN 978-0-936185-99-6

TEST PREP WORKBOOK FOR BASIC TCM THEORY
by Zhong Bai-song
ISBN 1-891845-43-8
ISBN 978-1-891845-43-7

TREATING PEDIATRIC BED-WETTING WITH
ACUPUNCTURE & CHINESE MEDICINE
by Robert Helmer
ISBN 1-891845-33-0
ISBN 978-1-891845-33-8

TREATISE on the SPLEEN & STOMACH: A
Translation and annotation of Li Dong-yuan's
Pi Wei Lun
by Bob Flaws
ISBN 0-936185-41-4
ISBN 978-0-936185-41-5

THE TREATMENT OF CARDIOVASCULAR
DISEASES WITH CHINESE MEDICINE
by Simon Becker, Bob Flaws &
Robert Casañas, MD
ISBN 1-891845-27-6
ISBN 978-1-891845-27-7

THE TREATMENT OF DIABETES MELLITUS
WITH CHINESE MEDICINE
by Bob Flaws, Lynn Kuchinski &
Robert Casañas, M.D.
ISBN 1-891845-21-7
ISBN 978-1-891845-21-5

THE TREATMENT OF DISEASE IN TCM, Vol. 1:
Diseases of the Head & Face, Including Mental &
Emotional Disorders
by Philippe Sionneau & Lü Gang
ISBN 0-936185-69-4
ISBN 978-0-936185-69-9

THE TREATMENT OF DISEASE IN TCM, Vol. II:
Diseases of the Eyes, Ears, Nose, & Throat
by Sionneau & Lü
ISBN 0-936185-73-2
ISBN 978-0-936185-73-6

THE TREATMENT OF DISEASE IN TCM, Vol. III:
Diseases of the Mouth, Lips, Tongue, Teeth & Gums
by Sionneau & Lü
ISBN 0-936185-79-1
ISBN 978-0-936185-79-8

THE TREATMENT OF DISEASE IN TCM, Vol IV:
Diseases of the Neck, Shoulders, Back, & Limbs
by Philippe Sionneau & Lü Gang
ISBN 0-936185-89-9
ISBN 978-0-936185-89-7

THE TREATMENT OF DISEASE IN TCM, Vol V:
Diseases of the Chest & Abdomen
by Philippe Sionneau & Lü Gang
ISBN 1-891845-02-0
ISBN 978-1-891845-02-4

THE TREATMENT OF DISEASE IN TCM, Vol VI:
Diseases of the Urogential System & Proctology
by Philippe Sionneau & Lü Gang
ISBN 1-891845-05-5
ISBN 978-1-891845-05-5

THE TREATMENT OF DISEASE IN TCM, Vol VII:
General Symptoms
by Philippe Sionneau & Lü Gang
ISBN 1-891845-14-4
ISBN 978-1-891845-14-7

THE TREATMENT OF EXTERNAL DISEASES
WITH ACUPUNCTURE & MOXIBUSTION
by Yan Cui-lan and Zhu Yun-long, trans. by Yang Shou-zhong
ISBN 0-936185-80-5
ISBN 978-0-936185-80-4

THE TREATMENT OF MODERN WESTERN
MEDICAL DISEASES WITH CHINESE MEDICINE
by Bob Flaws & Philippe Sionneau
ISBN 1-891845-20-9
ISBN 978-1-891845-20-8

UNDERSTANDING THE DIFFICULT PATIENT: A
Guide for Practitioners of Oriental Medicine
by Nancy Bilello, RN, L.ac.
ISBN 1-891845-32-2
ISBN 978-1-891845-32-1

YI LIN GAI CUO (Correcting the Errors in the Forest
of Medicine)
by Wang Qing-ren
ISBN 1-891845-39-X
ISBN 978-1-891845-39-0

70 ESSENTIAL CHINESE HERBAL FORMULAS
by Bob Flaws
ISBN 0-936185-59-7
ISBN 978-0-936185-59-0

160 ESSENTIAL CHINESE READY-MADE
MEDICINES
by Bob Flaws
ISBN 1-891945-12-8
ISBN 978-1-891945-12-3

630 QUESTIONS & ANSWERS ABOUT CHINESE
HERBAL MEDICINE:
A Workbook & Study Guide
by Bob Flaws
ISBN 1-891845-04-7
ISBN 978-1-891845-04-8

260 ESSENTIAL CHINESE MEDICINALS
by Bob Flaws
ISBN 1-891845-03-9
ISBN 978-1-891845-03-1

750 QUESTIONS & ANSWERS ABOUT
ACUPUNCTURE
Exam Preparation & Study Guide
by Fred Jennes
ISBN 1-891845-22-5
ISBN 978-1-891845-22-2